Child

A CLINICAL MANUAL

Neurology

Edited by

Bruce O. Berg, MD

*Professor of Neurology and Pediatrics; Director of Child Neurology,
University of California, San Francisco*

With Associate Authors

JONES MEDICAL PUBLICATIONS
Greenbrae, California

Copyright © 1984
JONES MEDICAL PUBLICATIONS
355 Los Cerros Drive, Greenbrae, CA 94904
(415) 461-3749

Library of Congress Catalog Card Number:84-080920

ISBN: 0-930010-05-1

Printed in the United States of America

9 8 7 6 5 4 3 2 1

Foreword

Child neurology has grown and has become firmly established as a specialty during the last 30 years. This period has seen an improved understanding of the nervous system and of many of the disorders that affect it. New diagnostic tools and therapeutic measures have been devised. Many neurologic diseases, once poorly understood and classified under the vague heading of degenerative disease, have now been recognized as being the result of inborn errors of metabolism and, in many of these, the enzymatic defects have been defined.

New diagnostic methods have made it possible to more readily and more accurately define abnormalities in the nervous system. Computerized axial tomography (CT scanning) and ultrasonography are noninvasive techniques that have revolutionized the localization of lesions in the brain and spinal cord. Neurologically impaired children have been benefited by some of the new methods of medical management that have been developed. For example, the ability to monitor and influence intracranial pressure has improved the survival rate of children with brain swelling secondary to trauma and to illnesses such as Reye's syndrome.

With the development of new drugs, infections of the nervous system including one viral illness can now be treated more effectively. New anticonvulsant agents and the development of drug monitoring have resulted in better seizure control in children with convulsive disorders. The judicious use of amniocentesis and prenatal diagnostic methods have led to the prevention of a number of neurologic disorders for which there are still no cures.

It is important that all physicians involved in the care of children be made aware of the dramatic changes that have resulted from this explosion of knowledge in neurology. In this book, Dr. Bruce Berg, a distinguished child neurologist and teacher, has made his specialty with much of its new information, available to these physicians by carefully selecting for discussion a limited number of topics encompassing both acute and chronic neurologic problems. Utilizing his own vast experience and that of some of his colleagues he has described in an informative, lucid, and concise manner with the liberal use of carefully conceived tables, a practical, clinical approach to the child with a suspected neurologic disorder.

Dr. Berg has pointed up the importance of the medical history and of the physical and neurologic examinations in making a diagnosis of neurologic disease at a time when there is a tendency to replace these basic tools and medical judgment by excessive and, at times, unthinking reliance on expensive diagnostic measures. All physicians who are responsible for the care of children will find this book extraordinarily informative and useful.

Sidney Carter, MD
March, 1984

To Linda,
Kate, and Sarah

Preface

This book is designed to be a readily available first reference on the practical matters of diagnosis, differential diagnosis, and treatment of disorders of the nervous system in infants and children. It is hoped that the book will be a useful guide for all physicians and house officers in pediatrics and neurology.

The book is organized into two interrelated parts. The first ten chapters deal with fundamental topics in child neurology; with neuroanatomic information included for a better understanding of the neurologic examination. The second part of the book is problem oriented and deals principally with major symptoms. Throughout, detailed tables are included for brevity and clarity of presentation. Key references are placed at the end of each chapter.

I thank the contributing authors for their ready enthusiasm and interest in the preparation of the text. Thanks also to all of my colleagues, from whom I have learned so much. I am particularly grateful to my wife, whose enduring patience and support enabled me to work during those precious hours when I should have been with my family.

I am indebted to Drs Robert A. Fishman and Michael J. Aminoff for their critical advice and continued support, to Dr Henry J. Ralston, III for his critical review of the sections on neuroanatomy, and to Mrs Lynda Levy and Ms Trish McGrath for their superb secretarial skills and remarkably good humor during the preparation of the manuscript.

Finally, I am indebted to Richard Jones of Jones Medical Publications for his knowledge, wisdom, and quiet patience in guiding the manuscript to its completion.

Bruce O. Berg, MD
San Francisco
April, 1984

Contents

Foreword *by Sidney Carter* iii

Preface v

1. Neurologic Examination *(Bruce O. Berg)* 1

2. Congenital Malformations *(Bruce O. Berg)* 28

3. Metabolic Encephalopathies *(Seymour Packman)* 51

4. Inborn Errors of Metabolism *(Bruce O. Berg)* 59

5. Neuromuscular Disorders *(Bruce O. Berg)* 85

6. Infections of the Nervous System *(James F. Schwartz)* 122

7. Trauma of the Brain and Spinal Cord *(Michael S. B. Edwards, Lawrence H. Pitts)* 135

8. Craniospinal Neoplasms *(Michael S. B. Edwards)* 146

9. Neurocutaneous Disorders *(Bruce O. Berg)* 166

10. Convulsive Disorders *(Bruce O. Berg)* 179

11. Problems of the Newborn *(Suzanne L. Davis)* 195

12. The Dysmorphic Child *(Bryan D. Hall)* 207

13. Ophthalmic Problems in Childhood *(Creig S. Hoyt)* 214

14. Problems in Language Acquisition *(Richard M. Flower)* 229

15. Headache *(Bruce O. Berg)* 241

16. The Hypotonic Infant *(Bruce O. Berg)* 250

17. Ataxia of Childhood *(Thomas K. Koch, Bruce O. Berg)* 257

18. Movement Disorders *(Bruce O. Berg)* 266

19. Intracranial Hypertension *(Lawrence H. Pitts, Michael S. B. Edwards)* 277

20. Coma *(Roger P. Simon)* 287

Appendix (Growth charts; head circumference charts) 302

Index 308

Authors

Bruce O. Berg, MD *Professor of Neurology and Pediatrics, Director of Child Neurology, University of California, San Francisco.*

Suzanne L. Davis, MB, ChB *Assistant Professor, Neurology and Pediatrics, University of California, San Francisco.*

Michael S. B. Edwards, MD *Associate Professor, Neurological Surgery, University of California, San Francisco.*

Richard M. Flower, PhD *Professor and Vice Chair, Otolaryngology, University of California, San Francisco.*

Bryan D. Hall, MD *Associate Professor of Pediatrics, University of Kentucky, Lexington, Kentucky.*

Creig S. Hoyt, MD *Professor of Ophthalmology and Pediatrics, University of California, San Francisco.*

Thomas K. Koch, MD *Instructor, Neurology and Pediatrics, University of California, San Francisco.*

Seymour Packman, MD *Assistant Professor, Pediatrics, University of California, San Francisco.*

Lawrence H. Pitts, MD *Chief, Neurosurgery Service, San Francisco General Hospital; Associate Professor, Neurosurgery, University of California, San Francisco.*

James F. Schwartz, MD *Professor of Pediatrics and Neurology, Emory University School of Medicine, Atlanta, Georgia.*

Roger P. Simon, MD *Associate Professor, Neurology, University of California, San Francisco; Chief, Neurology Service, San Francisco General Hospital.*

1

Neurologic Examination

Bruce O. Berg, MD

The clinical evaluation of children with symptoms referable to the nervous system demands complete attention to eliciting and interpreting historical details and performing a careful, complete neurologic examination. The history suggests the nature of the pathophysiologic process, and the examination localizes the site of the lesion.

There is a variety of clinical methods available, but each physician must develop his own method of performing the neurological assessment. One must be able to accommodate to and control each clinical situation— the loquacious historian as well as those of parsimonious prose. Above all *it is essential to listen to what the mother and child are telling you.*

The prenatal, perinatal, and developmental histories as well as the present illness are important to understand the nature of the patient's problem, and the wise clinician will not overlook the medical history of the biological family. The value of an accurate history in solving the clinical problem cannot be overemphasized.

The method of assessing the **mental status** of older children is similar to that of adults. In the case of very young patients, however, a developmental history will lend much pertinent information.

The patient's clothing should be removed so that abnormal physical findings are less likely to be overlooked. Allow the child to disrobe privately with his parents and have him wear an examining gown or remain in his underwear. A gentle but firm approach can be amazingly successful.

THE SKULL

The skull is readily available to inspection, palpation, auscultation, percussion, and measurement. The head circumference is a reliable indicator of intracranial volume. During the first 3 months of life, the full-term infant's head circumference should increase by 2 cm each month; from the third through sixth months, 1 cm each month; and from 7-12 months 0.5 cm each month (see Appendix).

Percussion of the skull is a useful diagnostic maneuver for in the presence of increased intracranial pressure an abnormally tympanitic sound may be elicited (McEwen's sign, 'cracked pot sound'). **Auscultation** of the skull may also provide useful information; cephalic bruits may be heard over the region of vascular malformations, tumors, or other space-occupying lesions that may compress large vessels. One should listen for bruits over the closed eye, the temporal fossae, and carotid arteries. Cephalic bruits are commonly heard in skulls of normal infants and young children; 60% of 4 to 5-year old and 10% of 10-year old children. One should be cautious, however, in their interpretation, particularly if the bruit is localized to one area of the skull or is obliterated by compression of the ipsilateral carotid artery.

Transillumination is a valuable examination technique that is performed with a Chun gun transilluminator or a flashlight utilizing two type D batteries. The Chun gun is preferred because it emits a standard light source of high intensity. Rubber adaptors are used with each of the light sources so that good contact is made between the rubber ring and the scalp. The procedure should be carried out in a darkened room after the examiner has accommodated to the darkness. Circumstances that may alter transillumination include the gestational age of the infant, extracranial and intracranial factors.

The degree of transillumination is greater in infants of decreased gestational age and there is about 1 cm decrease in frontal transillumination from about 26 weeks' gestation to term.

Extracranial conditions that increase transillumination include paucity of hair, decreased pigment of skin and hair or a collection of fluid between the skull and the light. Conditions that decrease transillumination include an abundance of hair with increased pigment of hair and skin, increased thickness of skull, or a subgaleal hematoma.

Intracranial conditions which increase transillumination include increased collections of fluid in the subdural or subarachnoid space or in those patients with thin cortical mantles and large ventricles.

Configuration of the skull may often lend a clue to the diagnosis, especially in patients with large or macrocephalic heads. The skull of a hydrocephalic child is commonly globular shaped; biparietal widening is often seen in patients with chronic subdural hematomas, and in patients with Dandy-Walker syndrome there is usually a ballooning of the posterior aspect of the skull. Other forms of skull irregularities are found in different types of craniostenoses, depending upon what sutures are prematurely fused.

Microcephaly is secondary to abnormally decreased brain growth and has been arbitrarily defined as a head circumference greater than 2 standard deviations below the mean for age, sex, and gestation. It does not always presage mental retardation, for about 2-7% of children who are considered microcephalic by definition have normal intelligence.

THE SPINE

The spine should be inspected for its configuration, such as abnormal curvature of scoliosis, khyphosis, or lordosis, and also for the presence of dermal sinus tracts. Dimples or dermal sinuses may overlie a vertebral anomaly that is otherwise asymptomatic. Areas of localized tenderness to percussion and/or palpation may indicate an intraspinal lesion.

Table 1-1 The Clinical History

Complaint (reason for referral) What is the problem as perceived by the parent and/or child.

Family history (biological family)

Mother's gestational history List each pregnancy in order; abortions still births, living children (ages, sex, medical status; if deceased, what was the cause of death).

Mother
Father
Maternal grandmother and grandfather
Mother's siblings (brothers, sisters)
Paternal grandmother and grandfather
Father's siblings (brothers, sisters)
} Age, medical status, occupation; if deceased, what was the cause of death.

Identify and describe any family member with neuromuscular disease, convulsive disorder or migraine, visual or hearing problems. Describe any family member who is mentally ill, mentally retarded, or who has a specific learning disability.

Past medical history

Birthdate. Birthweight

Describe gestational history: note duration of pregnancy — if there were trauma, infection, or vaginal bleeding. List medications taken during the pregnancy, including alcohol, and use of tobacco. Describe the labor, its duration, and whether the delivery was vaginal or by cesarian section.

Neonatal period Describe the infant's status at birth; note the Apgar score, condition while in nursery, and the duration of hospitalization.

Developmental history Age at which the following were achieved:

Head support; smiled; rolled over; sat alone; stood/cruised; walked alone; acquisition of language.

Diseases Describe illnesses; age at occurrence, duration, and possible sequelae.

Surgery List any operative procedure, the age of child when it occurred, and possible complications.

Trauma Describe what happened, the child's age when it occurred, and whether or not there was an alteration of consciousness, and if there were sequelae.

Present illness Describe the problem in appropriate chronology and detail.

Table 1-2 The Neurologic Examination

General Describe the physical habitus of the patient.

Weight: Height: Head circumference:
Blood pressure: Respiration: Pulse: Temperature:

Speech Describe the quality of speech — presence of dysarthria.

Skull Configuration, auscultation, percussion.

Spine Describe configuration, deformity, tenderness, or limitation of movement. Nuchal rigidity usually implies meningeal irritation. *Kernig's sign* is characterized by the involuntary flexion of the knees when the examiner gently flexes the thigh while the leg is in extension. *Brudzinski's sign* is the flexion of the knees and hips following the flexion of the head on the chest.

Mental status Note the method of assessment.

Cranial nerves

I. Olfaction Note the method of assessment.

II. Visual fields Note the method of assessment.

    Visual acuity O.D.   O.S.

    Fundi Describe media, disks, vessels, retina, and macula.

III, IV, VI. Pupils — size, configuration, reactivity to light and accommodation.

    Extraocular motility — abnormal eye movements.

V. Corneal reflex Motor and sensory components — describe method of testing.

VII. Facial mobility Symmetry of facial mobility.

    Taste Anterior 2/3 of tongue, note method of assessment.

VIII. Hearing Describe method of testing: Rinne test; Schwabach test; Weber test.

IX, X. Position and movement of palate and uvula; gag reflex. Describe sensation of posterior pharyngeal wall; phonation.

XI. Describe the bulk and power of sternocleidomastoid and upper fibers of trapezius muscles.

XII. Tongue — position, mobility, power, presence or absence of fasciculations.

Table 1-2 (cont'd) The Neurologic Examination

Motor system Describe the muscle bulk; presence or absence of fasciculations. Describe the muscle tone and power.

Tendon reflexes
  Biceps: C5-6
  Supinator: C5-6
  Triceps:C6-8
  Superficial abdominal:
    Upper: T7-9
    Lower: T11-12
  Patellar: L2-4
  Achilles reflex: L5-S2
  Plantar response (sign of Babinski): L4-S2

Station and gait Describe the quality of movement — whether there is truncal and/or limb ataxia or a specific disorder of movement.

Sensory system Pain and touch. Temperature. Vibration. Joint position sense. Higher cortical function: two-point discrimination; stereognosis; graphesthesia.

Sphincters

General examination

Cardiovascular system

Respiratory system

Abdomen

Skin

CRANIAL NERVES

I. OLFACTORY NERVE

Neural pathways The ability to perceive the vast array of smells in the environment is a primitive function dependent upon this first cranial nerve. First-order neurons are bipolar cells with ciliated distal processes located in the superior aspect of the nasal cavity. The axons penetrate the cribriform plate of the ethmoid bone and synapse within the olfactory bulbs. The axons of the next-order neurons traverse the olfactory tract to the olfactory tuberculum, dividing into medial and lateral striae with some fibers crossing the anterior commissure to the contralateral olfactory bulb. Fibers of the medial striae pursue a course to the medial hemispheric surface; whereas, those fibers of the lateral striae follow an oblique course around the anterior perforated substance to terminate in the prepiriform, periamygdaloid and entorhinal cortex. Because of bilateral hemispheric innervation, lesions proximal to neuronal decussation do not result in the loss of smell (anosmia). Olfactory impulses that reach the amygdala are thought to be related to maternal and sexual behavior but the full importance of these neurobehavioral relationships is not known.

Clinical evaluation of the olfactory nerve requires an unobstructed nasal cavity, free of mucus or inflammation. The common cold is the most frequent cause of impaired olfaction (hyposmia). Each nostril should be tested separately by gently compressing one nostril and presenting to the other a nonirritating volatile substance such as cinnamon, cloves, oil of wintergreen, or lavendar. Irritating substances such as camphor, ammonia, or formaldehyde should be avoided, for they may stimulate gustatory endorgans or fibers of the trigeminal nerve.

The ability to perceive smell appears in early infancy, as demonstrated by an infant's recognition of the odor of his mother's used breast pads, compared to breast pads of other mothers or unused pads. Infants also appear to recognize and sense differences between pleasant and unpleasant smells.

Causes of anosmia include trauma to the ethmoid bone or cribriform plate which may also result in a CSF leak. Other causes of impairment of smell include meningitis, hydrocephalus, the uncommon brain tumor of childhood located in this region of the olfactory neural pathway, and illicit drug sniffing.

II. OPTIC NERVE

This cranial nerve subserves the sense of vision and is the one cranial nerve that can be examined directly, at least in part by ophthalmoscopy. Primary modalities of optic nerve function include the visual fields, visual acuity, color vision as well as day and night vision. Each eye should be examined separately.

Neural pathway The site of the lesion causing a visual field defect is best understood by reviewing the neuroanatomy of the visual pathways (see Figure 1-1).

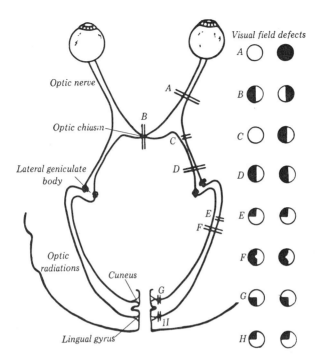

Fig. 1-1 The visual pathways. A-H show sites of potential lesions and associated deficits in the visual fields (black areas)

Clinical evaluation The *visual field* represents the perceived space subtended by one eye when that eye is fixed on some point. That point of fixation is projected on the macula while the other objects within that visual field are also percieved, particularly if in motion. In addition to white test objects, color test objects should be used to determine visual fields, for changes of the color field perimeter usually precede obvious changes of the visual fields (color desaturation).

The visual fields are examined by one of several methods including confrontation, using a tangent screen or by perimetry. Overlapping of the right and left visual fields enables one to have binocular vision; there is a crescentic monocular segment in each temporal field.

The method of confrontation compares the visual field of patient with that of the examiner, each of which is seated about 3 feet (1 meter) from the other. The patient closes the right eye while the examiner closes his left eye; each person gazes into the other's open eye. The examiner then introduces a white-headed pin, or similar object, into the peripheral visual field in a plane equidistant from both parties, documenting the point when the patient first sees that test object. This method, though somewhat crude, is very useful and can be readily accomplished at the bedside. The blind spot can also be demonstrated by this method.

When using a tangent (Bjerrum) screen, the three-dimensional visual field is projected upon a flat surface and that portion of central vision is examined. This method of examination is particularly useful in determining the overall dimensions of the visual fields, the configuration and size of the blind spot, as well as central visual defects (scotomata).

A variety of perimeters is available to determine visual fields. The patient sits before the instrument, looking at the fixation point; test objects are introduced into the visual field in one of the multiple meridians. When that object is first perceived by the patient, that point is recorded on a graph; the points of each meridian are connected for each test object and the perimeter of the visual field is established (the isopter). There are different isopters for each size of test objects.

Older infants and young children may be tested by introducing a dangling bright object, such as a shiny tape measure, from behind the patient's head and slowly introducing it into the field of vision. The child's eyes will quickly dart to the test object when initially seen. A normally intelligent child of 5 or 6 years can be tested by the confrontation method but it is usually not until the latter part of the first decade that perimeters are reliably used.

Visual acuity is a measure of the resolution power of each eye and should be evaluated for near and distant vision. Near vision is determined by presenting standard characters (Jaeger test) at a distance of 14 inches (35.5 cm) from the eyes. Distant vision is examined by presenting to the patient a set of standard letters of varying sizes (Snellen chart) that can be normally read at distances ranging from 10-200 feet. This examination is carried out by presenting the stimulus (letters) at 20 feet (6 meters) from the patient. Normal vision is determined arbitrarily as the ability to read standard letters at a distance of 20 feet; namely, 20/20 (6/6). The numerator is the distance of the patient from the chart and the denominator is the distance at which the smallest letter as read by the patient would be read by one with normal vision.

Color blindness, a heritable disorder primarily affecting males, may be total or partial. The usual method of examination of color vision is by presentation of pseudoisochromatic plates of Isahara, or other available standard test color cards. Day blindness (hemeralopia) and night blindness (nyctalopia) are considered in Chapter 13.

III, IV, VI. (OCULOMOTOR) NERVES

Neural pathways These cranial nerves are closely related functionally and neuronatomically. The *third nerve nuclei (oculomotor)* are located just below periaqueductal grey matter of the mesencephalon ventral to the aqueduct of Sylvius. This nerve innervates the inferior, medial, and superior recti muscles as well as the inferior oblique and levator palpebrae muscles. It contains parasympathetic fibers that innervate the intrinsic muscles of the eye, the ciliary muscle and sphincter of the pupil via the ciliary ganglia. The *fourth cranial nerve (trochlear) nuclei* are ventral to the aqueduct in the lower mesencephalic grey matter just rostral to the pons. This nerve, the smallest of all cranial nerves, innervates the superior oblique muscle. The *sixth nerve nuclei (abducens)* originate in the grey matter ventral to the fourth ventricle within the dorsal tegmentum of the

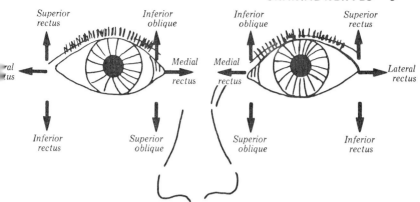

Fig. 1-2 The action of extraocular muscles attached to the globe in primary position, abduction, and adduction.

lower pons and innervate the lateral rectus muscles. These three cranial nerves regulate ocular motility, pupillary constriction, and some lid function (see Chapter 13).

V. TRIGEMINAL NERVE

Neural pathways The fifth and largest of all cranial nerves carries both sensory and motor fibers and has complex connections with other cranial nerves. The Gasserian ganglion, the cellular origin of sensory fibers, lies adjacent to the apex of the petrous bone in the middle fossa. Proximal fibers follow a course into the pons; the distal fibers are divided into three main sensory divisions — the ophthalmic, maxillary, and mandibular, which leave the skull through the superior orbital fissure, the foramen rotundum, and the foramen ovale, respectively. The motor root emerges from the pons below the Gasserian ganglion and leaves the skull through the foramen ovale, joining the mandibular root for a short distance and then divides to supply the muscles of mastication.

Sensory fibers carry impulses to three primary nuclei within the pons and medulla. Large diameter fibers primarily carry tactile information to the main sensory nucleus where, after synapse, axons ascend in the dorsal ascending trigeminal tract to the thalamus. The nucleus of the descending root (trigeminal spinal tract) extends caudally from the main sensory nucleus to a level of C4. Smaller diameter pain, temperature, and tactile fibers terminate on the cells of this nucleus. Fibers of the ophthalmic division are ventrolateral, mandibular fibers are dorsomedial, and maxillary fibers are in between. Exteroceptive fibers of VII, IX, and X join this descending tract at the levels at which they enter the brain stem, descend for varying distances, synapse, and neuraxons of the next order cross the midline to ascend in the ventral ascending trigeminal tract, and terminate in the thalamus. The course of the mesencephalic sensory root of the trigeminal nerve is closely associated with the motor root and carries proprioceptive impulses from muscle. Muscles innervated by the trigeminal nerve include the masseters, temporals, external and internal pterygoids, as well as smaller muscles including the myohyoid and anterior belly of the digastric muscles.

Clinical evaluation requires testing of the motor and sensory components of this nerve. The masseters, temporals, and internal pterygoid muscles elevate and extend the mandible; whereas, the external pterygoids with the assistance of smaller muscles depress the mandible. The pterygoids also effect side to side motion. As the patient clenches the jaw, the examiner should palpate the bulk of masseter and temporal muscles. Decreased bulk of one or both sides is usually apparent. External pterygoids are evaluated by having the patient open his mouth, noting any deviation of upper or lower incisor teeth. Asymmetrical movement is also detected by having the patient move the jaw from side to side. Masticatory muscles are tested by having the patient bite a wooden tongue blade with his teeth; normally one cannot readily pull the tongue blade from the mouth. Infant patients are examined by examining their suck and letting them bite the examiner's clean finger or rubber nipple. The tensor veli palatini, also supplied by this nerve, pulls the soft palate laterally and superiorly and the tensor tympani increases tension on the otic membrane.

The trigeminal nerve supplies sensory nerves to facial skin, mucous membranes of the conjunctivae, nostrils, gingivae, tongue, and inner cheek. The cornea also receives sensory fibers from this nerve. Sensory impairment of one of the three main sensory branches is readily distinguished from segmental (onion skin) sensory changes secondary to lesions of the spinal trigeminal tract which results in loss of pain and temperature but spares localized tactile sensation (Figure 1-3).

The trigeminal nerve also participates in a variety of reflexes. The *corneal reflex* demonstrates the integrity of both the fifth (afferent limb) and seventh (efferent limb) cranial nerves. The patient looks to one side while the examiner gently strokes the cornea with a few twisted strands of cotton wool. Normally, both eyelids blink simultaneously (orbicularis oculi muscles). The blink on the stimulated side is direct response and the contralateral blink is called the consensual response. In cases of unilateral trigeminal lesions, there is decreased or no direct or consensual response following ipsilateral stimulation; however, when the contralateral cornea is stimulated, there is normal bilateral lid blink. In cases of facial nerve lesions, there is decreased or absent lid blink on the involved side.

The jaw jerk is performed by placing the examiner's finger on the midpoint of the patient's chin, with the jaw slightly open. The examiner gently taps his finger with a percussion hammer and the jaw abruptly closes. Both afferent and efferent limbs of this reflex arc are components of the trigeminal nerve. The jaw jerk is absent in nuclear or peripheral lesions of the trigeminal nerve but is usually very brisk in lesions of supranuclear origin.

VII. FACIAL NERVE

The facial nerve, though primarily considered a motor nerve, has a significant sensory role, carrying exteroceptive fibers from the otic membrane and portions of the ear and mastoid, proprioceptive fibers from muscles it

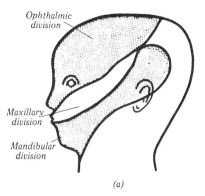
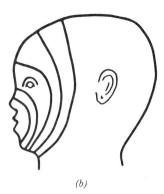

Fig. 1-3 Cutaneous distribution of the trigeminal nerve. (a) Peripheral distribution. (b) Segmental distribution.

innervates and parasympathetic fibers to the ganglion supplying the lacrimal gland, salivary glands as well as the nasopharyngeal mucosa. In addition, it carries fibers for taste from the anterior two thirds of the tongue.

Neural pathways The motor component originates in a nucleus within the lower pons from which fibers rise dorsally toward the floor of the fourth ventricle encircling the sixth nerve nucleus and then moving ventrolaterally, exiting from the lateral inferior aspect of the pons in the cerebellopontine angle. It enters the internal auditory meatus with its sensory root, the nervus intermedius, and the eighth cranial nerve, and follows the facial canal before moving downward, exiting from the skull through the stylomastoid foramen. The motor root pursues a course toward the parotid gland, dividing behind the mandible into the temporofacial and cervicofacial branches.

Supranuclear fibers for VII motor neurons supplying the lower two-thirds of the face originate in the inferior one-third of the contralateral precentral gyrus and follow a course in the genu of the internal capsule and basis pedunculus, terminating in the seventh nerve nucleus. The VII motor neurons that supply the upper face have bilateral cortical innervation which enables the frontalis and lid muscles to contract simultaneously. Closing one eye is actually learned behavior. Lower facial muscles are innervated by contralateral supranuclear fibers.

Cells of the sensory root, the nervus intermedius, are found in the geniculate ganglion which lies in the facial canal. The axons enter the pons with the motor root; distal fibers continue as the chorda tympani, carrying taste fibers, general visceral afferent as well as preganglionic parasympathetic fibers.

Afferent taste fibers follow the chorda tympani to the geniculate ganglion cell bodies. These fibers traverse the nervus intermedius to terminate in the nucleus solitarius. Secondary fibers are then relayed to the superior and inferior salivatory nuclei from which parasympathetic fibers are then directed to the salivary glands.

Exteroceptive fibers from the soft palate and uvula follow the posterior palatine nerve, the sphenopalatine junction, the greater superficial petrosal nerve, geniculate ganglion, and the nervus intermedius where, after entering the brain stem follow a caudal course in the spinal tract and nucleus of the trigeminal nerve.

Autonomic pathways subserve a secretory function to the lacrimal and salivary glands as well as the nasopharyngeal mucosa. Parasympathetic fibers originate in the superior salivatory nucleus in an area near the floor of the fourth ventricle, follow the nervus intermedius, pass through the geniculate ganglion without synapse, and then contact the cells of the submandibular ganglion (for salivary glands) or pterygopalatine ganglion (for nasal, palatine, and lacrimal glands). These glands also have a sympathetic nerve supply from the superior cervical ganglia via carotid plexus.

Clinical evaluation of the facial nerve requires an assessment of the motor and sensory components. Central facial weakness results in weakness of the contralateral lower facial muscles, sparing the upper facial muscles. Peripheral facial weakness, dependent upon what portion of the nerve is involved, is characterized by a widened palpebral fissure, the inability to bury the eyelashes, flattening of the nasolabial fold with drooping of that corner of the mouth, and decreased facial mobility. The facial muscles are deviated to the uninvolved side when speaking or smiling and commonly the patient cannot whistle, pronounce linguals, or puff out his cheeks. Food may accumulate between the teeth and the cheek and there is often drooling on the affected side. Patients with facial weakness may be unable to whistle or suck through a straw.

Most of these observations are made by inspection but are clearly evident when the patient is asked to close the eyes separately and together, smile, and whistle. A lag of lid closure is clearly evident while performing the corneal reflex.

Lacrimal function is usually determined by asking the patient if he is able to tear, but on occasion, one must observe whether there is normal tearing. This is readily done by placing a small piece of filter paper on the lower lid and observing the degree of moistening (Schirmer test). Another method of assessing lacrimal function is to stimulate the conjunctivae and/or nasal mucosa with some dilute noxious substance such as camphor or ammonia. *Submaxillary gland function* is similarly tested by placing a highly flavored material on the tongue and observing the degree of salivation.

Evaluation of taste requires that the tongue remains protruded during the testing situation. The four basic tastes are sweet, sour, salty, and bitter. Small volumes of the test substance from a cotton swab are placed on one side of the anterior two-thirds of the protruded tongue, one at a time. The tongue should be rinsed between each taste test. The posterior one-third of the tongue is innervated by the glossopharyngeal nerve. It is not surprising that taste is perceived in the newborn period as demonstrated by the longer periods of time an infant will suck from sweet solutions as compared to compounds that are bitter or salty.

VIII. ACOUSTIC NERVE

Cochlear Nerve

Neural pathways This eighth cranial nerve has two neural components, the cochlear nerve (hearing) and the vestibular nerve (position or orientation in space). The receptors of the cochlear nerve (the hair cells of the organ of Corti) are supplied by axons of the bipolar cells of the spiral ganglion from which rise the fibers of the cochlear nerve. This nerve enters the brain stem at the pontomedullary junction and the fibers bifurcate to terminate in the dorsal and ventral cochlear nuclei. Fibers from the dorsal cochlear nucleus cross the midline near the superior olivary nuclei and proceed to the lateral lemniscus. Some fibers of the ventral cochlear nucleus cross the midline as trapezoid fibers to the contralateral lemniscus, while others synapse with the bilateral olivary bodies and, through them, the nuclei of cranial nerves III, IV, and VI. A smaller number of fibers from both the dorsal and ventral cochlear nuclei ascend via the ipsilateral lateral lemnisci.

Nerve fibers from the lateral lemniscus project to the nucleus of the lateral lemniscus and then to the inferior colliculus and medial geniculate body from which auditory radiations ascend in the posterior aspect of the internal capsule to the temporal lobe (transverse gyri of Heschl). The human auditory system has bilateral hemispheric representation. Unilateral cortical lesions only mildly affect hearing in the contralateral auditory field; there is a decrement of ability to localize the origin of sounds. Deafness is rarely produced by cortical lesions.

Clinical evaluation of cochlear function requires the determination of the range of frequency and intensity of sound that the patient can perceive. Sound is perceived by air and bone conduction; both modalities should be assessed. The human can appreciate frequencies ranging from 16 to 25,000 Hz, with conversational speech in the range of 200-3000 Hz.

Hearing evaluations are carried out by a variety of methods. Examples include rubbing the thumb and forefinger outside the external auditory canal beyond the range of hearing and gradually bringing that sound stimulus closer to the patient's ear until it is heard. A ticking watch or vibrating tuning fork can also be used as a sound stimulus and in each of these methods a comparison is made with the examiner's hearing.

A tuning fork is most useful as the sound stimulus, for the frequency is known and both air and bone conduction can be tested. In the *Schwabach test* a tuning fork (512 Hz — conversational speech) is used. The base of the vibrating fork is placed against the patient's mastoid until it is no longer heard and then it is immediately placed against the examiner's mastoid for comparison. This same maneuver can be done to evaluate air conduction, but in this case a vibrating tuning fork is placed outside the external auditory canal.

The Weber test is performed by placing the base of the vibrating tuning fork on the patient's vertex. Normally, there is no lateralization of sound and it is heard equally well in both ears. If one canal is obstructed, the sound is heard better in that side; in conduction deafness, for example, the sound is lateralized to the involved side. Patients with sensorineural deafness may hear the fork best on the normal side.

The Rinne test compares air conduction with bone conduction. The base of the vibrating tuning fork is placed against the patient's mastoid process and when no longer heard by the patient, the vibrating tuning fork is brought outside the external auditory canal. Normally, air conduction is better than bone conduction and the Rinne test is positive. In cases where air conduction is decreased but bone conduction is unimpaired the test is called negative. Those patients with sensorineural deafness have impaired air conduction and bone conduction, but the relationship of the two modalities is retained and the Rinne test is considered positive. Patients with severe sensorineural deafness may have no bone conduction.

The most reliable method of evaluating hearing is using an *electronic audiometer* by which pure tones can be produced at specifically regulated frequencies and intensities. The patient is placed in a sound-proof room and after occluding one ear, a sound stimulus is presented to the other. The extent of hearing loss is expressed in decibels for each frequency tested and a range of hearing is plotted on a graph. Both air and bone conduction can be evaluated by this technique.

Vestibular Nerve

The vestibular system assists in regulating one's position in space and is composed of the semicircular canals, the utricle, saccule, and neural connections. This bony labyrinthine structure, enclosed within the petrous portion of the temporal bone, contains three membranous semicircular canals which are positioned at right angles to each other. Each canal is dilated at one end, the ampulla, and contains receptor hair cells. Endolymph is contained within the canals which are surrounded by perilymph. The receptor cells are stimulated by changes of direction or velocity of movement which, in turn, stimulates an appropriate motor response.

Neural pathways The saccule and utricle, membranous structures housed within the bony vestibule, contain receptor cells which are in contact with calcareous otoliths. The association of hair cells and otoliths varies with gravitational changes, and proprioceptive information is conveyed centrally regarding head-body position, and body movement. This neural system influences muscle tone, maintenance of position in space, tonic-neck, and neck righting reflexes.

Receptors of the vestibular nerve are supplied by the bipolar cells of Scarpa's ganglion within the internal auditory meatus; proximal fibers enter the upper medulla as the vestibular nerve. Most fibers terminate in the vestibular nuclei or go directly to the cerebellum. There are four vestibular nuclei — the medial, lateral, superior, and inferior (spinal), positioned in the lateral aspect of the floor of the fourth ventricle. Afferent fibers from the semicircular canals enter the brain stem, bifurcate and terminate in all four vestibular nuclei, but primarily in the superior and medial nuclei which are the major source of neural input to the medial longitudinal fasciculus. Through this fasciculus, fibers reach cranial nerves III, IV, VI, and IX, and the upper cervical cord. Some fibers ascend to the cerebellum, primarily to the flocculonodular lobe and the fastigial nuclei. Nerve fibers originating in these same cerebellar areas course to the ipsilateral fastigial nucleus and are then relayed back to the vestibular nuclei. By this feedback mechanism, the cerebellum has some inhibitory influence on vestibular function.

Afferent fibers from the utricle and saccule bifurcate after reaching the brain stem. Ascending fibers proceed to the lateral, inferior, and medial nuclei, and descending fibers terminate in the spinal vestibular nucleus. Some saccular afferent fibers go directly to the lateral nucleus. Neither saccular nor utricular fibers course to the cerebellum. The principal input of utricular fibers is to the lateral vestibular nucleus from which fibers course downward in the vestibulospinal tract which terminates on ipsilateral interneurons or motor neurons at all levels. By this mechanism the labyrinth is able to exert and influence posture and muscle tone.

IX. GLOSSOPHARYNGEAL NERVE

The glossopharyngeal and vagus nerves are intimately associated and have similar functions. Both have motor, sensory, and autonomic branches with nuclear origin in the medulla. Both nerves conduct exteroceptive, general, and special visceral sensation (Figure 1-4).

Neural pathways *Motor fibers* of the glossopharyngeal nerve arise from the nucleus ambiguus. Fibers are directed posteriorly and medially toward the floor of the fourth ventricle and then move laterally, emerging from the upper portion of the medulla as multiple nerve branches dorsal to the inferior olive. These motor filaments supply the stylopharyngeus muscle.

Sensory branches arise from the nucleus in the petrous ganglion located in the inferior aspect of the petrous bone, as well as in the jugular ganglion. Exteroceptive fibers (touch, pain, and temperature) supply part

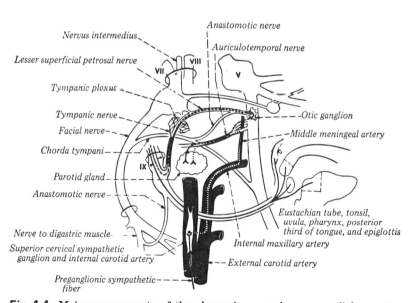

Fig. 1-4 Major components of the glossopharyngeal nerve, medial aspect. (Reproduced, with permission, from Haymaker W: *Bing's Local Diagnosis in Neurological Diseases.* Mosby, St. Louis, 1969.

of the posterior otic membrane and external auditory canal and course through the petrous ganglion, terminating in the trigeminal spinal tract and nucleus. General visceral fibers supply the mucosa of the pharynx, posterolateral aspect of the soft palate and uvula, fauces and tonsils, mastoid cells, eustachian tube, posterior one-third of the tongue, the carotid body, and terminate in the nucleus of the fasciculus solitarius.

Autonomic efferent fibers originate in the inferior salivatory nucleus. Preganglionic fibers course through the tympanic plexus and lesser superficial petrosal nerve to the otic ganglion; the postganglionic fibers are carried with the auriculotemporal branch of the trigeminal nerve to the parotid gland. The glossopharyngeal nerve also carries secretory and vasodilating fibers to the parotid gland and may stimulate secretions of the buccal and pharyngeal mucosa.

Clinical evaluation   Motor function of the glossopharyngeal nerve is limited to function of stylopharyngeus muscle. Abnormalities of these motor fibers result in lowering of the palatal curtain. This is difficult to evaluate because of associated vagal supply to these pharyngeal muscles. Sensory function of this nerve is also difficult to evaluate because not only do exteroceptive fibers supply inaccessible anatomical regions but these sites are also supplied by cranial nerves V, VII, and X. Special visceral sensory fibers supply taste to the posterior one-third of the tongue and with the vagus nerve, the hard and soft palate and posterior aspect of the pharynx. It is generally of no practical usefulness or importance to evaluate this function. Accessible regions of general visceral sensation include the fauces and tonsils, the posterior pharyngeal walls, the posterior one-third of the tongue, and parts of the soft palate. There is sensory overlap, however, from cranial nerves V and X.

X. VAGUS NERVE

Neural pathways   This nerve, the longest of all cranial nerves, is closely related in structure and function to the glossopharyngeal nerve. Motor fibers originate in the nucleus ambiguus, emerge from the brain stem as multiple roots, and leave the skull with the glossopharyngeal nerve through the jugular foramen. These motor fibers innervate striated muscles of the soft palate, pharynx, and the larynx, except for the tensor veli palatini (trigeminal), the stylopharyngeus (glossopharyngeal) muscle, and the upper third of the esophagus.

The sensory branches of this nerve have their cells of origin in the jugular ganglion and ganglion nodosum, found in the region of the jugular foramen. Exteroceptive fibers supply the external auditory canal and part of the otic membrane as well as a small area of the pinna. These afferent fibers course to jugular ganglion and terminate in the spinal trigeminal tract. These same areas are also innervated by cranial nerves VII and IX. Pain fibers from the dura mater of the posterior cranial fossa and transverse sinus traverse the jugular foramen and also terminate in the spinal trigeminal tract.

Afferent fibers of *general visceral sensation* from the inferior pharynx, larynx, and thoracic and abdominal viscera, course through the inferior (nodose) ganglion and terminate in the caudal aspect of the nucleus solitarius. Preganglionic general visceral efferent fibers arise from the dorsal motor nucleus of the vagus nerve and terminate in the thoracic and abdominal visceral postganglionic neurons. The postganglionic fibers innervate glands, as well as cardiac and smooth muscle.

Taste fibers, special visceral afferent fibers of the vagus nerve from the epiglottis and arytenoids, with branches of the glossopharyngeal nerve, terminate in the fasciculus solitarius and its nucleus. Visceral efferent fibers arise in the nucleus ambiguus and innervate the muscles of the soft palate, pharyngeal muscles and the larynx.

Clinical evaluation of the motor function of the vagus nerve is related to the soft palate, pharyngeal muscles, and larynx. Usually deviations of the soft palate and uvula are secondary to prior tonsillectomy. In unilateral vagal lesions, the palatal arch is lowered and pulled toward the normal side. Bilateral lesions result in the inability to elevate the palate and an absence of the palatal reflex.

Pharyngeal weakness may be difficult to demonstrate; but there is usually some impairment of swallowing and/or coughing. Impaired laryngeal function results in abnormality of articulation, respiration, and coughing. The vagus nerve also has a role in some reflex activity including a cough reflex, swallow and vomiting reflex, as well as a sternutatory reflex (nasal sneeze). Other reflexes include sucking and a carotid sinus reflex.

XI. SPINAL ACCESSORY NERVE

Neural pathways This cranial nerve is composed of two parts — the accessory or cranial root (the smaller of the two) and a spinal root. The *cranial segment* originates from neurons of the caudal aspect of the nucleus ambiguus and the dorsal efferent nucleus. Fibers exit from the medulla as rootlets, join the spinal root of this nerve and exit from the skull with the vagus nerve through the jugular foramen. The cranial root traverses the superior (jugular) ganglion and inferior (nodose) ganglion and is distributed with the vagus nerve.

The *spinal portion* originates from cells within the ventral horn of the spinal cord from the caudal medulla to C5-6. These rootlets emerge from the lateral aspect of the cord and ascend to enter the skull through the foramen magnum, join the cranial portion of the nerve and then leave the skull through the jugular foramen, descending the neck to supply the sternocleidomastoids and upper portion of the trapezius muscles.

Clinical evaluation of this nerve is limited to assessment of the sternocleidomastoid muscles which are readily available to inspection and palpation. They function with other cervical muscles to flex the neck and rotate the head. In unilateral weakness, there may be little alteration in head posture, but weakness of rotation is discerned by resisting rotation. Contraction of one muscle will result in the occiput pulled to the side of the contracting muscle and the head is drawn toward the ipsilateral shoulder.

The upper fibers of the trapezius muscle are evaluated by having the patient shrug his shoulders against resistance. In unilateral paralysis, the shoulder cannot be elevated or retracted. Muscle bulk can be appreciated by palpation and, on occasion, fasciculations are present.

XII. HYPOGLOSSAL NERVE

Neural pathways This cranial nerve originates from paired nuclei below the floor of the fourth ventricle and extends ventrolaterally, emerging from the medulla as multiple rootlets that are gathered into nerve bundles before leaving the skull through the hypoglossal foramen. This nerve has connections with the inferior (nodose) ganglion (X), the pharyngeal plexus, as well as branches to the cervical ganglia of the sympathetic trunk and fibers at C1 to C3.

The hypoglossal fibers supply the extrinsic and intrinsic tongue muscles, the styloglossus, hyoglossus, genioglossus, and geniohyoid muscles.

Clinical evaluation One must determine whether lingual muscle bulk is normal or if there is atrophy, with peripheral thinning. *Fasciculations,* found in lower motor neuron diseases, are characterized by fine wormian movements, commonly seen along the edge of the tongue. Careful inspection is particularly important in infants suspected of having progressive spinal muscular atrophy, because fasciculations may be observed in the tongue and not other skeletal muscles which are well covered by subcutaneous fat. It is important not to confuse the normally tremulous tongue of a crying infant with fasciculations.

Complete evaluation includes demonstration that the tongue moves up, down, and laterally. Power can be assessed by having the older patient push the tongue against a tongue blade. In unilateral weakness or paralysis, the protruded tongue deviates toward the involved side; whereas, if the tongue remains motionless on the floor of the mouth it will curl toward the normal side because of the unopposed action of the styloglossus muscle. In cases of **myotonia,** percussion of the protruded tongue results in localized contraction that only slowly dissipates. Impairment of rapid lingual movement may be secondary to weakness, incoordination, or a specific disorder of movement. Patients with **chorea and/or athetosis** may have difficulty in maintaining a protruded tongue and attempts to do so are notable for a 'tromboning' effect. Coarse irregular lingual movements are sometimes seen in dystonia or lingual apraxia.

MOTOR SYSTEM

The motor system is comprised of different parts of the central and peripheral nervous systems that are elegantly integrated in function, enabling one to stand erect, and to initiate and control movement. Evaluation requires assessment of each component's function, individually and together. There is no part of the neurological examination that so clearly demonstrates the importance of understanding normal development of structure and function of the nervous system as examination of the motor system, for what is normal at one age is clearly abnormal at another.

Terms commonly used in reference to the motor system include the pyramidal tract, corticospinal and corticobulbar tracts, upper motor neuron, lower motor neuron, and the motor unit.

The **pyramidal tract** refers to those fibers which traverse the pyramid in the medulla oblongata, regardless of their origin or destination. The majority of fibers comes from the cerebral cortex and continues into the spinal cord as part of the **corticospinal tract**. Some fibers from the cerebral cortex course to cranial motor nerve nuclei at, or above the level of the pyramid and comprise the **corticobulbar tract**. Although the pyramidal tract is well defined neuroanatomically, there is little justification for using the term 'pyramidal tract syndrome' for motor findings usually ascribed to pyramidal tract dysfunction are not those of an isolated pyramidal lesion, but result from lesions in the cerebral cortex and/or internal capsule. The term **upper motor neuron** refers collectively to corticospinal or corticobulbar tracts and several indirect pathways including the corticorubrospinal and corticoreticulospinal tracts.

The **lower motor neuron** refers to the large motor neurons of cranial nerve nuclei within the brain stem and/or anterior horn cells of the spinal cord. The **motor unit** is the lower motor neuron with its associated axon, neuromuscular junction and muscle fibers innervated by that axon. Characteristic physical findings of upper and lower motor lesions are noted in Table 1-3.

CLINICAL EVALUATION

Evaluation includes an assessment of muscle bulk (volume), tone, power, and tendon (stretch) reflexes. In addition, one must evaluate the quality of movement — whether or not there is truncal or limb ataxia or a specific disorder of movement. The presence or absence of fasciculations and myotonia should be determined as well as an evaluation of station and gait.

Muscle bulk There is normally great variability of muscle bulk from one patient to another; the limbs and torso should be carefully inspected for atrophy or hypertrophy. It is useful to inspect the standing, unclothed child for possible mild asymmetry of limbs or trunk that may otherwise pass undetected. Comparing the size of thumb nails is also helpful; a smaller thumb nail is consistent with a long-standing neuropathic process. The distribution of muscle atrophy may be useful in defining the clinical process, as in the case of atrophic muscles innervated by one motor nerve compared with hemiatrophy secondary to cerebral lesion. Comparative circumferential limb measurements have limited usefulness unless measured from the same bony landmarks. Palpation of muscle may provide useful information particularly in infant patients in whom an ample layer of subcutaneous fat conceals muscle bulk.

Fasciculations usually indicate an abnormality of the anterior horn cell. These are fine, irregular, wormian or twitching movements of groups of muscle fibers that are best seen when viewed from the side. They may be elicited when the muscle is slightly stretched or when gently percussed and usually do not move joints except in the case of small digital muscles. During infancy, fasciculations are most reliably detected in the tongue, which should be examined when both patient and physician are relaxed. The tongue of an irritable or crying baby is normally tremulous and easily mistaken for fasciculations. Fasciculations are sometimes seen in normal patients when under great stress.

Table 1-3   Comparison of Findings
in Upper and Lower Motor Neuron Lesions

	Upper motor neuron	Lower motor neuron
Muscle bulk	Normal to decreased	Decreased
Fasciculations	None	Present
Muscle tone	Decreased (infants) Increased (from early childhood)	Decreased
Power	Decreased	Decreased
Tendon reflexes	Increased	Decreased to absent
Plantar response	Extensor	Flexor to nonreactive

Muscle tone   The resistance of muscle to passive stretch is an essential part of the examination. Decreased tone (hypotonia) is typically found in lesions of the motor unit, cerebellum, or proprioceptive pathways, and is a common finding in chorea. Increased tone (hypertonia) is a characteristic feature of corticospinal or extrapyramidal tract lesions. Hypertonia of spastic type is greater during the initial phase of limb movement and then suddenly giving way, lending a quality of clasp-knife closure. Hypertonia secondary to extrapyramidal lesions has been described as uniform rigidity 'plastic,' 'lead-pipe,' or 'cog-wheel' — a stuttering rigidity.

Muscle power   There are two forms of muscle power that should be examined; namely, kinetic power in which the patient moves a limb against the resisting examiner, and static power in which the examiner attempts to move a stationary resistant limb of the patient. Both forms of muscle power are usually affected by a disease process except for some diseases of the extrapyramidal system in which static power is normal but kinetic power is impaired.

Major joints should be tested for flexion, extension, abduction, and adduction. Some joints should also be tested for internal and external rotation as well as supination and pronation. Grading muscle power is valuable, particularly when following a patient over a long period of time.

An assessment of muscle power in infants is primarily limited to inspection. Infants of 28-32 weeks' gestation move their limbs slowly with a writhing quality but sometimes demonstrate a rapid, coarse, limb movement. Infants of 32-36 weeks' gestation demonstrate increasing forcefulness of flexor movement, legs greater than arms. Full-term infants have limb movements that are quite vigorous often with alternating flexor movements of the legs.

Tendon reflexes (stretch reflexes), are elicited by tapping the tendon insertions of the muscle to be examined with a percussion hammer appropriate for the size of the child. One should tap gently, just enough to elicit a muscular contraction. In this way, one is better able to compare the relative reflex activity of both right and left reflexes. The muscle should be palpated during percussion of the tendon because in some patients the muscle contraction can be felt but not visualized. If the stretch reflexes cannot be elicited or they are strikingly decreased despite adequate tendon percussion, the patient should, at the count of three, either make a fist or forcefully squeeze the examiner's fingers while the examiner simultaneously percusses the muscle tendon (Jendrassik maneuver). Another method of increasing this proprioceptive input is to have the child pull his fingertips apart, again at the count of three, while the examiner simultaneously percusses the muscle tendon to be evaluated.

In full-term infants one may only elicit the biceps, patellar, and ankle jerks, and in about 10% of normal full-term infants no stretch reflexes can be elicited.

Plantar response (Babinski sign) is evaluated by scratching or stroking (with a key or similar pointed object) the lateral aspect of the sole of the foot from the heel to the distal metatarsals, moving medially toward the inferior aspect of the great toe. Dorsiflexion of that great toe, an extensor plantar response, particularly with fanning or separation of the toes, suggests corticospinal tract dysfunction. One must interpret dorsiflexion of the great toe in a skittish or resisting child with caution for it may represent withdrawal from a noxious stimulus and not true evidence of corticospinal tract dysfunction. In those patients where there is no movement of the toe following stimulus of the plantar surface of the foot, one must determine if the patient has normal power to dorsiflex or plantarflex that toe. A nonreactive plantar response may be as important as one that is obviuosly extensor.

The plantar response of the newborn and early infant has limited value. Gentle stroking or scratching of the plantar surface of the foot usually results in plantar flexion of the great toe; whereas, use of a noxious stimulus, such as a pin, results in an extensor plantar response. Dorsiflexion of the great toe, the extensor plantar response, will disappear in most infants during the first 12 months of life. There is no relationship between the disappearance of the infantile extensor plantar response and the ability to stand or walk.

Myotonia is a defect of the normal phase of muscle relaxation; the normal myotatic response to percussion is prolonged. This can be demonstrated by having the patient make a fist and then quickly relax the fingers and hand. Patients with myotonia have a delay in relaxation; the wrist is usually flexed with ulnar deviation and fingers are relaxed, often one at a time, beginning with the fifth digit. Other testing methods include abruptly opening forcefully closed eyelids, percussing the distal tendons of extensor muscles of the hand and fingers, or by percussing the protruded tongue that is supported by a tongue blade. In each case there is a delay of relaxation of muscle contraction: the eyelids open slowly, the hand and fingers are 'hung up,' and the tongue slowly returns to its usual quiet state.

Station refers to the posture or manner in which the patient stands. This involves inspection of the musculoskeletal system, so it is better to have the child undressed. Toddlers under the age of 3 or 4 years are normally lordotic with a prominent tummy. If lordosis persists beyond this period, however, one should be concerned about the possibility of weakness of the pelvic girdle muscles, agenesis of abdominal muscles, bony abnormalities of the pelvis and/or lumbosacral vertebrae, or some systemic diseases with associated prominent hepatosplenomegaly.

Children of 3 or 4 years should be able to stand erect with feet together and eyes open or closed. Those with cerebellar lesions of midline tend to sway back and forth, ultimately assuming a broad based stance to improve their stability. Those patients with cerebellar hemispheric lesions tend to sway or fall toward the side of the lesion. With the eyes closed the ataxia of cerebellar lesions is mildly increased; however, if there is a dramatic increase with the eyes closed, there is probably impairment of proprioception, or **sensory ataxia**. This markedly abnormal sway or falling with feet together and eyes closed is called a positive **Romberg sign**.

Abnormalities of station may be apparent in patients with muscular weakness of any cause; these patients tend to be tremulous and seek support from walls or available furniture, swaying from side to side. Unsteadiness may also have a psychogenic basis and one must cautiously look for inconsistencies in the neurological examination. Such unsteadiness may range from subtle to extreme and usually requires the elegant function of a normal nervous system in order to carry out such coordinated, incoordinate movements. Most patients do not hurt themselves even if they fall, but this is not always the case.

GAIT

Much is learned from observing and listening to the patient's gait. Integration of postural mechanisms as well as normal function of the entire neuromuscular system are needed to maintain an erect posture and then alternately shift weight from one leg to the other while moving forward. One gait cycle is the period of one heel-strike to the next heel-strike in the same leg.

Patients with **spastic hemiplegia** tend to maintain varying degrees of flexion of the hip and knee with equinovarus posture of the ankle and foot. There is an upward tilt of the pelvis on the affected side as the leg is swung up, out, around, and back to midline. Some patients are not able to clear the floor with their foot and the toes may be dragged along. There is decreased arm swing on the affected side.

Patients with **spastic diplegia** are usually toe-walkers from early childhood. Walking, characterized as a 'scissors gait,' is slow and shuffling with adduction of the lower limbs and flexion of the hips and knees. Commonly, toes are scraped along the floor with each step.

Ataxic gait, secondary to cerebellar dysfunction, is broad based, unsteady, sometimes lurching from side to side. Tremors of the head and trunk (titubation) may be present. Patients with lesions of one cerebellar hemisphere or unilateral vestibular lesions, tend to fall towards the side of that lesion. If proprioception is impaired, patients have a sensory ataxia and tend to look at the ground ahead, utilizing visual cues for foot placement. The gait has a slapping quality because of the separation of heel and sole strike.

When extrapyramidal function is impaired, patients are slightly bent over with flexion of shoulders, elbows, and wrists. The fingers may be extended at the metacarpophalangeal joints.

Steppage gait, typical of patients with weakness of dorsiflexion of the toes and feet, is characterized by raising the foot inordinately high to avoid scraping the toes on the ground, only to strike the heel, and then the anterior foot, producing a slapping sound.

Toe walking from time to time is normal for toddlers; it is usually not indicative of a disease process. However, if toe walking is persistent one should consider weakness of the pelvic girdle muscles as seen in Duchenne's muscular dystrophy, mild to moderate spastic diplegia, and occasionally some children with severe behavioral disturbances. Occasionally, transient toe walking is reported in family members of several generations, all of whom are normal.

ATAXIA

Ataxia generally refers to lack of coordination secondary to abnormal cerebellar modulation of movement and posture. However, impaired sensory input (proprioception) or weakness may also cause incoordination. It is useful to consider cerebellar function within a developmental frame of reference: the flocculonodular lobe, uvula, and nodulus (archicerebellum), concerned with maintenance of equilibrium; the midline anterior and posterior lobes (paleocerebellum) which regulate input and output from the spinal cord and vestibular nuclei; and the cerebellar hemispheres (neocerebellum) which have a reciprocal relationship with the cerebral cortex and ultimately the final motor pathway. Abnormal cerebellar function results in asynergia, dysmetria, inability to maintain the posture of a limb, and intention tremor.

Midline cerebellar lesions result in patients swaying back and forth, assuming a broad-based stance to maintain stability. Cerebellar hemispheric lesions may result in the patient's lurching or falling to the side of the lesion.

TEST METHODS

Abnormalities of posture and movement are demonstrated by a variety of tests. The examiner should have the patient stand with arms extended anteriorly and eyes open and closed. With closed eyes, the extended arm on the side of the lesion usually drifts downward and to the side. The Holmes rebound phenomenon may be assessed by having the patient stand with both arms extended anteriorly. The examiner applies mild to moderate downward force to the patient's arms and then suddenly releases that force. Abnormal rebound is demonstrated by the patient's inability to check that movement.

Nose-finger-nose-test   Here the examiner requests the patient to alternately touch the tip of his nose, the tip of the examiner's forefinger and back to the patient's nose. As the examiner moves his target forefinger from place to place, subtle abnormalities of coordination are readily apparent. The examiner may also have the patient (standing with extended arms and eyes closed) touch the tip of his nose. Ataxic patients will have a tremor, particularly as they approach the target.

Rapid alternating or rapid repetitive movements may demonstrate a decomposition of movement. Patients are asked to rapidly tap the tip of the forefinger against the thumb or tap the thigh with the hand. One should not confuse force with rapidity and coordination of movement.

SPECIFIC DISORDERS OF MOVEMENT

Such disorders are usually apparent at rest but are more obvious when the patient is anxious or under stress. Except for ballism or some patients with severe dystonia, these abnormal movements disappear during sleep. Though considered separately, these abnormal movements blend one into the other. Patients may manifest components of different movement types.

Athetosis is a slow, irregular, writhing or twisting movement, primarily distal, which may affect the trunk and/or limbs. There is usually alternating flexion, extension, or hyperextension of the wrist and digits, often one digit at a time; the thumb is usually flexed against the palm. Facial grimacing and incoordination of oropharyngeal muscles may be apparent, resulting in dysarthria and anarthria with drooling. A vacuous facial expression may belie a sound intelligence.

Ballism is a violent flailing of the limbs in which proximal muscles are affected more than distal and arms more than legs. The face, neck, and trunk may also be affected and, rarely, the severity of movement may catapult the patient from the bed. This movement may affect one limb (monoballismus), ipsilateral arm and leg (hemiballismus) and, rarely, bilateral limbs (biballismus).

Chorea is characterized by quick, uncoordinated movement that moves from place to place without semblance of regularity. At first glance, patients appear fidgety or restless. Commonly the face, neck, and distal muscles are affected; but any skeletal muscle can be involved. Choreic movement is often superimposed upon volitional movements which then seem exaggerated; hence the term chorea (Gr. = dance). Patients may try to mask the choreic movement by incorporating it with other pseudopurposeful movement; they have difficulty in sustaining muscular contraction as demonstrated by their squeezing the examiner's fingers (milk-maid's hand). Other methods of examination include having the seated patient protrude the tongue while simultaneously extending arms and legs. The tongue may slide back and forth, as a trombone, there is a 'spooning' of hand with a slight wrist flexion and hyperextension of metacarpophalangeal joints. Often patients have a tendency to pronate extended arms and hands.

Dystonia is an irregular, somewhat slow, twisting or torsion of limb and/or trunk muscles. Dystonia may be generalized or confined to a specific region such as the face, tongue, or neck. Dystonic posturing may last for hours or days and may be persistent during sleep. Long-lasting, permanent contractures may result. Tremors are sometimes present.

SENSORY EXAMINATION

This part of the examination is the most subjective, particularly in the case of children. Evaluation of exteroceptive and higher cortical function is the same in older children as in adults. However, when the patient is an infant or young child, one must be content with an assessment of response to pain

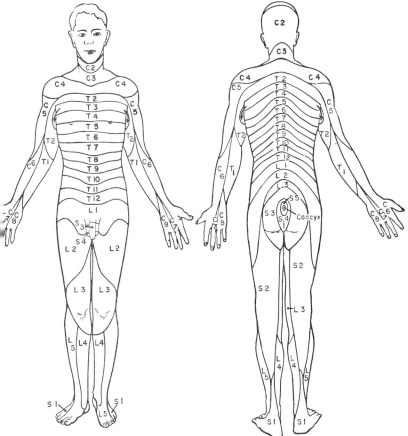

Fig. 1 5 Segmental distribution of the cutaneous nerves in man. (Reproduced with permission from Barr ML, Kiernan JA: *The Human Nervous System*, Harper & Row, Philadelphia, 1983.)

or in some cases, pain and touch. Instructions should be given clearly and the examiner should remain ever mindful of the patient's attentiveness. Children tend to become weary during sensory testing and are more easily distracted. On occasion, the sensory examination must be repeated several times before the findings are accepted.

TOUCH

Cotton wool is a good stimulus for evaluating touch. The child, with eyes closed, may respond either verbally or by raising a finger whenever touched by the cotton wool. It is rarely necessary to assess each of the spinal dermatomes or cutaneous areas of major superficial nerves unless there is good reason to suspect a sensory deficit (either from the history of sensory abnormality or a prior abnormal examination). Rather, the evaluation of major

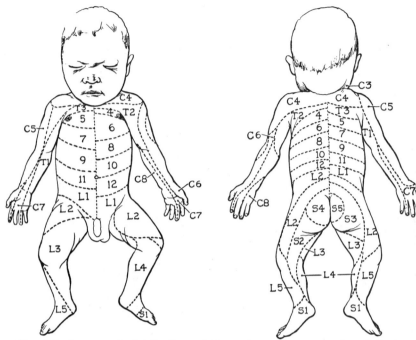

Fig. 1-6 Segmental distribution of the cutaneous nerves of an infant. (Reproduced with permission from Brann AW, Schwartz J: Central nervous system disturbances. *In* Fanaroff AA, Martin RJ (Eds) *Behrman's Neonatal-Perinatal Medicine*, 3rd ed. Mosby, St. Louis, 1983.)

areas of limbs and torso is generally sufficient. Because there is a normal variability of innervation and overlapping of several adjacent areas, one must be cautious in outlining areas of sensory loss. It may be useful to compare the distribution of weak muscles with areas of sensory loss (Figures 1-5, 1-6).

PAIN

Pain is best evaluated by using a clean pin but, since it may be alarming to the child, it is best done near the end of the examination. It is worthwhile to observe the child's facial expression during this testing, for young patients give indication of an unpleasant sensory perception. Infants withdraw from painful stimuli, but the examiner should present the stimulus a number of times to be assured the withdrawal is purposeful.

TEMPERATURE

The evaluation of temperature is usually not an integral part of the examination if the patient has responded normally to painful stimuli. However, when needed, either glass or metal tubes filled with cold (40 F) and warm (110 F) water are used as test stimuli; metal is better than glass, for it is a better conductor of heat.

PROPRIOCEPTION

Proprioceptive input arises from soft tissues other than the skin — the muscles, ligaments, and the tissues of the joints. Methods of examination include the ability to perceive position sense and the determination of the patient's perception of vibration. Children of 4 or 5 years are generally able to participate in tests of position sense. The examiner should gently grasp the lateral aspects of one of the child's great toes and demonstrate to the child with eyes open how the toe is moved up and down; then with the patient's eyes closed, the examiner moves the finger or toe up or down and the child must identify the direction of the movement.

Perception of vibration is assessed by placing the base of a vibrating tuning fork (128 Hz) against the bony prominence such as the malleolus or metatarsophalangeal joints. The patient's responsiveness is compared to the examiner's perception of the same vibration. Another test commonly used to demonstrate proprioception is to have the patient close his eyes, extend one forefinger somewhere in space and have the patient touch the tip of that finger with the tip of his other forefinger.

HIGHER CORTICAL SENSORY FUNCTION

Evaluation includes tests for two-point discrimination, stereognosis, the ability to perceive symbols 'written' on the skin, localization of stimulated cutaneous areas, and discrimination between sizes and shapes of objects.

Two-point discrimination is evaluated by using a discriminator much like a compass or caliper. The patient is instructed with eyes closed to distinguish if touched by one or two points. It is usually best to demonstrate his being touched by one and then two points before proceeding with his eyes closed. Normally, one can perceive points 1 mm apart on the tip of the tongue; 2-4 mm on the fingertips; and 8-12 mm on the palm of the hand.

Stereognosis is the ability to perceive the form of objects by touch. The patient with closed eyes is asked to identify a small object placed in his palm. In clinical practice, common objects used include coins, key, button, or a paper clip. The patient should be familiar with the test objects before being examined.

Graphesthesia is the ability to perceive letters or numbers written on the skin. Impairment or loss of graphesthesia, in the presence of an intact sensory system, implies a cortical lesion. A variety of other tests of higher cortical function are available.

REFERENCES

Denny-Brown D: *Handbook of Neurological Examination and Case Recording.* Harvard University Press, Cambridge, 1960.

De Jong RN: *The Neurologic Examination.* Harper and Row, Hagerstown, 1979.

Haymaker W: *Bing's Local Diagnosis in Neurological Diseases*, 15th ed. Mosby, St. Louis, 1969.

Paine RS, Oppe TE: *Neurological Examination of Children.* Spastics Society Medical Education and Information Unit, London, 1966.

2

Congenital Malformations

Bruce O. Berg, MD

EMBRYOLOGIC DEVELOPMENT

Familiarity with the normal embryologic development of the human nervous system will enable one to better understand the occurrence and nature of malformations. There is a well established, orderly pattern of development; some events seem to occur spontaneously and at the same time, while others are triggered by a recognized antecedent biological event. There is an embryologic timetable of development with critical or vulnerable periods when exposure of the embryo to noxious or inimical agents results in specific malformations. It is the time of insult rather than the type of noxious agent that is the important factor

Problems of nervous system malformations are not without significance; about 3% of living neonates and 7% of still-births have malformations of the nervous system. About 75% of fetal deaths and 40% of infant deaths have associated malformations of the nervous system.

The first gestational month is considered the period of induction. By the 18th gestational day, the embryonic disk is composed of ectoderm, mesoderm, and endoderm and by the end of the third week the neural plate, neural tube, and axial skeleton have been formed (see Figure 2-1).

The notochord (formed by the third week) and the mesoderm serve as primary inductors that determine the differentiation of ectoderm into the neural plate. The neuroectoderm develops into the central nervous system — the brain and spinal cord. By the close of the third week, major components of the forebrain are apparent and by the end of the fourth week, there is a tubular configuration with dilated vesicles at the rostral end. The anterior neuropore, located at the rostral aspect of the neural groove and corresponding to the site of the lamina terminalis, closes at 24-26 days of gestation and the site of the caudal neuropore, generally in the lumbar region, closes at 26-28 days. When the caudal neuropore has closed there is no longer any communication between the central canal and the amniotic fluid (Figure 2-1).

After the induction of neuroectoderm by mesodermal elements, the neural tube assumes an inductive influence on mesodermal components which become the skull and vertebral column. From the end of the first month of gestation, major neural processes have been formed and **cellular proliferation and differentiation** begin. Areas of cellular proliferation are

28

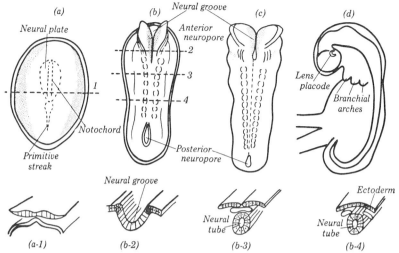

Fig. 2-1 Formation of the neural crest and neural tube. *(a)* Dorsal aspect of the developing embryo at about 18 days' gestation. *(b)* Dorsal view of developing embryo at 21 days' gestation, with transverse sections *(b 2-4)* demonstrating formation of the neural tube. *(c)* Dorsal view of developing embryo at 23 days'. *(d)* Lateral aspect of a 26-day embryo.

found in the thickened regions of cells around the periphery of the ventricular system. The majority of these cells are destined to become neuroblasts that migrate laterally. Processes from these cells pursue a course to the external surface.

From the eighth gestational week, there is a secondary migration of neuroblasts to form the cerebral cortex. This process does not end until after birth. Neuronal proliferation and migration result in the rostral aspect of the tubular structure resembling the human brain. Migration and cellular differentiation continue; cortical gyri are apparent during the second trimester and secondary sulci are apparent in the third trimester; tertiary sulci are present by the sixth postnatal month. The last trimester and the first several years show increasing cellular differentiation and elaboration of neuropil (Figure 2-2).

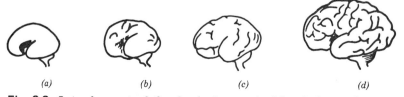

Fig. 2-2 Lateral aspect of the developing cerebral hemispheres, demonstrating increasing gyral and sulcal complexity. *(a)* 12 weeks. *(b)* 26 weeks. *(c)* 32 weeks. *(d)* 36 weeks.

DISORDERS OF NEURULATION

Malformations of neural tube closure are severe anomalies and, except for meningoceles or meningomyeloceles, are generally incompatible with any significant survival. Defects are usually associated with failure of closure of the rostral and/or caudal neuropore, although there may be skipped areas of abnormalities of neural tube closure. **Rachischisis** refers to a congenital fissure of the spinal column, or failure of neural tube closure, and **dysraphism** refers to incomplete neural tube closure.

Alpha-fetoprotein (AFP), a fetal serum globulin, is initially produced in the yolk sac and then the fetal liver and gut. A portion of that protein moves from the fetal urine to the amniotic fluid and appears in the maternal serum as well as the amniotic fluid. In cases of neural tube defects, there is a leak of fetal blood components into the amniotic fluid and, hence, an increase in maternal serum and amniotic fluid levels of this protein. Elevations of maternal AFP appear during the first 20 weeks of gestation period and then decline. If the serum AFP is abnormally elevated, ultrasonographic examination must be performed to delineate possible fetal structural abnormalities if amniocentesis and abortion are contemplated. One collaborative study of AFP maternal screening in Great Britain reported an 80% detection rate of the fetuses with neural tube defects. Elevations of amniotic fluid AFP have also been reported in some cases of omphalocele, gastrointestinal obstruction, sacrococcygeal teratoma, and Turner syndrome.

ANENCEPHALY

This is a relatively common malformation, incompatible with life, characterized by partial or complete absence of the brain with associated defects of the cranial vault and scalp. The frontal bones above the supraorbital ridge, parietal and squamous portion of the occipital bones are absent and there are commonly bony defects through the foramen magnum with rachischisis of the cervical spine. Exposed tissue is an angiofibromatous mass containing degenerated neural and glial tissue. The cerebellum, brain stem, and spinal cord are present but often malformed and small. The eyes are well developed but the optic nerves are usually absent. The pituitary gland is markedly hypoplastic or absent and the adrenal glands are usually hypoplastic, containing mostly medullary tissue.

Associated malformations of virtually every organ system have been reported. The trunk and limbs are usually well developed but the arms are relatively large compared with the legs. Patients may suck and swallow but their deformities are lethal and they die within hours to several days and at most a matter of weeks.

This malformation is seen most commonly in the Western world with the highest prevalence rate in Great Britain and Ireland and the lowest in Africa, Asia, and South America. The incidence varies from 1:1000 live births in the USA to 5:1000 in Wales and Ireland. There is a preponderance of females affected and whites are 3-6 times more commonly affected than blacks. It has been generally accepted that anencephaly is a defect of neural tube closure during the most critical gestational period of

21-26 days. However, more recently an alternative view of etiology is that the closed neural tube is opened, and previously formed portions of the brain degenerate. There is no universally accepted cause of this anomaly although a wide variety of possible causes have been proposed. The defect, as other open neural tubular defects, can be detected prenatally by demonstrating an elevation of AFP in the maternal serum.

During their short lifetime, these patients may have spontaneous limb movements and withdraw from noxious stimuli. Primitive reflexes including suck, root, and righting reflexes are usually present.

ENCEPHALOCELES

Encephaloceles are characterized by associated defects of cranium and cerebral substance. The bony defect, or cleft, without protrusion of meninges or brain, is called cranium bifida occulta. When the meninges protrude through the defect it is a meningocele and if the protrusion includes brain substance it is called an encephalocele. In cases where the ventricle extends through the bony cleft into the herniated sac the defect is called a hydranencephalocele. Sixty to 75% are located in the occipital region, with others occurring in the frontal, nasofrontal, nasopharyngeal, parietal, or temporoorbital regions. Encephaloceles affecting the anterior part of the skull, though rare in the Western world, are relatively common in Southeast Asia and have been called sincipital encephaloceles.

The **pathogenesis** of encephaloceles is unknown although similar malformations have been produced experimentally by exposure to teratogens. The **diagnosis** is usually readily apparent because of the obvious protruding sac. Those few cases wherein the defect affects the sphenoid and/or ethmoid bones are less apparent but should be suspected in a short child with hypertelorism. Neurologic findings are variable and depend upon the extent of the defect. Mental retardation is common with varying degrees of corticospinal tract dysfunction. Other anomalies are commonly associated with the encephalocele.

Surgical removal is usually readily accomplished, but there is a potential risk of infection. The prognosis depends upon the site and extent of the malformation although it is usually unfavorable.

EXENCEPHALY

This is a rare malformation in which the brain is outside the skull. As the gestation progresses, neural tissue gradually degenerates. It is unusual that such infants are carried to term.

CRANIUM BIFIDA AND SPINA BIFIDA

These conditions result from the failure of closure of the midline of the skull and posterior vertebral arches, respectively. These bony defects allow protrusion of the brain and/or spinal cord, resulting in a variety of nervous tissue malformations. Defects of the skull are usually midline, primarily affecting the occipital region but can occur in other sites. There may only be the bony defect or an associated protrusion of brain tissue and meninges (encephalocele). Defects of fusion of the posterior vertebral arches alone are called **spina bifida occulta**.

Spina bifida with protrusion of meninges are considered **meningoceles** and those patients with protrusion of meninges and neural tissue have **meningomyeloceles**. A spectrum of fusion abnormalities ranges from one segment to partial or complete dysraphism. However, patients with complete dysraphism are usually spontaneously aborted early in the pregnancy.

About 75% of patients with spina bifida have meningomyeloceles. They are most commonly found in the lumbar region and least commonly in the cervical region. Anterior midline defects are uncommon but are sometimes found in patients with neurofibromatosis. Approximately 75% of patients with lumbosacral meningomyeloceles have associated hydrocephalus secondary to Chiari malformations of the hind brain.

Management of patients with meningomyeloceles requires the expertise of different specialists, for it may involve surgical repair of the lesion and control of hydrocephalus by shunting, orthopedic management of paralysis and potential hip dislocation, observation and treatment of genitourinary abnormalities, and control of any infectious process such as meningitis and/or ventriculitis. Above all, there should be one physician (a child neurologist or a skilled pediatrician) who is the primary physician in charge of the patient's total treatment.

About 75% of children who have had no surgical repair of their lesion die within the first year of life. One study of all patients treated early and nonselectively, indicated that regardless of vigorous medical and surgical treatment (some cases requiring many repeated operations) over one-half of patients died before the age of 2 years. Associated problems included chronic urinary abnormalities, severe paralysis, kyphosis, and other associated anomalies.

In order to identify patients who would have some reasonable chance for quality life, if vigorously treated, a list of adverse criteria were developed (Lorber). These criteria include: severe paraplegia (below L1); gross head enlargement with a head circumference greater than 2 cm over the 90th percentile corrected for birth weight; kyphosis; associated gross congenital anomalies or major birth injuries.

Though it is difficult to obtain reliable, comparative results of different studies, about 80% of patients untreated are dead by the age of 3 years; whereas, 75% of selected patients treated early were alive, though significantly handicapped, at 6 years. Physicians in the USA have been more inclined to aggressively treat children with these multiple difficult problems. Patients with thoracolumbar meningomyeloceles and/or severe hydrocephalus have a particularly poor prognosis. One of the key factors in deciding a treatment plan depends upon the assessment of the patient's future mental ability, a difficult task, rather tenuously related to the thickness of cortical mantle as determined by CT brain scan.

The family must be fully informed about the status of the infant — what are the malformations and what do they mean to the infant in terms of survival, future development, and requirement for frequent future medical and surgical care.

ARNOLD - CHIARI MALFORMATIONS

These are more appropriately called Chiari malformations, and are characterized by protrusion of the cerebellum through the foramen magnum; they are usually associated with hind-brain abnormalities (Figure 2-3). **Chiari type I** consists of the hind brain displaced into the spinal canal with protrusion of the cerebellar tonsils through the foramen magnum. Associated abnormalities include those of the basilar-occipital bones, the atlas/axis, platybasia or basilar impression, small foramen magnum, and occasionally abnormalities of cervical vertebrae. Hydromyelia or syringomyelia may be present.

Clinical manifestations of Chiari type I, if apparent, are usually found in older patients and include head tilt, paralysis of lower cranial nerves, or ataxia. Some patients complain of headache and/or vertigo.

Patients with Chiari type I, usually but not always, improve following cervical laminectomy and removal of the posterior aspect of the foramen magnum. A ventriculoperitoneal (VP) or ventriculoatrial (VA) shunt may be required.

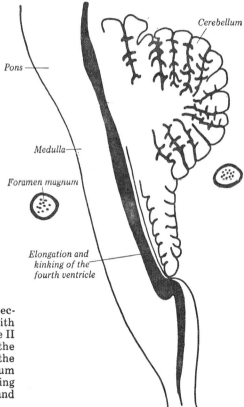

Fig. 2-3 Median sagittal section of a brain stem with Chiari malformation, type II showing protrusion of the cerebellar tonsils below the level of the foramen magnum with elongation and kinking of the fourth ventricle and hind brain.

Chiari type II is the most common of this group of malformations and is frequently associated with lumbosacral meningomyeloceles. This malformation is characterized by the findings of type I but, in addition, the hind brain and fourth ventricle are elongated and often kinked, protruding through the foramen magnum into the spinal canal. The lower cranial nerves may be stretched within the spinal canal as they ascend to traverse the foramen magnum and reach their muscles of innervation. Hydrocephalus is usually present because of abnormalities of the aqueduct of Sylvius. Hydromyelia or syringomyelia are occasionally seen.

The clinical manifestations of Chiari type II malformation are primarily those of hydrocephalus; cerebellar signs are not usually apparent. Abnormalities of cranial nerve function, particularly the lower cranial nerves, may be present and include laryngeal stridor, dysphagia, weakness of the sternocleidomastoid muscles, or lingual fasciculations.

The treatment of Chiari type II malformation with hydrocephalus is a VP or VA shunt.

Chiari type III malformation is an occipital encephalocele; hydrocephalus is a commonly associated finding. **Chiari type IV** is a variant of these malformations in which the cerebellum is hypoplastic. Some patients have an occipital encephalocele. Patients with an occipital encephalocele as part of the Chiari types III or IV may benefit from surgical removal of the abnormal extruded tissue. The outlook for the quality of life and survival is generally poor.

DIASTEMATOMYELIA

This is a cleft, or duplication of the spinal cord around an associated bony and cartilagenous septum originating from the posterior vertebral arch and extending anteriorly. Most patients have lesions confined to the lower thoracic and/or lumbar regions but the lesions may extend for many spinal segments. The anomaly occurs three times more frequently in females than males and the majority of patients have a patch of hypertrichosis overlying the dysraphic area. Less commonly associated abnormalities include a nevus, angioma, lipoma, or dermal sinus. Abnormalities of spinal curvature are not rare.

There may be no neurologic abnormality recognized in early life, although one lower limb, usually below the knee, is often deformed. The arch of the foot is abnormally high and the forefoot is adducted and inverted; commonly the growing child has a peculiar gait or posture.

Patients may have impairment of pain and temperature as well as light touch. There may be findings of upper motor neuron and lower motor neuron lesions and some patients have bladder dysfunction. The diagnosis is well demonstrated by metrizamide myelography and CT scan.

The bony septum should be surgically removed but the existing neurologic deficit persists. Any progressive spinal cord damage following the surgical procedure probably results from repeated trauma secondary to movement of the vertebral column. The septum should be removed, if detected, in relatively asymptomatic patients.

DIPLOMYELIA

Diplomyelia is characterized by duplication of the spinal cord. It may occur without other anomalies but is sometimes associated with spina bifida or spinal cord tumors.

HYDROMYELIA

This is a congenital abnormality of the spinal cord notable for abnormal dilation of the central canal which compromises the surrounding spinal cord structures including the anterior horn cells. It occurs almost entirely in the cervical or lumbar region but may traverse the entire length of the cord. The etiology remains unclear. Onset of symptoms is usually in the second decade or later and characterized by sensory loss, muscular atrophy, and incoordination. There is no specific treatment.

SYRINGOMYELIA

Syringomyelia is an anomaly characterized by cavitation of the spinal cord. The cavities are lined by ependyma and/or glial tissue and sometimes communicate with the central canal. They are primarily found in the cervical cord but may extend cephalad into the brain stem. Abnormalities of the basilar skull bones with hydrocephalus are frequently associated, and intramedullary tumors are found in 20-30% of patients.

Since the cavities are usually central, crossed fiber tracts are commonly affected, resulting in abnormalities of pain and temperature, but sparing the posterior columns. Some patients have trophic ulcers of the fingers and/or vasomotor instability. If the cavity extends cephalad, anterior horn cells and corticospinal tracts can be affected resulting in asymmetrical lower motor neuron findings in the arms and concomitant spasticity in lower limbs.

Diagnosis is established by metrizamide myelography and CT scan. A variety of surgical therapeutic methods have been utilized but more recently shunting of the central canal to the subarachnoid space has been of great benefit.

SYRINGOBULBIA

Syringobulbia is characterized by anomalous cavitation extending to the brain stem, disrupting lower cranial nerve nuclei and resulting in stridor, hoarseness, or lingual weakness. The clinical diagnosis is confirmed by CT scan and myelography.

SACRAL AGENESIS

A range of sacrococcygeal anomalies is included in this diagnostic category. Both partial and complete forms are recognized and lumbar vertebrae may be included as part of the malformation. Partial sacral agenesis includes those conditions in which only a part of the sacrum and coccyx are missing. Complete sacral agenesis is considered as that condition where the iliac bones are directly fused. Several other associated malformations of different organ systems have been reported. Patients may have a neurogenic bladder with urinary incontinence. Recurring urinary tract infections may be a problem and a delay in diagnosis may result in hydronephrosis.

The rare **caudal regression syndrome** found in infants of some diabetic mothers has been characterized by agenesis of the sacrum and coccyx and/or malformation of lower extremities. Other associated malformations have included renal agenesis, skeletal defects of the tibia and fibula, hip dislocation, clubbed feet, cleft palate, and congenital heart disease. The relationship of prediabetic state and frank diabetes to this syndrome is unclear.

DISORDERS OF CELL MIGRATION

Abnormalities of cell migration may be partial or complete, resulting in localized or generalized areas of cortical malformation wherein neurons do not reach the cortical surface.

LISSENCEPHALY AND PACHYGYRIA

These abnormalities are considered together because of their similar features. **Lissencephaly** refers to a smooth cortical surface without sulci, similar to the embryonic cerebrum at the end of the first trimester. **Pachygyria** refers to a brain with primitive development of sulci. The majority of neuroblasts do not reach the external cortical surface and may be left behind as heterotopia. There are decreased secondary sulci and in some cases only the sylvian fissures are apparent. **Micropolygyria** refers to abnormally small convolutions with increased secondary sulci, and may be a prenatal malformation or secondary to postnatal infection.

Lissencephaly and pachygyria are usually clinically manifested by microcephaly, varying degrees of corticospinal tract dysfunction, most commonly spastic quadriplegia, convulsions, and severe mental retardation. Micropolygyria is often associated with mental retardation and corticospinal tract dysfunction.

SCHIZENCEPHALY

This is a term used to describe symmetrical clefts in the cortical surface that may extend from the ventricles to the external cerebral surface. There may be significant absence of brain substance.

AGENESIS OF THE CORPUS CALLOSUM

This is a rare cerebral malformation of unknown etiology. Though usually sporadic, there are reports of variable inheritance including autosomal dominant, autosomal recessive, and x-linked recessive traits. Males and females are equally affected.

The corpus callosum is one of the major neopallial commissures that develops from the region of the closed rostral neuropore during the end of the third gestational month. Normal callosal development proceeds in a rostral-caudal direction and the interhemispheric fibers begin to cross during the fourth gestational month. Defects of the corpus callosum vary from partial to complete absence and are usually, but not always, associated with abnormalities of the septum pellucidum.

There is no one clinical syndrome that is typical of agenesis of the corpus callosum; the malformation is usually detected unexpectedly on CT brain scans during the investigation of patients for a variety of seemingly unrelated neurologic signs and symptoms. The fact that this anomaly has been found at autopsy in asymptomatic patients suggests that its absence is not necessarily associated with recognized nervous system dysfunction.

Commonly, identified patients with agenesis of the corpus callosum have enlarged heads; however, normal and abnormally small heads have also been found. Seizures and mental retardation are common.

Aicardi syndrome is characterized by absence of the corpus callosum infantile spasms, mental retardation, lacunar chorioretinopathy, and commonly, abnormalities of the vertebral bodies. The syndrome appears to be limited to females. An absent corpus callosum is also found in arhinencephaly, cyclopia, and a rare syndrome with associated anterior horn cell disease.

Agenesis of the corpus callosum has been associated with other nervous system malformations as well as skin, ocular, cardiac, endocrine, and renal abnormalities. Vertebral column and extremities may be malformed. There is no specific treatment.

HYDRANENCEPHALY

Hydranencephaly is a condition in which most of the cerebral hemispheres have been destroyed and the residua are contained within a membranous sac which is attached to the basilar structures of the skull. The fluid contained within this sac may be clear, cloudy, or blood stained and has increased protein. The main cerebral areas affected are in the distribution of the internal carotid artery; whereas, that cerebral substance supplied by the vertebral arteries tends to be spared. It should not be presumed, however, that this condition is simply one of vascular occlusion of the anterior cerebral vascular supply for it has been identified following maternal prenatal infection, trauma, or drug ingestion.

The gestation and birth are usually unremarkable and the head may be of normal size, small, or abnormally large. In patients with normal head circumference, fontanelles may be large. Occasionally, the skull bones seem a bit 'loose.' Primitive reflex activity is usually present and the first several months of life may seem normal, unless there is increased intracranial pressure. As time passes it becomes apparent that the infant is inordinately irritable, quiet, or alternating between the two states. The stretch reflexes become increased and the infant becomes spastic. Profound developmental delay becomes readily apparent. Convulsive activity is common, but is not always present. The structure of the eyes is usually normal; pupils are reactive to light, albeit sluggishly, but most patients have abnormal extraocular motility. Associated malformations are uncommon. Most patients survive a matter of months but there are scattered case reports of patients living for several years.

MICROCEPHALY

Microcephaly is a condition in which the head circumference (OFC) is greater than minus 2 standard deviations below the mean for age, sex, race, and gestation. Neuropathologists usually define the term as patients with a brain weight less than 900 gm (adult). Dwarfs are not considered as microcephalic if their mentality is normal and limb-torso measurements are of normal proportions.

Although microcephaly is commonly considered as primary (genetic) or secondary (environmental), such classification is inherently inaccurate, as exemplified by children of mothers with phenylketonuria. Nevertheless. this dichotomy has some practical clinical value and is frequently used. Primary microcephaly indicates abnormal prenatal development and secondary microcephaly is the result of an insult during the perinatal and/or early postnatal life. The etiology of primary microcephaly usually includes a genetic defect, chromosomal abnormalities, or environmental insult. Microcephaly may be inherited as an autosomal recessive trait. These patients are generally free of other associated malformations. There appears to be incomplete penetrance for there is a relatively high incidence of mental subnormality in family members who are not microcephalic.

The patient's small head becomes more apparent with age; there is a receding forehead and abnormal scalp hair whorls are common. The weight and height are frequently decreased, presumably because of hypopituitarism and decreased growth hormone. Developmental milestones are delayed but there is variability of mentality and behavior with 2-7% of microcephalic patients, by definition, having normal intelligence. Hyperactivity is common and about one-third of patients have convulsions. Motor ability is also variable, ranging from clumsiness to spastic quadriplegia.

Microcephaly is often a characteristic feature of a variety of syndromes associated with chromosomal abnormalities including deletions, translocations, and trisomies. It has been reported in other syndromes, however, in which chromosomal karyotypes are normal.

Environmental factors include exposure to a radiation particularly during the fourth through the 20th week, but has also resulted following exposure to radiation as late as the 24th week. Other environmental factors include intrauterine infections and biochemical abnormalities.

Maternal in-utero infections that may result in congenital microcephaly include cytomegalic inclusion disease, genital herpes infection, lues, rubella, and toxoplasmosis. The developing nervous system is also vulnerable to exposure to noxious chemical agents including maternal PKU, alcohol, phenytoin, trimethadione, carbon monoxide, and methyl mercury.

MACROCEPHALY

Macrocephaly is a term that refers to patients with a head circumference (OFC) greater than 2 standard deviations over the mean for age, sex, race, and gestation. It contrasts with **megalencephaly** which refers to brains of unusually large size and weight. The average brain weight (male) of newborns is 370 gm ; 1080 gm by the age of 3 years; and 1350 gm from 6-14 years. Some patients with megalencephaly have brains weighing 1½-2 times greater than average; males are more commonly macrocephalic than females.

Table 2-1 Differential Diagnosis of Macrocephaly

Hydrocephalus
Hydranencephaly
Subdural effusions
Primary macrocephaly
Benign intracranial hypertension
Megalencephaly
    Primary megalencephaly
        Normal variant
        Abnormal cerebral cytoarchitectonics
    Metabolic diseases of the CNS
        Leucodystrophies
        Lipidoses
        Histiocytosis
        Mucopolysaccharidoses
    Neurocutaneous syndromes
        Tuberose sclerosis
        Neurofibromatosis
        Sturge-Weber syndrome
        Klippel-Trenaunay-Weber syndrome
Primary diseases of bone
        Achondroplasia
        Bone dysplasias
        Hyperphosphatemia
        Osteogenesis imperfecta
        Osteopetrosis
        Rickets
Soto syndrome (cerebral gigantism)
Riley-Smith syndrome (macrocephaly, pseudopapilledema
   and multiple hemangiomas)
Abnormal chromosomal karyotype

Macrocephaly is a physical sign found in a variety of pathophysiologic states as well as in some normal persons (Table 2-1). Despite the wonders of CT and NMR brain scans, it is not always easy to sort out a credible differential diagnosis and one must carefully apply the principles of clinical neurology: viz, obtaining a careful and complete history and performing a complete examination.

HYDROCEPHALUS

This condition is characterized by increased volume of cerebrospinal fluid (CSF) associated with ventricular dilation. The process is considered **active** when there is a progressive increased intracranial pressure and **arrested** when the intracranial pressure has stabilized and no longer causes increasing ventricular enlargement.

The terms **communicating and noncommunicating hydrocephalus** originated from studies in which phenolsulfonphthalein (PSP) was injected into one lateral ventricle. If the dye was found in the lumbar subarachnoid fluid within 20 minutes following ventricular injection, it was thought to be communicating hydrocephalus; whereas, if the lumbar subarachnoid fluid contained no dye, it was thought to be noncommunicating. This concept of communicating or noncommunicating hydrocephalus has been found useful in clinical practice.

Closure of the neural tube occurs at about 28 days, separating that tube from the amniotic fluid. About the same time the roof of the fourth ventricle dilates and the ependymal lining forms a single epithelial layer. The roof of the fourth ventricle is perforated by an active process of differentiation that begins before the development of choroid plexus function. Three critical and related events have now begun: perforation of the roof of the fourth ventricle; development of secretory epithelium in the choroid plexuses; and the differentiation of the leptomeninges into arachnoid trabeculae with formation of the subarachnoid space.

The ventricular system parallels the growth of each segment of the CNS but the central canal of the spinal cord is usually obliterated after birth because of growth of neuronal and glial elements. The ventricular system then terminates at the level of the obex.

Choroid plexus fluid formation involves two processes: filtration across the choroidal capillary wall and fluid produced by secretion of the choroidal epithelium. There is also transependymal CSF formation. The relative contribution of choroidal and transependymal formation of CSF in the human is not universally accepted at this time. The formation rate of CSF is about 0.35 ml/minute or about 500 ml/day. The CSF volume of an infant is about 5 ml, and 150 ml in the adult. Sites of reabsorption of the CSF are the arachnoidal villi and the cranial and spinal subarachnoid spaces (Figure 2-4).

Causes of hydrocephalus are many, and are generally considered as an excessive production of CSF, obstructive processes in the CSF circulatory pathway, or impaired absorption. There has been controversy regarding whether a choroid plexus papilloma can cause hydrocephalus by excessive production of CSF or the tumor mass obstructs the CSF circulation. There are now several reports of patients with choroid plexus papillomas and hydrocephalus without evidence of any obstructive process.

There have been questions regarding venous insufficiency as a cause of hydrocephalus. Under normal conditions the CSF pressure exceeds the pressure within the sagittal sinus; however, in hydrocephalic children the pressure of the sagittal sinus is equal or exceeds the intracranial pressure. While in some cases venous insufficiency plays a role in the pathogenesis of hydrocephalus, impaired absorption by arachnoid villi and obstruction of the CSF pathways are considered to be of much greater significance. The quantitative importance of spinal absorption in humans in not known (see Table 2-3).

Two important factors determine the **clinical course** and manner of presentation of patients with hydrocephalus; viz, the patient's age and the specific cause of hydrocephalus. Age is important because if cranial sutures are not closed, an active hydrocephalic process usually causes abnormal enlargement of the head. Hydrocephalus occurring before 2 years of age often

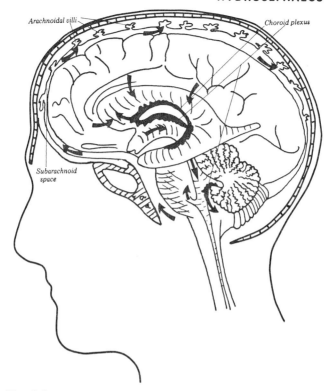

Arachnoidal villi

Choroid plexus

Subarachnoid
space

Fig. 2-4 Pathways of the CSF, showing transependymal
formation and that produced by the choroid plexuses,
circulation within the subarachnoid space, and absorption into the venous system via the arachnoid villi.

results in an abnormally large, somewhat globular skull. MacEwen's sign is
present and frontotemporal scalp veins become prominent. The child may
have impairment of upward gaze (sunset sign) secondary to dilation of the
suprapineal recess of the third ventricle compressing the mesencephalic
tectum. Unilateral or bilateral sixth nerve palsies are common and other
abnormalities of external ocular motility may be seen. Commonly, there is
increased tone of the lower limbs compared to the upper limbs, presumably because corticospinal fibers from the cortical leg area are stretched
around the distended lateral ventricles to reach the brain stem and spinal
cord. Some patients may have corticobulbar dysfunction with phonation
and feeding difficulties. Optic nerves may become atrophic secondary to
compression of dilated third ventricles.

Older children and adolescents with active hydrocephalus, may have
intermittent headache and occasional vomiting after postural changes,
particularly early in the morning. Papilledema and/or sixth nerve palsies
are sometimes seen. Changes of muscle tone are similar to that seen in

younger patients. Older patients may also have manifestations of abnormal endocrine function including menstrual irregularities or amenorrhea, delayed acquisition of secondary sex characteristics, diabetes insipidus, hypothyroidism, and occasionally abnormalities of growth.

The **diagnosis of hydrocephalus** is usually evident from the clinical evaluation. Appropriate growth charts to plot head measurements must be used, particularly for infants of varying gestational ages and sex. This is exemplified by preterm infants of appropriate weight for date who have a growth spurt in head circumference during the first month of life. When unequivocally abnormal head growth is documented, further diagnostic study is required. The CT brain scan is the neurodiagnostic study of choice for so much information is obtained regarding brain substance, ventricular size, and configuration. Every attempt should be made to delineate the etiology of hydrocephalus before any surgical procedure is undertaken.

Information regarding the flow of CSF may be obtained following injection of one of a number of radioactive agents into the lumbar subarachnoid space. The material is detected in the basilar cisterns within 1 hour and then rises over the hemispheres to the parasagittal regions. Some reflux of the radioactive material has been found within the ventricles in some patients with communicating hydrocephalus, including normal pressure hydrocephalus. More recently, metrizamide used in conjunction with computerized tomography has been most useful in demonstrating CSF circulation in normal patients as well as those with hydrocephalus. These studies are particularly useful in patients who are suspected of having **normal pressure hydrocephalus** or children who have abnormally large head circumferences but remain within the same percentile.

Treatment of hydrocephalus Since Torkildsen introduced the ventriculocisternostomy, neurosurgeons have directed the CSF into a variety of body cavities (Figure 2-5). At this time, the most common shunting procedures are the VA and VP shunt.

The VA shunt, as in the case of any hardware placed within body cavities, has inherent complications with an incidence ranging from 15-30%, consisting of thromboembolic phenomena, bacteremia, and shunt obstruction. The VP shunt is probably more commonly used at this time and may have associated complications of bacteremia or obstruction. On occasion, bacteremia cannot be cleared with antibiotics alone, and the shunt must be removed until the infection has been cleared. It is then replaced at a later time. Other uncommon complications include dislodgement of the shunt from its mooring.

It is difficult, if not impossible, to compare the wide variety of shunting procedures and their complications. Some patients require one shunt without revision and others require many revisions. In one study of the results of shunting infant patients, the survival rate after 15 years was about 50%, with 15% of survivors mentally subnormal.

NORMAL PRESSURE HYDROCEPHALUS

This is a form of communicating hydrocephalus in which there is an abnormality of the subarachnoid spaces, resulting in obstruction to normal CSF flow and its reabsorption. Patients have ventriculomegaly but without

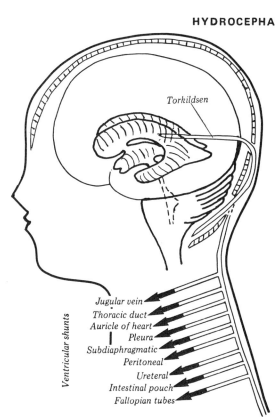

Fig. 2-5 Surgical shunting procedures that have been used in the treatment of hydrocephalus. (Modified and reproduced with permission from Ransohoff J, et al: J Pediatr 56:399-411, 1960).

obvious clinical signs of increased intracranial pressure; normal pressures are recorded at the lumbar subarachnoid space. This clinical entity primarily occurs in older patients with a gradual onset of mild loss of intellect and memory with slowing of mental processes, gait apraxia, and urinary incontinence. Experience with normal pressure hydrocephalus in childhood is limited but should be considered in a child who is slowly dementing and has a gait disturbance. The pathogenesis is not yet fully understood.

CONGENITAL COMMUNICATING HYDROCEPHALUS

There is a small group of infants who, though development and behavior are normal, have an abnormally large head circumference. CT brain scans show dilated subarachnoid spaces and ventriculomegaly. It is not uncommon that the capacious subarachnoid spaces and, in some cases, marked ventriculomegaly, suggest cortical atrophy, and grave predictions regarding the future are inappropriately given to the parents.

Table 2-2   Pathogenesis of Hydrocephalus

Lateral ventricles	Arachnoidal or subependymal cysts Subependymal hemorrhage Tumor
Foramen of Monro	Colloid cyst Tumor Inflammation (ventriculitis)
Third ventricle	Tumor Colloid cyst Hemorrhage

Aqueduct of Sylvius	Chiari malformations
	Inflammation (in-utero infection
	    meningitis)
	Tumor
	Septum, congenital
	'Stenosis' — genetic (x-linked) trait
	Vascular malformation — aneurysm
	    (AVM) of vein of Galen

Fourth ventricle	Chiari malformations Inflammation (meningitis) Dandy-Walker syndrome Tumor Vascular malformation Hemorrhage
Subarachnoid space	Inflammation Subarachnoid hemorrhage Leptomeningeal cysts
Arachnoid villi	Congenital decrease or absence of villi Obstruction from hemorrhage Inflammation

Modified and reproduced with permission from Lemire RJ, et al: *Normal and Abnormal Development of the Human Nervous System.* Harper & Row, Hagerstown, 1975.

If the patient is otherwise asymptomatic, has normal developmental milestones, and aside from the head circumference, has a normal neurological examination, it is generally prudent to observe that patient carefully on an outpatient basis over a period of months and repeat the brain scan rather than immediately implanting a shunt. Most of these patients are normal and over a period of months the CT brain scan also becomes normal.

DANDY - WALKER SYNDROME

This syndrome is characterized by developmental abnormalities of the fourth ventricle and cerebellum. There is a cystic dilation of the fourth ventricle, the aqueduct, the third and both lateral ventricles. The foramen of Magendie is atretic or absent and there is a failure of development of one or both foramina of Luschka. Although it has been suggested that the obstructive hydrocephalus is secondary to atresia or absence of the foramina of Magendie and Luschka, the constellation of structural abnormalities imply an insult to the developing nervous system before the time of development of the fourth ventricle. All foramina of the fourth ventricle may be closed or one may be open. Other associated malformations include agenesis of the corpus callosum, heterotopia, gyral abnormalities, as well as anomalies of the cerebellum and brain stem.

The head circumference is increased and there is a 'ballooning' of the occipital region. Plain skull films demonstrate an enlarged posterior fossa with elevation of the torcular Herophili. Air injected into the lumbar subarachnoid space seldom fills the ventricular system but ventriculography using a 'hanging-head position' is usually diagnostic. The current neurodiagnostic studies of choice include CT or NMR brain scans.

Patients commonly first see a physician because of an abnormally enlarged head with a prominent occiput. They may have delayed acquisition of motor skills and an occasional patient may have a sixth-nerve palsy. There is varying abnormality of corticospinal tract function. Older children may have symptoms and signs of increased intracranial pressure with vomiting and headache. Ataxia is usually a late finding. Therapy usually consists of surgical excision of the cyst wall; however, a shunting procedure may be required.

CRANIOSYNOSTOSIS

Craniosynostosis is the premature closure of cranial sutures, resulting in a variety of skull deformities, or craniostenoses. The pathogenesis is not known, although a variety of hypotheses have been presented, primarily emphasizing abnormalities of the mesenchymal layer of ossification centers. It is generally believed there is a primary abnormality of the basilar skull bones at dural attachment sites and that premature closure of sutures is a secondary phenomenon. Bone growth is impeded in a plane perpendicular to the suture line; hence, the skull size increases in a plane parallel to the suture line. Clinical terms related to craniostenosis are listed in Table 2-3.

The most common form of craniosynostosis is that affecting the sagittal suture, resulting in scaphocephaly. Premature closure of the coronal suture results in widening of the skull, and other skull deformities are secondary to differing combinations of prematurely fused sutures. Syndromes associated with craniosynostosis are noted in Table 2-4.

There is only one form of **treatment** at this time; namely, the surgical excision of the fused suture and application of silastic or similar material to the edges of the craniectomy to avoid formation of bridges of reossification. Reasons for surgical intervention depend upon the presence or the possibility of developing chronic increased intracranial pressure which may cause brain injury, and/or the need for reconstructive surgery.

Table 2-3 The Craniostenoses

Clinical term	Suture(s) prematurely fused
Scaphocephaly	Sagittal suture
Dolichocephaly	Sagittal suture
Brachycephaly	Coronal suture
Plagiocephaly	Unilateral or bilateral lambdoid and/or coronal sutures. Sagittal suture may be involved
Trigonocephaly	Metopic suture
Oxycephaly (acrocephaly, hysicephaly, turricephaly, tower head)	All sutures

Patients with multiple sutures prematurely fused have greater potential for developing chronic increased intracranial pressure and must be carefully evaluated regarding the need for surgical treatment.

Those patients with only the sagittal suture prematurely fused rarely have any associated neurologic dysfunction or intellectual impairment. Nonetheless, there are compelling reasons to carry out reconstructive surgery in these cases early in life, during the first 6 months of age, to avoid an increasing deformity of the skull. The mortality and morbidity for surgical correction of craniosynostosis is less than 1%.

VASCULAR MALFORMATIONS

This group of congenital cerebrovascular malformations usually does not make its presence known until after the second decade of life. They have been arbitrarily classified as arteriovenous malformations, venous malformations, cryptic or occult malformations, and aneurysms.

ARTERIOVENOUS MALFORMATIONS

These lesions are composed of both normal and abnormal arteries and veins and are surrounded by fibrous tissue and often inflammatory cells. There are usually feeding arterial vessels and prominent draining veins. The majority of patients have AVMs involving the hemispheric convexities or the parasagittal cortex and are supplied principally by branches of the middle cerebral artery. Apical AVMs are commonly supplied by the anterior cerebral artery and those lesions of the posterior hemisphere are

Table 2-4 Syndromes Associated with Craniosynostosis

	Head	Face	Limbs	CNS
Apert's syndrome	Forehead is broad and high; the occiput is somewhat flattened. Skull may be tower shaped. Coronal and lambdoid sutures usually prematurely fused. Other facial sutures may also fuse prematurely.	Prominent, sometimes protruding, eyes with reversed slant of palpebral fissures. Hypoplastic maxillae with flat nasal bridge, lending 'beak-like' appearance to nose. Palate narrow and high arched.	Syndactyly of all limbs which may affect soft tissue and/or bone. Upper limbs are often shortened.	Usually moderately to severely mentally subnormal. Some patients have increased ICP. Associated malformations of other organ systems are not uncommon.
Carpenter's syndrome	Premature closure of coronal and lambdoid sutures as in Apert's syndrome; however, all sutures may be fused prematurely.	Flat nasal bridge associated with a flat face. Reversed palpebral fissure with lateral displacement of medial canthi. Epicanthic folds, microcornea and micrognathia have been reported.	Partial syndactyly of 3rd & 4th fingers. Polysyndactyly of toes with duplication of 1st or 2nd toes.	Most patients are mentally subnormal.
Chotzen's syndrome	Flat forehead and occiput with increase in vertical dimensions. Usually coronal sutures are prematurely fused.	Forehead is wide and flat with ocular hypertelorism present. Prominent, broad nose and mandible; ptosis is sometimes seen.	Syndactyly of proximal soft tissue of fingers. Occasionally, syndactyly of toes is present.	Reported patients have been mentally subnormal.
Crouzon's disease	Skull configurations vary. Commonly the forehead is broad and flat with decreased A-P diameter. Those patients with multiple sutures fused may be microcephalic. Orbits are generally small.	Eyes are proptotic and widely spaced with a reversed slant of palpebral fissures. Maxillae and zygoma are hypoplastic and the nose is 'beak-like.' Palate is narrow and high-arched; occasional malformations of auditory canals are present.	Limb abnormalities are usually not seen.	Mild to moderate mental subnormality often present. When multiple sutures are closed, increased ICP, optic atrophy and blindness may develop.
Pfeiffer's syndrome	Broad prominent forehead with flat occiput, lending a tower-like appearance to skull. Hypoplastic maxillae.	Ocular hypertelorism with protruding eyes. Flat nose with prominent mandible. Divergent strabismus is common.	Thumbs and great toes are abnormally wide, short and deviate medially. There is usually syndactyly of 2nd & 4th fingers and varying combinations of syndactyly of toes.	Intelligence is usually within normal limits.

NOTE: *Inheritance* of all syndromes listed here is autosomal dominant, with the exception of Carpenter's syndrome which is an autosomal recessive trait.

supplied by the posterior cerebral artery. Deep hemispheric AVMs are less common but may occur anywhere within the cerebral substance, brain stem, and spinal cord.

The most common clinical presentation is intracranial hemorrhage which may be limited to the subarachnoid space; whereas, other patients have bleeding into the cerebral parenchyma producing focal neurologic deficits with intracranial hypertension. Cerebellar hematomas are usually secondary to arteriovenous malformations. Some patients may have recurring fits, headaches, or visual loss before the hemorrhage.

Computerized tomography with and without contrast enhancement is of great diagnostic usefulness but cerebral angiography is the diagnostic procedure of choice.

It is ideal that the child with a ruptured AVM has fully recovered from the acute insult before an elective surgical procedure is undertaken. **Treatment** methods include complete excision, ligation of the feeding artery(ies), or embolization with isobutyl-2-cyanoacrylate (IBCA). There is some controversy regarding the use of IBCA to 'glue' the lesion because use of such substances does not necessarily guarantee protection against future hemorrhage and in no way replaces surgical excision as the definitive treatment for arteriovenous malformations.

The mortality of the first bleed is high, about 25%, and there is a 25% chance of rebleeding during the next 5 years. The child's brain, however, is remarkably resilient and an aggressive attempt should be made to excise the lesion if the procedure can be done safely.

Malformations of the vein of Galen   Although commonly considered an 'aneurysm of the vein of Galen' these lesions are arteriovenous malformations, accounting for 10% or less of all intracerebral arteriovenous malformations.

The clinical presentation is age-related, with different clinical signs and symptoms occurring in the neonatal period, in infancy, and in childhood.

Neonates with malformations of the vein of Galen demonstrate signs and symptoms of congestive heart failure secondary to a large arteriovenous shunt and increased cardiac output. They have cardiomegaly with left axis deviation on ECG. A loud intracranial bruit is commonly heard. The outlook is poor and most patients succumb to heart failure within the first few months of life.

Infants with malformations of the vein of Galen usually present with hydrocephalus, seizures, congestive heart failure, and sometimes a subarachnoid hemorrhage. Hydrocephalus is secondary to narrowing or obstruction of the aqueduct of Sylvius by the vein of Galen. An intracranial bruit is loud and synchronous with the pulse. The outlook for these children is generally poor, with mortality approaching 80%, and death secondary to intracranial hypertension, subarachnoid hemorrhage, and/or heart failure.

Older children have a subarachnoid hemorrhage accompanied by convulsive activity and focal neurologic signs. Diagnosis is made by computerized tomography but specifically confirmed by angiography. The mortality of children with this malformation approaches 50%.

OCCULT ARTERIOVENOUS MALFORMATIONS

Most arteriovenous malformations are demonstrated by angiography but there is a small group that is occult or 'cryptic.' These lesions are usually not demonstrated by angiography either because of partial thrombosis, slow blood flow, or compression of the vessels by a hematoma.

Occult arteriovenous malformations may present with fits and are typically demonstrated at CT scan as an unenhanced dense lesion that will enhance after contrast injection. Occasionally, intracranial hemorrhage can result in neurologic deficits.

To obviate the risk of future hemorrhage, it is suggested that patients suspected of having occult arteriovenous malformations have those lesions surgically removed.

VENOUS 'ANGIOMAS'

The natural history of venous malformations has not been well understood because the lesions are typically asymptomatic. Venous malformations have no arterial component, and are comprised of small veins that drain into dilated venous channels. They were earlier considered to be angiomas but really have no characteristics of tumors and are, rather, congenital malformations of cerebral veins.

CT scan has improved the capability to demonstrate cerebral venous malformations but angiography is the preferred neuroradiologic technique to show the radially arranged veins draining into the dilated venous channel.

Differentiation of arteriovenous malformations from venous malformations is important because the latter is an uncommon cause of a vascular event. In the relatively few reported patients with symptomatic venous malformations, the severity of the intracerebral hemorrhage was mild and there were no deaths. Venous malformations of the posterior fossa represent a greater risk of hemorrhage than those located in other areas of the brain. Since the risk of hemorrhage from venous malformations is relatively small, it seems prudent to withhold surgery except for those patients who have already bled from that lesion.

ANEURYSMS

An aneurysm is the dilation of the wall of an artery. Cerebral aneurysms are rare in childhood. Despite their increased incidence in children with coarctation of the aorta and those with renal polycystic disease, they occur in less than 1% of patients under 20 years of age. There is no known relationship of aneurysmal rupture to gender, race, or physical activity.

Since major factors related to the rupture of an aneurysm include increasing age, arterial hypertension, and atheromatous lesions, it is no surprise that there is a significant increase in frequency after the second decade of life. These saccular (berry) vascular lesions arise at the junction of dividing arteries, where there is a defect in the media of the arterial wall, usually covered by the internal elastic membrane which often has degenerative changes, and layers of the external elastic membrane. The integrity of the vessel at this point is dependent on the internal elastic lamina.

Common sites for aneurysms to occur are at the junction of the anterior cerebral and anterior communicating arteries and the distal aspect of the internal carotid artery. If multiple aneurysms occur they are more probably mycotic in nature.

The most common **clinical expression** of intracranial aneurysms is spontaneous hemorrhage, and with the sudden release of blood into the subarachnoid space and/or intracerebral substance, an abrupt increase in intracranial pressure. This sudden intracranial hypertension is generally manifested by severe headache, vomiting, confusion, stupor, or coma. The event may result in death.

In cases of lesser degrees of intracranial hemorrhage, a variety of abnormal neurologic deficits will result, depending upon the location of the aneurysm and the extent of the bleed. In cases of subarachnoid hemorrhage, signs of meningeal irritation are apparent as manifested by severe headache, nuchal rigidity, and fever.

When subarachnoid hemorrhage is suspected, a CT scan should be immediately performed; and in those patients without evidence of increased intracranial pressure or focal neurologic deficit, a lumbar puncture should be carried out. Angiography may be required to define the details of the vascular lesion.

The patient must receive meticulous supportive care to stabilize vital signs and to avoid, if possible, cerebral edema. It is generally imprudent to attempt the immediate surgical removal of an intracerebral hematoma except in extreme emergencies. It is, rather, more reasonable to delay any surgical procedure until such time when local factors such as vascular spasm and edema have decreased. The risk of rebleeding from an intracranial aneurysm has been reported to be as high as 50%.

REFERENCES

Adams RD, Sidman RL: *Introduction to Neuropathology.* McGraw-Hill, New York, 1968.

Fishman RA: *Cerebrospinal Fluid in Diseases of the Nervous System.* Saunders, Philadelphia, 1980.

Lemire RJ, Loeser JD, Leech RW, Alvord EC: *Normal and Abnormal Development of the Human Nervous System.* Harper & Row, Hagerstown, 1975.

Lorber J: Spina bifida cystica: results of treatment of 270 consecutive cases with criteria for selection for the future. Arch Dis Childh 47:854, 1972.

Martin NA, Edwards MSB, Wilson CB: Management of intracranial vascular malformations in children and adolescents. *Concepts in Pediatric Neurosurgery,* :ol 4, Karger, Basel. In press.

Moore KL: *The Developing Human.* Saunders, Philadelphia, 1973.

Warkany J, Lemire RJ, Cohen MM: *Mental Retardation and Congenital Malformations of the Central Nervous System.* Year Book, Chicago, 1981.

3

Metabolic Encephalopathies

Seymour Packman, MD

Recent emphasis has been placed upon the identification, treatment, and prevention of morbidity and mortality of the metabolic encephalopathies. Therapeutic approaches to a variety of inborn errors of metabolism have been systematized and some conditions may now be viewed as treatable disorders. Successful treatment regimens have been based upon an understanding of fundamental disease mechanisms, and have benefited from refinements in the use of special diets.

INCIDENCE

Although individually rare, the aggregate incidence of inborn errors is relatively high. In one newborn screening program, an inborn error of metabolism or transport was found in 1/3000 newborns, almost certainly an underestimate of total incidence. A different estimate was derived from considering that undiagnosed inborn errors of metabolism account for a significant fraction of neonatal seizures. By that calculation, as many as 1/1000 newborns have an inborn error of metabolism leading to seizures, and more than 3500 babies/year in the USA are at risk for an inherited metabolic disorder leading to seizures in the newborn period. Since at least 20% of neonates with convulsions die, and since an additional 20% are permanently handicapped, it is clear that this is a major health problem for a significant number of babies across the nation. Accordingly, every clinician should understand the application of and the principles underlying the protocol of this section (Figure 3-1).

INHERITANCE

These disorders are inherited either as an autosomal recessive trait, or as in the case of ornithine transcarbamylase deficiency, are x-linked. The existence of an affected relative with a similar pattern of illness is therefore of great diagnostic importance. This relative will most often be a sibling of either sex but, in the case of x-linked disease, may be a maternal uncle, a male sibling or a mildly affected mother or other female relative. A careful family history (see Chapter 1) must be obtained, with attention given to stillbirths, unexplained deaths, and unexplained neurologic diseases or delayed development of any kind or degree of severity. Hospital records and data of postmortem examinations should be studied when available.

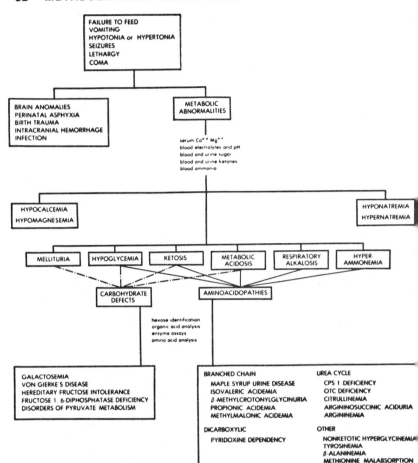

Fig. 3-1 Approach to a newborn or infant with acute encephalopathy due to inherited metabolic disease. (Reproduced with permission from Rudolph AM, Hoffman JIE (Eds) *Pediatrics*, 17th ed, Appleton-Century-Crofts, New York, 1982.)

DIAGNOSIS

The most fundamental aid to diagnosis is a high index of suspicion. Inherited metabolic disorders must be considered by the physician who is called upon to formulate a list of possible causes for the observed abnormalities in a neurologically impaired child. Once inborn errors of metabolism are considered, there is a relatively simple diagnostic sequence (Figure 3-1) for approaching disorders of carbohydrate and amino acid metabolism. Metabolic diseases affecting the biosynthesis and degradation of macromolecules, namely, storage diseases (lysosomal hydrolase deficiencies) are more slowly progressive encephalopathies and are discussed in Chapter 4.

Any child who presents acutely with failure to feed, vomiting, hypotonia or hypertonia, seizures, lethargy, or coma should be thought of as suffering from one of two general etiologic categories: (1) disorders resulting from infection, cardiopulmonary dysfunction, congenital structural abnormalities, or perinatal trauma; (2) disorders due to a metabolic abnormality.

Of particular importance in diagnosing inborn errors of metabolism is the recognition that the onset of disease manifestations is, with rare exception, postnatal, with symptoms appearing after a period of apparent good health. This interval may be quite short and directly follow the start of feedings in the newborn period. On the other hand, the interval may be longer, and directly follow a catabolic insult such as infection, dehydration or an excessive protein or carbohydrate load later in life. Given the variable patterns of progression of illness in older infants and children, a history of postnatal onset of symptoms after a definite interval period of good health can serve as a critical historical marker directing attention to metabolic disorder as the cause of an acute encephalopathic episode.

SYMPTOMS

There are patterns of illness which will identify the neonate, infant, or older child whose neurologic dysfunction may well be due to an inborn error of metabolism. In spite of a large number and diversity of heritable biochemical lesions causing encephalopathic states, the nonspecific symptoms are strikingly similar from one disease to the next.

In the neonatal period, symptoms should be viewed within the context of the limited repertory of responses to illness by infants of that age group. Irritability and failure to feed may be accompanied by incoordinated sucking and swallowing and/or by abnormalities of muscle tone, namely, hypertonia or hypotonia (see Chapter 16). Persistent and severe vomiting and/or convulsions may become part of the clinical course. In mildly affected patients, symptoms may disappear only to recur within days or weeks. In more severely affected infants there will be inexorable progression from lethargy to coma, episodes of apnea and, finally, death.

Neonates with metabolic diseases sometimes evince more delimited acute CNS symptoms, most often in the form of generalized or partial seizures. These may include staring spells, eye rolling, or myoclonus, accompanied variously by hypotonia, tremulousness, lethargy, and/or a feeble cry. Typical EEG patterns described include slow frequency waves, bursts of random spike discharges or hypsarrhythmia.

In the infant and older child, acute clinical manifestations are quite similar, but neurologic symptoms are characteristically intermittent. The child often shows poor growth or 'failure to thrive,' significant developmental delay, and specific neurologic deficits such as ataxia or visual dysfunction.

PHYSICAL FINDINGS

A paucity of abnormal physical findings is the rule in heritable metabolic diseases; nevertheless, certain components of the physical examination deserve emphasis. Complete ocular examination is essential; ophthalmoscopy allows direct observation of the neural tissue of the fundus. Corneal clouding, cataracts, and macular or retinal pigmentary changes may also be helpful in the differential diagnosis. Hepatomegaly may be present in galactosemia, von Gierke's disease, fructose intolerance, and some forms of congenital lactic acidosis. Abnormal hair structure (trichorrhexis nodosa) may be present in certain urea cycle defects. Finally, an unusual odor of the child's body or urine has been the key to identification of several aminoacidopathies, including branched-chain ketoaciduria (maple syrup), isovalericacidemia (sweaty feet), and 3-methylcrotonyl glycinuria (cat-like). Ketosis accompanies many of the illnesses under consideration and will cause the sweet odor of ketone bodies in the urine.

LABORATORY STUDIES

Since there is no reliable clinical specificity offered by the many conditions grouped in the metabolic category, laboratory studies must be performed. Measurement of serum calcium, magnesium and electrolytes, blood pH, glucose, ketones and ammonia, and urine pH, sugar, and ketones, provide a simple, rapid and generally available screening battery (see Figure 3-1).

The evaluation and treatment of neonates with hypocalcemia, hypomagnesemia, and hyper- or hyponatremia are discussed in Chapter 11. Mellituria, hypoglycemia, ketosis, metabolic acidosis, respiratory alkalosis, and hyperammonemia are clinical chemical aberrations that suggest disorders of carbohydrate or amino acid metabolism and allow a preliminary categorization of the patient.

Disorders of carbohydrate metabolism should be considered in a sick neonate or infant with any combination of mellituria, hypoglycemia, ketosis, or metabolic acidosis. Similarly, hypoglycemia, ketosis, metabolic acidosis, respiratory alkalosis or hyperammonemia should lead to the consideration of a primary inherited disorder of amino acid metabolism. Further definition will usually require more directed analytical procedures. These include specific colorimetric and flocculation screening tests on urine specimens, qualitative and quantitative amino acid and carbohydrate analysis, and organic acid analysis.

Whenever feasible, a specific metabolic defect should be confirmed by enzyme assay, in order to insure accuracy of diagnosis and treatment, proper genetic counseling, and accurate prenatal diagnosis. It is important to emphasize that treatment of acute symptoms must be started immediately, often well before the results of screening and specialized studies are available.

DIFFERENTIAL DIAGNOSIS

Aminoacidopathies Two large subgroups — disorders of branched-chain amino acid catabolism and disorders of the urea cycle — account for a majority of disorders of amino acid metabolism presenting with acute symptoms in the neonate or infant (Figure 3-1). Disorders of the distal urea cycle can be identified according to the accumulation in urine or plasma of products proximal to the enzyme block: arginine (arginase deficiency), argininosuccinic acid (argininosuccinate lyase deficiency), and citrulline (argininosuccinate synthetase deficiency) (Figure 3-2). Orotic acid secondarily accumulates in the urine in ornithine transcarbamylase

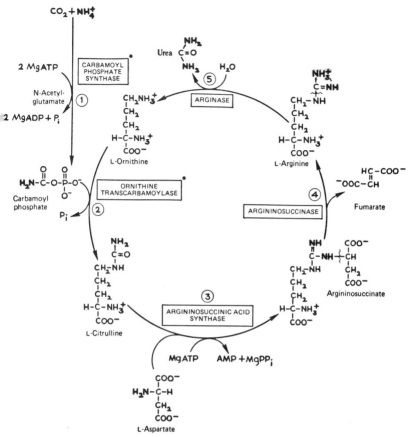

Fig. 3-2   Reaction sequence of the urea cycle. (Reproduced with permission from Martin DW Jr, Mayes PA, Rodwell VW: *Harper's Review of Biochemistry*, 19th ed. Copyright 1983 by Lange Medical Publications, Los Altos, CA.)

deficiency. Carbamyl phosphate synthetase deficiency can be suspected on the basis of the total picture of clinical and chemical aberrations, but may be difficult to differentiate from transient hyperammonemia of the newborn or certain of the organic acidemias.

Hyperammonemia is the chemical hallmark of these disorders, but such hyperammonemia can occur in other disorders of lysine and ornithine metabolism, and in several of the organic acidemias (methylmalonic acidemia, propionic acidemia and β-ketothiolase deficiency). The acid-base status can be a major discriminant between disorders of urea cycle and organic acidemias. Patients with organic acidemias suffer from metabolic acidosis with varying degrees of ketosis. In contrast, patients with urea cycle defects characteristically present with respiratory alkalosis, resulting from central stimulation of hyperventilation by the elevated ammonia.

The organic acidemias of primary concern are defects in the catabolic pathways of the branched-chain amino acids, leucine, isoleucine, and valine. The most important chemical aberration is a metabolic acidosis, due to the accumulation of organic acids. Additionally, secondary biochemical changes in the organic acidemias can occur, including hyperglycinemia, hypoglycemia, hyperammonemia, lactic acidemia, and ketonuria. Such chemical findings should then be taken as clues to include defects of branched-chain amino acid catabolism in the differential diagnosis. It should be noted that an inappropriately high urine pH, in the face of metabolic acidosis, should suggest the diagnosis of renal tubular acidosis, a disorder which may clinically mimic organic acidemia and other conditions discussed in this chapter.

Carbohydrate defects Inborn errors of carbohydrate metabolism can be divided into two broad categories: defects in pyruvate disposition, and 'other' (Figure 3-1). Each involves a particular step in the catabolism of a single hexose, and each is inherited as an autosomal recessive trait. Hypoglycemia is an important chemical clue in these diseases and may be delayed in appearance until age 3 days or later. Hypoglycemia combined with hepatomegaly and acidosis are seen in von Gierke's disease, hereditary fructose intolerance, and galactosemia.

The clinical picture in classical galactosemia may include cataracts (even in the newborn period) and jaundice. Jaundice may also be seen in hereditary fructose intolerance. Nonglucose mellituria (i.e., positive Clinitest, negative glucose oxidase test) is a valuable, simple laboratory clue to the diagnosis of both hereditary fructose intolerance and galactosemia.

Defects in pyruvate metabolism include pyruvate dehydrogenase complex deficiency states and disorders of gluconeogenesis (including von Gierke's disease). Such primary lactic acidoses must be distinguished from the secondary lactic acidoses of organic acidemias, and from the secondary lactic acidosis caused by drugs, malignancy, or hypoxemic states. Similarly the hypoglycemia due directly to defects in gluconeogenesis must be distinguished from that occurring secondarily in organic acidemias. While distinctions can sometimes be made on clinical grounds, differentiation often requires urine organic acid quantitation.

TREATMENT

Among the disorders of carbohydrate or amino acid metabolism noted in Figure 3-1 are many examples in which prevention of death or disability follows prompt diagnosis and treatment. The treatment modalities used in aminoacidopathies and disorders of carbohydrate metabolism are few and conceptually simple. The success of any of these approaches is clearly a function of time — the longer the neurologic derangement persists before treatment, the poorer the prognosis.

Since acidosis or alkalosis is commonly observed in these disorders, **correction of acid-base status** is essential and of immediate importance. Appropriate adjustments in electrolyte balance and hydration should, of course, be performed.

Selective avoidance of a particular nutrient or class of nutrients is more specific and most crucial. Restriction of galactose in galactosemia, of fructose in hereditary fructose intolerance, of branched-chain amino acids in maple syrup urine disease, and of protein in propionicacidemia, methyl-malonicacidemia, and urea cycle defects can often mean the difference between life and death. Avoidance of protein should be widely employed for a short time in any child who presents with a significant acute neuro-logic dysfunction, especially as a clinical response to protein avoidance may also be of diagnostic help. Cessation of protein feedings for a few days is harmless; whereas, continuation of dietary protein in a child with an aminoacidopathy is often lethal. It is of major importance when insti-tuting nutritional restrictions that attention be directed to total caloric intake. Maintenance of an adequate caloric intake (often utilizing glucose, glucose polymers, and lipid preparations) is essential for prevention of tissue catabolism, and must be achieved by whatever route of administra-tion is feasible or available, namely parenteral or oral.

Chemical supplementation has also been shown to be quite valuable in a growing number of these disorders. Glucose infusions will, of course, control hypoglycemia regardless of the cause. The use of pyridoxine in pyridoxine-dependent seizures, and of vitamin B_{12} in vitamin B_{12} respon-sive methylmalonicacidemia may be life-saving. In addition to vitamin B_{12} and pyridoxine, inborn errors of metabolism have been described which respond to thiamine, biotin, folate, and niacin in pharmacologic doses. In a child who is gravely ill, and whose course has been one of inexorable de-cline, it is not inappropriate to administer a battery of rationally chosen cofactors in the hope that the baby's biochemical lesion will respond to one of the vitamins.

Exchange transfusion or peritoneal dialysis has been reported to yield prompt improvement in some patients with disorders of amino acid metabolism, including maple syrup urine disease and hyperammonemic states.

GENETIC COUNSELING

Treatment of heritable metabolic disorders involves considerations beyond the acute phase of the illness, and even beyond the progress of the pro-band. Identification of the disorders will be followed by the ability to counsel families about their recurrence risks. All but one of the disorders noted in Figure 3-1 are inherited as autosomal recessive traits, meaning that such families are faced with a recurrence risk of one in four. In cases of x-linked ornithine transcarbamylase deficiency the counseling is more complex, and attention must be given to differential risks in males versus females.

Many of the conditions in question can be diagnosed prenatally, thereby offering families the option of therapeutic abortion. Furthermore, at least two disorders, vitamin B_{12} responsive methylmalonicacidemia and a biotin responsive organic aciduria, have responded to prenatal treatment by maternal vitamin supplementation. Because of the importance of genetic counseling to the family, the physician has an obligation to try to arrive at a diagnosis, however grave the prognosis in the proband, and to explain the importance of requisite studies to parents.

REFERENCES

Danks DM: Plan of management for newborn babies in whom metabolic disease is anticipated or suspected. Clin Perinatal 3:241, 1976.

Milunsky A: *The Prenatal Diagnosis of Hereditary Disorders.* Charles C. Thomas, Springfield, 1973.

O'Brien D, Goodman SI: The critically ill child: acute metabolic disease in infancy and early childhood. Pediatrics 46:620-626, 1970.

Packman S: Approach to inherited metabolic disorders presenting in the newborn period. *In* Rudolph AM, Hoffman JIE (Eds) *Pediatrics,* 17th ed, Appleton-Century-Crofts, New York, 1982, pp 256-258.

Rosenberg LE: Diagnosis and management of inherited aminoacidopathies. Clin Endocrin Metabol 3:145, 1974.

Scriver CR, Rosenberg LE: *Amino Acid Metabolism and its Disorders.* Saunders, Philadelphia, 1973.

Special Diets for Infants with Inborn Errors of Metabolism (American Academy of Pediatrics Committee on Nutrition) Pediatrics 57:783, 1976.

4

Inborn Errors of
Metabolism

Bruce O. Berg, MD

During the last several decades, an abundance of information has been learned regarding the structure and particularly the function of the nervous system. A variety of aminoacidurias has been described, and there is much more information available regarding the glycogen storage diseases, mucopolysaccharidoses, and other storage diseases.

It is recognized that these diseases are uncommon and it is a rare circumstance when a specific therapy is available. At the same time, new therapeutic modalities are being continually introduced and some with gratifying results. It is most important to establish the diagnosis because many metabolic defects are heritable, and the parents of an affected child should have as much information as possible regarding the likelihood of having another child similarly affected.

THE AMINOACIDURIAS

PHENYLKETONURIA

Phenylketonuria (PKU), inherited as an autosomal recessive trait, is a metabolic abnormality in which phenylalanine, an essential amino acid, is not converted to tyrosine, resulting in significant elevations of serum phenylalanine and urinary excretion of phenylpyruvic acid. The basic defect in 'classic PKU' is the absence of phenylalanine hydroxylase, an enzyme comprised of two fractions, a labile form found only in the liver, and a heat stable form found in other tissues, which is essential to convert phenylalanine to tyrosine.

In cases where phenylalanine cannot be converted to tyrosine there is a transamination of phenylalanine to phenylpyruvic acid which is then metabolized to phenyllactic and phenylacetic acids (see Figure 4-1). Normal serum concentrations of phenylalanine during infancy may range from 1.1-2.5 mg/dl; whereas, patients with PKU have serum phenylalanine concentrations as high as 50-60 mg/dl. Patients with typical PKU have normal levels of dihydropteridine reductase but this may be decreased to absent in other forms of the disease (see Table 4-1). The frequency of PKU is approximately 1 in 14,000.

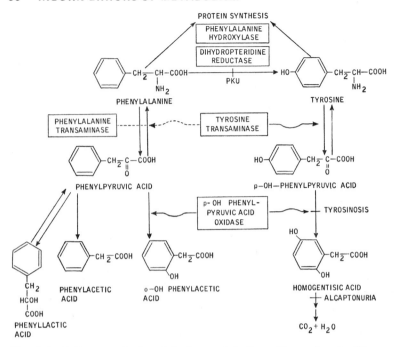

Fig. 4-1 Pathways of phenylalanine metabolism. (Reproduced with permission from Carpenter GG, Auerbach VH, DiGeorge AM: Phenylketonuria. Pediatr Clin N Amer 15:313, 1968.)

Clinical characteristics   Affected infants usually appear quite normal at birth but within several months become irritable and may have recurring vomiting. Though milestones may be reached at a normal time, they are usually delayed in both motor and intellectual skills. Acquisition of speech and language is delayed.

Patients are usually less than standard height and weight and about 25% of patients have eczema. Typically, the child is of fair complexion, blond with blue eyes. A lingering, musty odor sometimes described as 'mousey,' 'barnlike,' 'old urine,' is commonly present and is secondary to the urinary excretion of phenylacetic acid.

Seizures occur in at least 25% of patients and in early life are typically infantile spasms. As the patients become older, the convulsions assume other forms of the generalized epilepsies (see Chapter 10).

Microcephaly is common and increased muscle tone with hyperreflexia is generally present. Patients often assume an unusual seated position, 'schneidersitz' (tailor's position) and many children have a fine, rapid and irregular tremor at rest as well as with outstretched arms. The plantar responses are variable.

Electroencephalograms are usually abnormal and hypsarrhythmia is commonly found, sometimes when no clinical convulsive activity has been noted. Most untreated patients have an IQ less than 20 with the remainder

Table 4-1   The Hyperphenylalaninemic Traits of Man

Trait identified	Enzyme defect	Urine tests	Clinical features
'Classical' phenylketonuria	Trace of phenylalanine hydroxylase activity	FeCl$_3$ (+) (not always in newborn period)	Mental retardation and other signs; preventable by early treatment. Phe tolerance 250-500 mg/day
Phenylketonuria ('mild' variant with relaxed phenylalanine tolerance)	Unknown	FeCl$_3$ (+) (not always in newborn period)	Mental retardation without early treatment; high tolerance for dietary phenylalanine during treatment (>500 mg/day)
Phenylketonuria ('transient' variant)	Partial phenylalanine hydroxylase deficiency	FeCl$_3$ (+)/(—) (not always (+) in newborn period)	Mental retardation without early treatment; changing status affects treatment need (< 500 mg/day → normal tolerance)
Hyperphenylalaninemia (without phenylketone excretion)	Partial phenylalanine hydroxylase deficiency	Negative	Plasma phenylalanine is consistently less than 1 mM. Asymptomatic trait.
Neonatal hyperphenylalaninemia	Presumed phenylalanine hydroxylase deficiency	Usually negative	Often associated with hypertyrosinemia; normal adaptive phenomenon predominantly in prematures
Offspring of maternal phenylketonuria	No significant deficiency in (heterozygous) offspring	Expected to be negative after birth	Transient falling postnatal hyperphenylalaninemia. Congenital malformation, somatic, and cognitive development impaired

Reproduced with permission from Scriver CR, Rosenberg LE, *Amino Acid Metabolism and its Disorders*, Saunders, Philadelphia, 1973.

under 50; however, about 4% of untreated patients have IQ determinations greater than 60.

Diagnosis should be made in the first month of life. All newborns should be routinely screened after several days of life and after the beginning of feeding. This is generally done by obtaining a drop of blood by heel stick on a standard filter paper and determining the serum phenylalanine content by the Guthrie test. By this test, the serum phenylalanine content is determined by assessing the ability to inhibit the inhibition of *Bacillus subtilis* growth by 2-thienylalanine. A fluorometric method of determining phenylalanine content is also available. All patients with positive screening tests must have a quantitative determination of serum phenylalanine and tyrosine.

With the introduction of newborn screening programs a ferric chloride test is used less often. In this test 6 drops of FeCl$_3$ (5% FeCl$_3$ in water) are added to 0.5 ml of urine. There will be a color change to dark green within the next several minutes (see Table 4-2).

Treatment   Serum phenylalanine concentration can be controlled by restriction of dietary intake of phenylalanine with preparations such as Lofenalac. There is a concomitant decrease of urinary excretion of phenylpyruvic acid and other metabolic end-products. There is also improvement in neurologic abnormalities, behavior, and other typical signs and symptoms of disease.

The management of patients with PKU is not easy and should be directed by those who have experience with this disease and the many problems of dietary control. Duration of treatment is not universally accepted and although it has generally been the practice to discontinue the diet at the age of 5 years, there are suggestions that patients may have a decline in intellect following the cessation of dietary restriction of phenylalanine.

HISTIDINEMIA

Histidinemia is a rare metabolic disorder in which there is great increase of histidine in the urine, blood, and often the cerebrospinal fluid. The true incidence of the disease is not known although it has been suggested that it is similar to that of PKU. There may be no clinical abnormality noted in the patient's early life but after a few years it is apparent that about one-half of patients have delayed acquisition of speech, considered by some to be an impairment of auditory memory. Mental and growth retardation have been reported.

Histidase, which facilitates conversion of histidine to urocanic acid, is absent from the liver and skin in affected patients. The diagnosis is established by finding an elevation of histidine in the blood and no urocanic acid or histidase in the skin. Some patients have hyperalaninemia. A positive urinary ferric chloride test is commonly present.

MAPLE SYRUP URINE DISEASE

This branched chain ketoaciduria is notable for presentation of signs and symptoms in the early newborn period and a urinary aroma of maple syrup. The branched chain amino acids, leucine, isoleucine, and valine, are significantly increased in the urine and blood.

Infants appear normal at birth but within several days manifest respiratory irregularity, feeding problems, fits, intermittent rigidity, and hypotonia. Patients may be hypoglycemic. In this severe form of the disease, death usually occurs before the end of the first year.

There is a milder form with similar, though intermittent, biochemical characteristics and manifested by ataxia and lethargy which may progress to stupor and/or coma. Neurologic signs and symptoms may be provoked by infection, anesthesia/surgery, immunizations, or stress. There have been efforts to control diet by attempting to maintain serum concentrations of leucine, isoleucine, and valine within normal limits. Unfortunately, it is difficult to maintain such control over extended periods of time and most patients have repeated cerebral insults. It must be noted, however, that in some patients in whom the diagnosis is made early, and where therapeutic dietary control is meticulously maintained, the intellectual status may approach normal.

DISORDERS OF SULPHUR - CONTAINING AMINO ACIDS

Homocystinurea is a metabolic abnormality of sulphur-containing amino acids in which there is a defect of the enzyme cystathionine synthetase that catalyzes the production of cystathionine from homocystine and serine. Patients are generally normal at birth, though some manifest signs of failure to thrive and/or seizures during the first year of life. The disorder is progressive. Typically, patients have ectopic lens, and myopia and/or glaucoma may occur.

Table 4-2 Screening Tests for Metabolic Defects

Condition	Ferric chloride	DNPH	Bene-dict's	Nitro-prusside	CTAB
Phenylketonuria	Green	+	—	—	—
Maple syrup disease	Navy blue	+	—	—	—
Tyrosinosis	Pale green (transient)	+	±	—	—
Histidinemia	Green brown	±	—	—	—
Hyperglycinemia	Purple	+	—	—	—
Methylmalconic aciduria	Purple	+	—	—	—
Homocystinuria	—	—	—	+	—
Cystinuria	—	—	—	+	—
Gargoylisms	—	—	—	—	+
Galactosemia	—	—	+	—	—
Fructose intolerance	—	—	+	—	—
Cystathioninuria	—	—	—	+	—

Reproduced with permission from Menkes JH, Eviator L: Biochemical methods in the diagnosis of neurological disorders. *In* Plum F (Ed): *Recent Advances in Neurology*, Davis, Philadelphia, 1969.

Ferric chloride test Add 6 drops of $FeCl_3$ (5% $FeCl_3$ in water) to 0.5 ml of urine. The color change occurs quickly and continues over the ensuing 3-4 minutes.

Dinitrophenylhydrazine reaction (DNPH) Add 0.5 ml of DNPH reagent to 0.5 ml of urine. A positive reaction is bright yellow, cloudy, precipitate.

Benedict's test Clinitest tablets are suitable for this test. Add 1 Clinitest to 5 drops of urine and 10 drops of water. Wait for about 15 seconds and then shake the tube. Blue is negative and green to orange is positive (compare with color change accompanying Clinitest tablets).

Cyanide-nitroprusside test Add 2 ml of urine to 1 ml of NaCn. This solution is allowed to mix and a few drops of NH_4OH are added. Wait for 5-10 minutes before adding several drops of sodium nitroprusside. A positive test is a deep purple color found in the presence of a homocystine, cystine, and acetone.

CTAB test 1 ml of 5% solution cetyltrimethylammonium bromide in 1 molar citrate buffer (pH 6.0) is added to 5 ml of filtered urine. The mixture is incubated at 37 C for about 30 minutes. A heavy flocculation indicates positive reaction. The test is positive in patients with varying forms of mucopolysaccharidosis.

The older patient is usually of fair complexion with dry, somewhat friable hair. A malar flush is common and livido reticularis is usually present. Patients have a 'gangly' appearance with long extremities and digits, a wide carrying angle, genu valgum, and often pes cavus. Osteoporosis is common and some patients have thoracic abnormalities, either pectus excavatum or carinum.

Vascular occlusions, arterial and/or venous, are common and may occur in one or multiple vessels; cerebral, cardiopulmonary, and renal vessels are often affected.

The diagnosis is established by demonstrating increased levels of urinary homocystine, plasma methionine, and a positive urinary cyanide-nitroprusside test (see Table 4-2). Some patients have benefited from diets in which methionine is restricted. Another method of reducing homocystine excretion is by the administration of large doses of pyridoxine up to 100-500 mg/day. Though seemingly beneficial, the long-term effects of diet restriction are not well known.

Cystathioninuria is a rare metabolic abnormality characterized by increased urinary excretion of cystathionine, resulting from a deficiency of cystathionase. Though initially reported in several patients who were mentally subnormal, the metabolic abnormality has been found in normal persons, suggesting there is no clear association with signs of neurologic dysfunction. Cystathioninuria has been reported in patients with galactosemia neuroblastoma, pyridoxine deficiency, and liver disease.

DISORDERS OF AMINO ACID TRANSPORT

HARTNUP DISEASE

This is a rare disease, characterized by an erythematous, photosensitive, scaly rash on exposed skin surfaces, intermittent ataxia, behavioral disturbances, and renal aminoaciduria. It was named after the first family described with the typical signs and symptoms, and is inherited as an autosomal recessive trait.

Neurologic signs and symptoms may appear before or without the skin rash and include intermittent headache (reminiscent of migraine), photophobia, mental retardation, episodic bouts of psychosis, and intermittent ataxia. During the attack patients have an unsteady broad-based gait, jerky movements, and an intention tremor. Commonly, an inadequate diet will precipitate the symptoms.

Plasma concentrations of amino acids are normal or decreased, but certain urinary amino acids are increased from five to ten times; namely, alanine, asparagine, glutamine, histidine, isoleucine, leucine, phenylalanine, serine, threonine, tryptophane, tyrosine, and valine.

Symptoms are often present during periods of malnutrition but seem to lessen or disappear with time and improvement of diet. Because of the similarity to the clinical features of pellagra, patients have been treated with nicotinic acid. However, there is commonly a lessening or disappearance of signs and symptoms with time. The efficacy of treatment with nicotinic acid is difficult to evaluate.

CYSTINURIA

This disease is an inherited abnormality of amino acid transport which affects the epithelial cells of the renal tubule and gut. The reabsorption of arginine, cystine, lysine, and ornithine is impaired, resulting in formation of renal calculi composed primarily of cystine, the least soluble of these amino acids.

Newborn screening programs suggest that cystinuria is one of the more commonly inherited metabolic abnormalities, with an incidence ranging from 1 in 7000 to 1 in 20,000 births. Though the disease occurs in both sexes, males are more severely affected. Signs and symptoms of renal calculi may be present in early life but are more likely to appear in early adult life. Urinary tract infections are common and renal failure may occur.

Management of patients is directed to avoidance of formation of renal calculi. The likelihood of cystine calculi formation can be lessened by increasing fluid intake and, hence, urine volume.

IMINOGLYCINURIA

Renal iminoglycinuria is a benign metabolic abnormality in which there is increased urinary excretion of proline, hydroxyproline, and glycine that is secondary to a specific impairment of renal transport. The reabsorption of the amino acids is approximately 80% and glycine 60% of normal. A transient iminoglycinuria occurs normally during the early period of infancy.

UREA CYCLE DISORDERS

These disorders are secondary to enzyme deficiencies at different steps of the urea cycle (see Figure 3-2). Although there is some variability of clinical presentations, the clinical courses are remarkably similar. Patients usually appear normal at birth but once feedings begin there is the onset of symptoms including lethargy, tachypnea or labored respirations, poor feeding, seizures, stupor, coma, and sometimes death. There may be a history of a sibling who expired in early life of unknown causes.

One common finding in affected patients is hyperammonemia that is generally related to the amount of protein ingested. Those patients with complete enzyme defect usually do not survive; whereas, those with partial defect may ultimately achieve near-normal or normal urea synthesis. It is believed that signs of neurologic dysfunction are secondary to long-standing hyperammonemia. The clinical features are summarized in Table 4-3.

Table 4-3 Urea Cycle Disorders

Type	Clinical characteristics	Enzyme defect
Citrullinemia (autosomal recessive)	A range of severity of signs and symptoms dependent upon the enzyme defect. Neonatal form is the most severe, resulting in death. An intermediate form is characterized by paroxysmal recurring vomiting, often with fits and coma. A mild form exists in which there are no abnormal signs or symptoms.	Arginosuccinic acid synthetase (liver, skin fibroblasts).
Argininosuccinic aciduria (probable autosomal recessive)	One of the more common defects of the urea cycle; characterized by mental retardation, fits, intermittent ataxia, and hepatomegaly. There are 3 identified types: neonatal, subacute, and that of later onset. The neonatal type is characterized by lethargy, anorexia, tachypnea, respiratory alkalosis, fits, coma, and death. The subacute type is characterized by anorexia, failure to thrive, and fits; the hair is dry, friable, and short. The Late onset type is notable for irritability, feeding difficulties, recurring vomiting, and developmental delay; seizures are common and intermittent ataxia and cranial nerve palsies may occur. Hair is dry, short, and friable.	Argininosuccinase
Carbamyl phosphate synthetase deficiency (heritability not determined)	Few patients are reported — symptoms common to all in varying combinations include irritability, lethargy, hypotonia, recurring vomiting, failure to thrive, respiratory distress, and seizures. Symptoms are often precipitated after eating high protein meal. Demise within the first few years of life is common.	Carbamyl phosphate synthetase.

Disorder	Clinical features	Enzyme/defect
Ornithine carbamyl transferase deficiency (probable x-linked dominant)	Patients appear normal at birth but within hours to several days become lethargic and feed poorly. Tachypnea, seizures, unresponsiveness, and death. Apparently males more frequently succumb within the neonatal period; whereas females usually live but are physically and mentally retarded. During periods of hyperammonemia, patients may become lethargic and ataxic, have headaches, vomiting, seizures (reminiscent of migraine), and possibly coma. Similar signs and symptoms may be provoked by anesthesia/surgery.	Ornithine carbamyl transferase.
Argininemia (hyperargininemia) (probable autosomal recessive)	Patients present in childhood with hyperammonemia, episodic vomiting, seizures, hepatomegaly, and mental retardation. Spastic diplegia and ataxia have been reported.	Arginase.
Ornithinemia	There are at least 3 types of ornithinemia:	
	1. Variably characterized by poor feeding, irritability, ataxia, and recurring seizures.	Defect of ornithine decarboxylase reported.
	2. Characterized by liver disease and renal tubular dysfunction; mental retardation may occur.	Ornithine ketoacid transaminase (liver).
	3. Represented by a group of reported Finnish patients who had gyrate atrophy of the retina and choroid. Not associated with hyperammonemia or homocitrullinemia.	Ornithine aminotransferase

DISORDERS OF CARBOHYDRATE METABOLISM

GALACTOSEMIA

The syndrome of galactosemia is the result of administration of galactose, given primarily as lactose, to persons who have an inherited inability to normally metabolize galactose, resulting in failure to thrive, mental retardation, liver disease, and cataracts. There are at least two recognized metabolic defects and potentially others.

The more common abnormality is the deficiency of galactose 1-phosphate uridyl transferase; however, another syndrome characterized by elevated serum galactose, galactosuria, cataracts, and pseudotumor cerebri has been associated with deficiency of galactokinase, an enzyme necessary to phosphorylate galactose, enabling it to proceed in the normal galactose metabolic pathways. In both types of enzyme deficiency, cataracts appear to be caused by increased levels of galactitol, formed in the lens from D-galactose by aldose reductase.

Clinical manifestations The types of disease inherited as autosomal recessive traits are characterized by hepatosplenomegaly, failure to thrive, cataracts, and pseudotumor cerebri. Patients with galactose-1-phosphate uridyl transferase deficiency commonly appear normal at birth although some have cirrhosis and cataracts at that time. The most common clinical presentation in virtually all patients with transferase deficiency is failure to thrive occurring shortly after the introduction of milk. Vomiting and/or diarrhea are present. Usually within 1 week there is evidence of impaired liver function manifested by jaundice and/or hepatomegaly. Cataracts are present at birth or soon after but may be observed only at slit-lamp examination. Developmental delay is usually apparent within several months after birth.

Some infants with transferase deficiency have milder symptoms, occurring after 3 or 4 months and manifested as growth retardation and developmental delay. Pertinent laboratory findings include, in addition to abnormal liver function tests, increased serum galactose, galactosuria (a urinary reducing substance which does not react to glucose oxidase test), aminoaciduria, and proteinuria. The aminoaciduria and proteinuria are secondary to toxic effects on the kidneys.

The clinical characteristics of patients with galactokinase deficiency are less well defined. Though palpable, there is little or no enlargement of the liver or spleen and no suggestion of failure to thrive. Cataracts have been detected and an occasional patient has pseudotumor cerebri. Without apparent evidence of failure to thrive, hepatosplenomegaly, or notable cataracts, these patients are detected only by routine screening of the urine and/or blood.

Diagnosis The demonstration that galactose 1-phosphate was elevated in red blood cells suggested an abnormality in the subsequent metabolic chain. It was later shown that the erythrocytes were deficient in galactose 1-phosphate uridyl transferase. This enzyme deficiency is also present in white blood cells, liver, gut, and skin fibroblasts.

In patients with elevated serum galactose, the diagnosis of galactokinase defect is made by finding normal galactose 1-phosphate uridyl transferase and an absence of galactokinase in the red cells. All children with cataracts should have their urine examined for sugars by methods other than glucose oxidase.

Treatment   The management of patients with galactosemia depends upon the elimination of all galactose-containing foods from the diet. Formulas including soybean milks and Nutramigen are useful. As the child ages, other foods that can be safely eaten are listed in certain nutritional guides.

It is essential to establish a close relationship with the child and parents to effect the best adherence to the dietary regimen. There is no substantive evidence that chronic administration of the diet is harmful.

Patients improve remarkably well while on the diet, and if treated from shortly after birth most patients will have normal mentality, albeit some will have specific learning disabilities.

THE GLYCOGEN STORAGE DISEASES

Glycogen is the primary biochemical structure, an intricately branched, compact polymer, in which glucose can be stored. It is a large molecule but because of differing physiological needs from moment to moment, there is no one established molecular weight, but rather a range from 1 to 5 or 6 million. Glycogen is found in virtually all cells, particularly in the liver, and to a lesser extent the skeletal muscle. Two groups of enzymes are required to cleave units of glucose from the glycogen polymer. Deficiencies of individual enzymes result in a variety of disease states (see Table 4-4).

THE MUCOPOLYSACCHARIDOSES (MPS)

The MPS are inherited diseases characterized by the progressive deposition of a heterogeneous group of mucopolysaccharides (glycosaminoglycans) in multiple organs. Affected patients, initially described by Hunter, were mentally and physically retarded, had bony deformities and corneal clouding. As additional patients were identified, their dysmorphic features became more apparent and the term 'gargoylism' was introduced.

Generally, the disorders though varying widely in severity, are progressive and are characterized by coarse physical features, dysostosis multiplex, joint stiffness and/or contractures, corneal clouding, hepatosplenomegaly, cardiac and vascular abnormalities, and most patients are mentally subnormal.

Table 4-4 The Glycogen Storage Diseases

Type	Clinical characteristics	Enzyme defect
I **von Gierke's disease** (autosomal recessive)	Short stature with remarkably protuberant abdomen secondary to liver enlargement. Patients have tendency to become obese but there is a paucity of skeletal muscle bulk with hypotonia. Kidneys are enlarged and occasionally there is splenomegaly. Xanthoma are common with increasing age. Variable degrees of hypoglycemia occur. Hypoglycemic convulsions are common during the first few years of life; however, asymptomatic hypoglycemia is not uncommon in later years. Patients have a near-normal lifespan.	Glucose-6-phosphatase
II **Pompe's disease** (autosomal recessive)	Generalized glycogenosis usually presenting as hypotonia with firm skeletal muscles of normal mass. Cardiomegaly is common in infancy with congestive heart failure. Death usually from cardiorespiratory failure during infancy. Different types have been described that may begin during early childhood but the disease progresses more slowly. Muscular weakness is striking in all forms and death comes by the end of the second decade. Deposition of glycogen is found not only in skeletal muscles, heart and liver but also in CNS and peripheral nerves.	α-1, 4-glucosidase
III **Cori's disease** (autosomal recessive)	Generally less severe than type I. Hypoglycemic convulsions occur. Growth retardation and hepatomegaly are found in early life and occasionally splenomegaly. Liver returns to normal size during puberty. Hepatitis has been reported in older patients and some may have mild cirrhosis. Muscle cramps, weakness, and atrophy are common.	Amylo-1, 6-glucosidase

Type	Clinical manifestations	Enzyme deficiency
IV Andersen's disease (heritability undetermined)	Occurs rarely and is manifested by failure to thrive, hypotonia, hepatomegaly, and splenomegaly. Cirrhosis appears early and death occurs before 4 years.	α-1, 4-glucan α-1, 4-glucan 6-glucosyl transferase
V McArdle's disease (probable autosomal recessive)	Normal at rest but patients have cramping and painful contractures on exertion and occasionally myoglobinuria. Symptoms are either mild or not present during childhood. Myoglobinuria reported in about one-half of patients.	Phosphorylase (muscle)
VI Hers' disease (heritability undetermined)	Mild symptoms similar to type I. In addition to decreased liver phosphorylase there may be reduction of leucocyte phosphorylase.	Phosphorylase (liver)
VII (Autosomal recessive trait suggested)	Clinical manifestations similar to McArdle's disease with muscle weakness and cramping following exercise; myoglobinuria has been reported. Reduced phosphofructokinase found in muscle and erythrocytes.	Phosphofructokinase (muscle)
VIII (Heritability undetermined)	No recognized abnormal clinical manifestations except for enlarged liver; there are no signs of muscle weakness, cramping, or atrophy.	Hepatic phosphorylase, kinase

The known MPS are secondary to a deficiency of a lysosomal enzyme needed to break down two mucopolysaccharides — dermatan sulfate and/or heparan sulfate. The clinical features of known MPS are noted in Table 4-5.

Diagnosis The clinical evaluation of each patient is of great benefit in distinguishing the type of MPS. However, the specific diagnosis is confirmed only by enzyme assay of fibroblasts and/or leucocytes.

THE MUCOLIPIDOSES

This is a rare group of disorders, inherited as an autosomal recessive trait, and presenting as widely differing clinical problems which have some biochemical similarities. The two recognized disorders of this disease category are categorized by the deposition of MPS without excessive urinary excretion of MPS.

ML II (I-cell disease) is characterized by early onset, sometimes at birth, of bony lesions similar to dysostosis multiplex with congenital hip dislocation and chest deformities. Patients are macrocephalic, there is no corneal clouding and there appears to be progressive intellectual deterioration. Cultured fibroblasts contain inclusions seen on phase microscopy; hence, the term 'I-cell disease.' The inclusions are enlarged lysosomes filled with MPS.

ML III is usually apparent by 2 or 3 years of age and is characterized by progressive stiffness of the shoulders and hands. Later in the first decade, patients manifest dwarfism, coarse facies, and dysostosis multiplex. Corneal clouding may be apparent on slit-lamp examination; aortic and mitral valvular disease may be present.

A number of enzymes are involved in this group of mucolipidoses. Determination of N acetyl-hexosaminidase or arylsulfatase A activity in the serum which are increased two or three times has proven to be an effective screening test.

DISORDERS OF LIPID METABOLISM

One notable feature of nervous tissue is the high concentration of lipids contained primarily in myelin. Principal lipid components of myelin include cerebrosides, cholesterol, ethanolamine phosphatides, and lecithin. Abnormalities of lipid metabolism have been classified in a variety of ways; however, it seems most reasonable to utilize a classification that considers the nature of the storage material and the enzyme deficiency (see Figure 4-2)

$$\begin{array}{l} \text{SPHINGOSIN} \\ \qquad | \qquad = \text{CERAMIDE} \\ \text{FATTY ACID} \end{array}$$

CERAMIDE – P – CHOLINE   = SPHINGOMYELIN

CERAMIDE – GLUCOSE   = GLUCOCEREBROSIDE

CERAMIDE – GALACTOSE   = GALACTOCEREBROSIDE

CERAMIDE – GALACTOSE – SULFATE   = SULFATIDE

The most complex sphingolipids, the gangliosides, have a number of hexoses and sialic acids (n-acetylneuraminic acid, NANA) attached to ceramide.

Example: Gm_1

$$\begin{array}{l} \text{CERAMIDE – GLUCOSE – GALACTOSE –} \\ \qquad\qquad\qquad \text{n-ACETYLGALACTOSEAMINE – GALACTOSE} \\ \qquad\qquad\qquad\qquad\qquad\qquad\qquad\quad | \\ \qquad\qquad\qquad\qquad\qquad\qquad\qquad \text{NANA} \end{array}$$

Fig. 4-2 The sphingolipids

THE GANGLIOSIDOSES

Gangliosides are glycosphingolipids which contain sialic acid attached to the short chain of hexoses. There are at least ten gangliosides in brain but four comprise about 90% of the total brain ganglioside concentration. They are catabolized by the cleavage of individual sugar molecules but should there be a deficiency of one hydrolase, further catabolism is blocked; hence, the basis of the ganglioside storage diseases (gangliosidoses).

Generally, the five most common gangliosidoses, each inherited as an autosomal recessive trait, are characterized by progressive deterioration of intellectual and motor function (see Table 4-6).

FABRY'S DISEASE (a-GALACTOSIDASE A DEFICIENCY)

This disease is rare, inherited as an x-linked trait, and characterized by deposition of glycosphingolipids in tissue. Affected patients usually complain first of episodic pain in the extremities; cutaneous vascular lesions and corneal dystrophy are apparent. The most striking symptom is recurring episodic pain which may last from minutes to several days and characterized as 'burning—excruciating—needle-like' pain in the palms or soles, sometimes radiating to the proximal extremities.

Patients have unusual skin lesions, angiokeratoma corporis diffusum universalis, which may also be present in other diseases; it is characterized as punctate angiectasiae. The lesions are flat or raised and most often found on the hips, thighs, buttocks, and scrotum. The conjunctivae and oral mucosae may also be involved.

Phenytoin or carbamazepine may alleviate the recurring pain.

Table 4-5 The Mucopolysaccharidoses (MPS)

Type	Clinical characteristics	Increased urine MPS	Enzyme defect
MPS I Hurler syndrome (autosomal recessive)	Severe dysostosis multiplex; dwarfism with joint stiffness and contractures (particularly of the elbows) and claw hands; marked lumbar lordosis. Corneal clouding is severe. Protruding abdomen with enlarged liver and spleen. Deafness and mental deterioration are common. Cardiac valves are involved, with death usually occurring during the first decade.	Dermatan sulfate Heparan sulfate	α-L-iduronidase
MPS II Hunter's syndrome x-linked recessive)	Two forms — one mild, one severe. Dwarfism with coarse facial features and stiff joints. Progressive deafness occurs but no corneal clouding. Heart disease with valvular abnormality and myocardial ischemia. In severe form, death occurs by 15-20 years; those with milder signs and symptoms may live 5 or 6 decades.	Dermatan sulfate Heparan sulfate	Iduronate sulfatase
MPS III Sanfilippo's syndrome (autosomal recessive)	Two biochemical forms exist: types A and B are not clinically distinguishable. Moderate dwarfism with mild dysostosis multiplex and joint stiffness. Mild to moderate enlargement of liver and spleen; corneal clouding does not occur. Progressive severe mental retardation is present. A third biochemical type has been considered.	Heparan sulfate	Type A: heparan N-sulfatase Type B: N-acetyl -α-D-glucosaminidase

MPS IV Morquio's syndrome (autosomal recessive)	Primary features are skeletal abnormalities and their effects on the CNS. Patients have coarse features with a short neck, pigeon chest, dwarfism with genu valgum. Fingers are stiff but wrists often 'loose,' Mild corneal clouding present. Os odontium absent or hypoplastic. Cervical myelopathy develops with secondary hemi/quadriplegia. Patients usually succumb before 3rd or 4th decades.	Keratan sulfate — Hexosamine 6-sulfatase
MPS V Scheie's syndrome (autosomal recessive)	Severe clouding of cornea; retinal pigmentary degeneration and/or glaucoma may be seen. Coarse facies but dwarfism not present. Stiff joints with claw hands. Deafness may occur. Abnormal cardiac function particularly affecting aortic valves. Normal intellect with full life span. Recently classified as MPS-1-S.	Dermatan sulfate Heparan sulfate — α-L-iduronidase
MPS VI Maroteaux-Lamy (autosomal recessive)	Similar appearance to MPS 1 but normal intellect. Spectrum of severity from mild, intermediate, to severe with varying degrees of genu valgum and lumbar kyphosis. Corneal clouding and cardiac valvular abnormalities. Hydrocephalus sometimes occurs and hypoplastic os odontium sometimes present. Patients with severe form may survive to the 3rd decade.	Dermatan sulfate — N-acetylgalactosamine 4-sulfatase
MPS VII (Autosomal recessive)	Variably coarse facies, corneal clouding, dysostosis multiplex, protuberant abdomen with enlarged liver and spleen. Normal intellect as well as mental retardation have been reported.	Dermatan sulfate Heparan sulfate — B-glucuronidase

As patients become older there is progressive involvement of the heart, vessels, and kidneys from deposition of glycosphingolipid. There is commonly progressive renal failure; renal transplantation may be necessary.

Diagnosis is made by renal biopsy and is confirmed by demonstration of deficiency of a-galactosidase A in plasma or serum.

NIEMANN - PICK DISEASE (SPHINGOMYELIN LIPIDOSIS)

The clinical features of this disease, most commonly present in Ashkenazim, include intellectual deterioration, progressive neurologic deterioration, manifested by spasticity and/or ataxia, fits, and hepatomegaly. Macular degeneration with 'cherry-red spot' may be present.

The basis of the disease process is a deficiency of sphingomyelinase, resulting in the storage of sphingomyelin in 'foam cells' of the reticuloendothelial system; namely, the liver, spleen, lymph nodes, lung, and bone marrow. The disorder of lipid metabolism, inherited as an autosomal recessive trait, has been classified into five types (see Table 4-7).

KRABBE'S DISEASE (GLOBOID CELL LEUCODYSTROPHY)

Krabbe's disease, inherited as an autosomal recessive trait, is characterized by a severe decrease of white matter galactolipids. The genetic defect is a decreased to absent galactosylceramide β-galactosidase.

The onset of symptoms is usually between 3 and 6 months of age and is notable for irritability, recurring fevers of unknown cause, and increased muscle tone. The infant cries excessively, often with exaggerated responses to auditory, tactile, or visual stimuli. Vomiting is common and patients feed poorly. Seizures are usually present early in the disease.

Within weeks to months, there is significant increase in muscle tone and an occasional patient remains in an opisthotonic posture. Microcephaly is sometimes present. Stretch reflexes are abnormally brisk until such time that spasticity will dampen their excursion. Optic atrophy occurs with pupils responding only sluggishly to light and some patients become deaf. Most patients do not survive more than several years although a small number will live a longer period of time.

Diagnosis The clinical features of Krabbe's disease are suggestive of a number of neurodegenerative diseases; however, certain laboratory studies enable one to confirm the diagnosis. The peripheral nerves are involved with delayed nerve conduction velocity. The CSF protein concentration is usually significantly elevated with a normal cell count. Confirmation of the diagnosis is attained by finding decreased to absent cerebrosidase in leucocytes and skin fibroblasts. The enzyme can be assayed in amniotic fluid cells enabling prenatal diagnosis.

GAUCHER'S DISEASE

Gaucher's disease, inherited as an autosomal recessive trait, is one of the most commonly recognized sphingolipid storage diseases and is manifested by three presently recognized separate types. The one characteristic pathologic feature of the disease is a large histiocyte, the Gaucher cell, filled with a lipid that stains for carbohydrate with periodic acid Schiff (PAS) reagent. These cells are found in the reticuloendothelial system. namely, the spleen, lymph nodes, liver, and bone marrow. Electron microscopy has demonstrated within the storage material, inclusion bodies of tubular configuration. The clinical types are:

I — adult form This disease is commonly noted during the second decade when patients complain of episodic bone pain, splenomegaly, and a tendency to bruise easily. Some patients have fever. Splenomegaly has been noted in the first decade, but no further symptoms occur until the second decade. Hepatomegaly is common and the lungs may be involved resulting in pulmonary dysfunction. Recurring pneumonia is often the cause of death.

II — acute infantile form Signs and symptoms of neurologic dysfunction are apparent by 3-6 months including opisthotonus, strabismus, increased muscle tone with hyperreflexia. Dysphagia, laryngeal stridor are common and some have seizures. Serum acid phosphatase is elevated and Gaucher cells are demonstrated in bone marrow aspirate. Pulmonary function is impaired and infection is common. Death comes before the end of the first year.

III — subacute juvenile form Relatively uncommon form of disease, characterized by hepatosplenomegaly; some patients have increased muscle tone, hyperreflexia, and ataxia. Seizures are common. Identified patients may live to the fifth or sixth decade.

Diagnosis of Gaucher's disease should be considered in patients with abnormal enlargement of the liver and/or spleen and neurologic dysfunction. The demonstration of Gaucher cells from bone marrow aspirate is suggestive of the diagnosis; however, the diagnosis can only be confirmed by demonstration of decreased to absent glucocerebrosidase in fibroblasts and/or leucocytes.

METACHROMATIC LEUCODYSTROPHY (MLD) (Sulfatide Lipidosis)

The clinicopathologic features of this disease were initially described as an hereditary demyelination (leucodystrophy), but it was not until 30 years later when that same tissue was reexamined that metachromasia was demonstrated. MLD is a sphingolipid storage disease which is secondary to a deficiency or absence of an enzyme that desulfates the galactoceramide, cerebroside sulfate, and prevents conversion of the sulfate to a cerebroside. The enzyme, arylsulfatase A, is decreased to absent in leucocytes, fibroblasts, and urine. It can be assayed from cells of the amniotic fluid and, hence, is an important prenatal diagnostic test.

There are at least four forms of the disease (see Table 4-8): the late infantile MLD, a juvenile form, and an adult form have a decreased arylsulfatase A. The fourth type, multiple sulfatase deficiency, is a rare form of the disease in which onset of clinical signs and symptoms resembles late infantile MLD and occurs during the first few years of life. Patients have rather coarse features that are reminiscent of the mucopolysaccharidoses. These patients have decreased activity of at least five enzymes: arylsulfatase A, B, C, and of steroid sulfatases.

Diagnosis When the diagnosis of one form of MLD is considered, certain laboratory studies are of great usefulness to confirm that diagnosis.

Table 4-6 The Gangliosidoses

Type	Clinical characteristics	Enzyme type
Gm₁ gangliosidosis infantile form type I	Symptoms begin at birth or shortly thereafter. Poor feeding with weak suck and swallow. Patients appear dull and may never sit alone. Irregular respirations and recurrent pneumonia are common. Generalized epilepsy with tonic/clonic activity occurs frequently. If the patient survives the first year, he ultimately becomes decerebrate, blind, deaf, and spastic quadriplegic. Patients have coarse features, large tongue, and a macular cherry-red spot found in about one-half of patients. Hepatosplenomegaly present shortly after birth.	β-galactosidase
Gm₁ gangliosidosis juvenile form type 2	Appear normal during infancy; however, ataxia becomes apparent at about 1 year of age. Dysarthria, followed by loss of speech, and generalized muscle weakness. Progressive deterioration of intellectual and motor function, and within months patients assume posture of decerebrate rigidity. Seizures occur between 1 and 2 years. Recurring infections occur and are the usual cause of death. There are generally no coarse features and no hepatomegaly. Blindness may occur.	β-galactosidase
Gm₂ gangliosidosis Tay-Sachs disease	Weakness and acoustimotor response present by 6 months of age. Patients may sit alone but are usually not able to stand or walk. Progressive and rapid deterioration of intellectual and motor function. Skin has a pale translucent quality much like Dresden china. Increasing problems with feeding, hypotonia, and weakness; macular cherry-red spot is present in over 90% of cases. Patients manifest gelastic as well as myoclonic fits. As time passes, macrocephaly is apparent; patients usually die before the age of 5 years. The disease is particularly common in the Ashkenazim which comprise about 70% of known cases; 30% of patients are non-Jews.	Hexosaminidase A

Gm$_2$ gangliosidosis type 2 (Sandhoff's disease)	Clinical findings similar to Tay-Sachs disease. Generalized progressive weakness and intellectual deterioration present during the first 6 months of life. Acousti-motor response, cherry-red spots, macrocephaly become apparent and death usually occurs by the age of 3 years, secondary to recurring pulmonary infection.	Hexosaminidases A & B
Gm$_2$ gangliosidosis type 3 juvenile form	Symptoms usually occur between 2 and 6 years of age as ataxia with progressive spasticity, dystonic posturing, and loss of speech. Seizures may occur. Blindness occurs late and most patients succumb between 5 and 15 years most often from pulmonary infections.	Hexosaminidase A
Gm$_2$ gangliosidosis adult (chronic form)	Slowly progressive deterioration of gait and posture beginning in childhood. There is loss of muscle bulk, mild ataxia and pes cavus. Optic fundi were normal and reported patients were of normal intelligence.	Hexosaminidase A (decreased)

Table 4-7 Types of Niemann-Pick Disease

Type	Clinical characteristics	Enzyme defect
A (acute type) autosomal recessive	Most described as having Niemann-Pick disease belong to this group. There is early involvement of the CNS, liver, and spleen during first year. Hypotonia usually appears early but is replaced by spasticity. About 50% have macular degeneration with a cherry-red spot. Seizures are sometimes present. Feeding is increasingly difficult and patients appear emaciated with a remarkably protuberant tummy secondary to hepatosplenomegaly.	Sphingomyelinase
B (chronic type) autosomal recessive	May have hepatosplenomegaly early in life without evidence of CNS involvement. There is increasing pulmonary dysfunction secondary to infiltration of lung. The typical foam cells are found in liver, spleen, bone marrow, and lymph nodes.	Sphingomyelinase
C (chronic type) autosomal recessive	Patients appear normal until about 2 or 3 years old and occasionally longer. They have generalized epilepsy, usually tonic/clonic and/or myoclonic fits and become increasingly spastic and ataxic. Hepatosplenomegaly is less prominent than in types A and B but there is progressive neurologic deterioration, and patients die near the end of 1st decade or shortly thereafter.	Sphingomyelinase
D (Nova Scotia) autosomal recessive	These patients have common ancestry in Nova Scotia and generally do well until 5-10 years old. Hepatosplenomegaly becomes apparent and patients have increasing motor incoordination, seizures, and mental deterioration. Foam cells are present in spleen and lymph nodes. Some survive to the end of 2nd decade.	Not determined
E (adult form)	Adults have been described with hepatomegaly but no neurologic abnormalities. Foam cells have been identified in their bone marrow.	Not determined

Table 4-8 Metachromatic Leucodystrophy

Type	Clinical characteristics	Enzyme defect
Late infantile Stage 1	During the first several years of life, a child who is able to sit, stand, and walk, becomes weak, hypotonic, and genu recurvatum may be present. They are unsteady and fall easily. Occasionally, muscle tone is increased without increased stretch reflexes. Peripheral neuropathy with delayed nerve conduction velocity.	Arylsulfatase A (cerebroside sulfatase)
Stage 2	Shortly thereafter, the child can sit but is no longer able to stand or walk. Dementia becomes apparent with concomitant dysarthria and loss of speech. Some complain of aches and pains in their legs.	
Stage 3	The child becomes quadriplegic and muscle tone is increased or decreased. There is progressive dementia and speech is lost. Some patients assume a dystonic, decerebrate, or decorticcate posture. Stretch reflexes are absent.	
Stage 4	Patients remain in a vegetative state, requiring tube feeding. During the late stages of MLD, macular degeneration is apparent with grey-brown discoloration.	
Juvenile	Clinical course similar to late infantile MLD. Early signs and symptoms are behavioral; children may seem lackadaisical, lose interest and do poorly in school. Emotional disturbances are common; it is assumed they have a specific learning disability. Later, motor dysfunction becomes apparent with gait disturbance, ataxia, and/or signs of extrapyramidal abnormalities. Delayed nerve conduction velocities with reduced action potentials. CSF protein is elevated with normal cells; marked reduction of arylsulfatase A activity in urine, leucoctyes, fibroblasts.	Arylsulfatase A
Adult	Arbitrarily defined as signs and symptoms that begin after age of 21. Behavioral and intellectual deterioration associated with increasing motor impairment is common. Muscle tone is increased with hyperreflexia. Greater impairment of corticospinal and extrapyramidal systems than that of the peripheral nerves. Ataxia and tremor may be present; seizures may occur later. CSF protein levels are normal. Nerve conduction velocities are diminished. Decrease arylsulfatase A demonstrated in urine, leucocytes, fibroblasts. Protracted course is usual and patients are often thought to have schizophrenia or an organic dementia.	Arylsulfatase A

Table 4-9 Lipid Disorders of Unknown Cause

Disease form	Clinical characteristics	Ultrastructural features
Infantile neuronal ceroid lipo-fuscinosis	Onset occurs in latter part of first year, characterized by myoclonic and/or tonic/clonic fits, optic atrophy, and blindness. Rapid mental deterioration resulting in spastic quadriplegia.	Intraneuronal deposition of osmophilic granular material.
Late infantile form (Jansky-Bielschowsky-Batten) (curvilinear bodies)	Normal mental and motor development for several years; abrupt onset of generalized seizures, usually myoclonic and/or akinetic; an apparent ataxia develops. Progressive dementia and loss of vision with optic atrophy and retinal pigmentary degeneration. Progressive neurologic deterioration until patient remains in a decerebrate or decorticate posture and ultimately a vegetative state.	Intraneuronal inclusions described as 'curvilinear bodies' with granular and lamellated cytosomes.
Late infantile form (lipofuscin storage)	Clinical characteristics are generally similar to those described above.	Membrane-bound granular osmophilic material. Similar inclusions may be demonstrated in skeletal muscle and Schwann cells.
Juvenile form (Spielmeyer-Vogt)	Loss of vision followed by intellectual deterioration becomes apparent between the middle of the 1st and 2nd decades. It is commonly presumed the child has a learning disability and is frequently moved to the front of the class to 'see better.' Retinal pigmentary degeneration is apparent and ultimately optic atrophy. Impairment of motor function becomes apparent and some patients are ataxic. Generalized seizures of tonic/clonic type may be present.	Cytoplasmic inclusions described as granular osmophilic deposits. Other inclusions have also been described including 'fingerprint' and/or rectilinear profiles.
Juvenile dystonic lipidosis	This type is rare and characterized by progressive intellectual deterioration, impairment of upward gaze, ataxia, and dystonia. Attentional deficit, behavioral abnormalities, and visual loss is apparent. Clinical course is somewhat protracted and, in time, patients have seizures. Decerebrate or decorticate postures occur before death.	Intraneuronal storage of lipopigment as well as phospholipids. Storage material not completely identified.
Adult form	Progressive cerebellar ataxia, corticospinal and extrapyramidal dysfunction. Choreoathetosis has been reported and myoclonic fits are common.	Intraneuronal storage of cytosomes containing lipofuscin-lipid material.

Table 4-10 Disorders of White Matter

LIPID DISORDERS 83

Diffuse sclerosis (Schilder's disease)	There has been much confusion regarding this condition, and there is controversy whether or not the entity actually exists. The present view is that it is an acute demyelinating process that occurs sporadically and whose pathological changes are similar to multiple sclerosis. Patients have a relentlessly progressive deterioration of intellectual, motor, and visual function. Seizures may occur at any time during course.
Adrenoleuco-dystrophy Considered x-linked recessive	Probably patients earlier thought to have Schilder's disease had ALD. Early development is usually normal until latter part of 1st decade when behavioral changes occur and there is an impairment of memory. Progressive gait disturbances become apparent and dysarthria followed by dysphagia occurs. Impairment of auditory perception and ultimately deafness and blindness with optic atrophy. Seizures occur late in the course of disease. Patients manifest overt signs of adrenal insufficiency including fatiguability, recurring vomiting, and melanoderma. Some have mild signs and symptoms of adrenal insufficiency that may be overlooked. CSF protein is commonly elevated with normal cells. Biochemical studies of brain, adrenal gland, and skin fibroblasts have shown increased long chain (C_{22}-C_{26}) fatty acids. Diagnosis is established by typical clinical course with adrenal insufficiency and characteristic changes on CT head scan. Determination of fatty acid profile may be done.
Adrenomyelo-neuropathy (? x-linked)	Considered variant of ALD. Usually signs of adrenal insufficiency are present in childhood, and several decades later neurologic signs of spastic paraparesis and polyneuropathy are apparent. Dementia and ataxia have been reported. Similar profile of fatty acids.
Canavan's disease (spongy degeneration of CNS) autosomal recessive	A rare disease with onset of symptoms during first 6 months of life, characterized by lack of development hypotonia, optic atrophy, and seizures. Choreoathetosis has been reported. Typically a progressive marked enlargement of head during 1st year. The hypotonia disappears and the patient becomes spastic. Death occurs within several years. Marked edema of the cortex; demyelination is secondary.
Alexander's disease	Notable for macrocephaly, progressive intellectual deterioration, spasticity, and seizures. Onset of signs and symptoms during 1st year and most children are dead by age of 5. Some may survive longer. Cause is unknown and no treatment is available. Eosinophilic material, resembling neurokeratin, is found in subpial and subependymal region.
Pelizaeus-Merzbacher disease x-linked recessive/ autosomal dominant	Rare, slowly progressive demyelinating disease of which there are at least 2 types. Signs and symptoms are present during the 1st few months of life. Patients have striking, unusual nonrhythmic ocular quivering and wandering movements. Head control is poor and development slow. Microcephaly, ataxia, and tremor soon become apparent. Knee contractures may be present and eventually increasing muscle tone. There are no laboratory studies of specific value. Patients may survive for several decades.

There is elevation of CSF protein with normal cells, except in the adult form of the disease. Motor nerve conduction velocities are delayed. Sural nerve biopsies when appropriately obtained and stained with either cresyl violet or toluidine blue will show metachromatic material within the neural sheath. Confirmation of diagnosis is by assay of arylsulfatase A from leucocytes, fibroblasts, and urine.

LIPIDOSES OF UNKNOWN CAUSE

This group of progressive neurodegenerative diseases is characterized by deposition of intraneural material which appears by histochemical reaction to be glycolipids and/or gangliosides. There is no identifiable neurochemical abnormality that has been detected thus far. These diseases have been categorized, however, on a clinicopathologic basis (see Table 4-9).

DISORDERS OF WHITE MATTER

There is a group of disorders of unknown etiology in which white matter is primarily involved. At this time, there is no known association of an enzyme defect and neurologic abnormalities. These major white matter disorders are noted in Table 4-10.

REFERENCES

Lehninger AL: *Biochemistry*, Worth, New York, 1975.

Scriver CR, Rosenberg LE: *Amino Acid Metabolism and its Disorders*, Saunders, Philadelphia, 1973.

Stanbury JB, Wyngaarden JB, Frederickson DS: *The Metabolic Basis of Inherited Disease*, McGraw-Hill, New York, 1978.

5

Neuromuscular Disorders

Bruce O. Berg, MD

GENERAL CONSIDERATIONS

Neuromuscular diseases are relatively common in childhood. The clinical presentation depends upon what part of the motor pathway is involved, the pathophysiologic process, and the age of the child (see Chapter 1).

WEAKNESS

It is essential to document the **quality of weakness** within a developmental frame of reference and determine if the weakness is static or progressive. Weakness in infancy can be manifested by a feeble cry, weak suck, little or no movement; and in severe weakness, respiratory embarrassment secondary to involvement of thoracic muscles. Older infants may be delayed in sitting, standing, and walking or they may never reach these milestones. Toddlers are normally lordotic, but persistent lordosis may indicate weakness of the pelvic girdle as seen in Duchenne's muscular dystrophy. Unilateral shoulder drooping or decreased arm swing may indicate a brachial plexus injury or hemiparesis. Older children may have difficulty in hopping, jumping, or climbing stairs; the gait may be broad-based or waddling.
Weakness of acute onset suggests a vascular or traumatic etiology, whereas a subacute onset is more consistent with an inflammatory process, such as dermatomyositis. If the onset is insidious, it is more likely to be a degenerative or a metabolic disease affecting nerve or muscle. Intermittent weakness is seen in metabolic processes such as periodic paralysis, and if there is fluctuating weakness, worse after activity or at day's end, myasthenia gravis must be considered.

EXAMINATION OF THE MOTOR SYSTEM

The changes of muscle tone must be considered in relation to the age of the patient (see Chapters 1 and 16). Muscle bulk of infants may be difficult to assess because of prominent subcutaneous fat, which also masks the presence of fasciculations. During infancy, fasciculations are most reliably detected in the tongue, which should be examined when both infant and examiner are relaxed. The tongue of an irritable or crying baby is normally tremulous and easily mistaken for fasciculation. In normal infants and young children, stretch reflexes are often less active in the arms than legs. Asymmetrical or nonreactive plantar responses may be as significant as unequivocally extensor plantar responses. A complete neurologic examination must be performed.

Most diseases in which weakness is the primary symptom are caused by abnormalities of the motor unit. Upper motor, or corticospinal tract lesions, also cause weakness but the neurological findings are such that there is little cause for uncertainty. It is useful to consider the differential diagnosis of weakness in terms of the motor unit. (Table 5-1.)

USEFUL LABORATORY TESTS

Serum enzymes When serum aldolase was found to be increased in patients with Duchenne's muscular dystrophy, other enzymes were studied in reference to neuromuscular diseases. Serum levels of creatine phosphokinase (CPK), glutamic-oxaloacetic transaminase (GOT), and aldolase were elevated, but the CPK was particularly useful in correlating with muscle diseases. Muscle contains significant quantities of creatine and creatinine. Most of the creatine exists as a high energy compound, creatine phosphate. When needed, the creatine phosphate can be used to replenish decreased stores of ATP; the reaction is catalyzed by creatine phosphokinase.

$$\text{Adenosine diphosphate} + \text{creatine phosphate} \xrightarrow{\text{CPK}}$$
$$\text{adenosine triphosphate} + \text{creatine}$$

CPK is found primarily in skeletal muscle, smooth muscle, and brain. It has three isoenzymes including MM found almost entirely in skeletal muscle, BB found primarily in brain, and MB found in cardiac muscle with a smaller fraction of MM. The MM isoenzyme is of primary importance in the diagnosis of diseases of skeletal muscle.

Serum CPK is particularly useful in distinguishing neurogenic diseases from myopathies; however, mild elevations of serum CPK can be found in neurogenic processes and normal serum levels found in some congenital myopathies. Marked elevations are noted in Duchenne's muscular dystrophy

Table 5-1   Neurologic Findings in Lesions of the Motor Unit

	Anterior horn cell	Axon	Myoneural junction	Muscle
Muscle bulk	Decreased	Normal to decreased	Normal to decreased	Decreased
Fasciculations	Present	Absent*	Absent	Absent
Tone	Decreased	Decreased	Normal to decreased	Decreased
Power	Decreased	Normal to decreased	Fluctuating weakness	Decreased
Stretch reflexes	Decreased to absent	Decreased	Normal to decreased	Decreased
Plantar response	Flexor to nonreactive	Flexor to nonreactive	Flexor	Flexor to nonreactive

* May be present during recovery from nerve injury.

and significant elevations of CPK have been found in cases of trauma, status epilepticus, and severe anoxia. Less notable elevations are found in facioscapulohumeral, limb-girdle muscular dystrophies, and myositis. To avoid spurious elevations of serum CPK, blood should be obtained for enzyme assay at first venepuncture and before muscle biopsy or EMG. Serum CPK may be increased for several days following venepuncture. Serum levels of CPK are normally elevated for at least the first several months of life. The enzyme has not been useful in prenatal detection of myopathies.

Muscle biopsy is very helpful in the diagnosis of neuromuscular diseases. Muscle to be biopsied should be moderately rather than severely weak to increase the likelihood of demonstrating meaningful pathological changes. It should be performed under local anesthesia and preferably before EMG. If this is not possible, the muscle selected for biopsy should be marked so that multiple needle insertions of EMG are prevented and misleading areas of focal inflammation and/or necrosis from needle tracks are avoided. It is best to have the person directly involved in the patient evaluation perform the biopsy. Muscle tissue should be obtained for light microscopy, histochemical studies, and electron microscopy.

Stains commonly used for light-microscopic evaluation include hematoxylin and eosin (H & E), hematoxylin van Gieson (HVG), Gomori trichrome, PAS for glycogen and Oil-Red-O to demonstrate lipids.

The light-microscopic changes of muscle in **neurogenic atrophy** include decreased volume (atrophy) of affected motor unit fibers. The fascicular atrophy is seen in cross section as groups of uniformly small fibers with dark nuclei and little change in connective tissue.

The changes seen at light microscopy in a **myopathic process** are characterized by abnormal variability of fiber size diameter, migration of nuclei from their normal subsarcolemmal position toward the center of the fiber as 'row' (longitudinal section) or 'central' (transverse section) nuclei, increased connective tissue and fat, and fiber degeneration. Several types of muscle fiber degeneration have been described including hyaline, granular, or fatty. Infiltration of inflammatory cells is seen in 50-75% of biopsies of patients with myositis. Other distinguishing structural abnormalities are demonstrated in congenital myopathies.

Skeletal muscle is composed of light and dark fibers reflecting myoglobin concentration. The dark, or red fibers, contract slowly and maintain steady tension; whereas the light, or white fibers, contract quickly (twitch). The oxidative metabolic activity is high in white fibers (type I) and a lesser degree of oxidative activity is found in red fibers (type II), although they demonstrate high glycolytic activity. Intermediate fiber types have been identified.

Histochemical methods have been used to demonstrate muscle fiber types on the basis of a variety of enzyme reactions. The primary enzymes used include nicotinamide adenine dinucleotide, reduced - tetrazolium reductase (NADH - TR), adenosine triphosphate (ATPase), phosphatase, and phosphorylase, which is useful in suspected cases of type II glycogenosis (Pompe's disease). Some myologists prefer to use myofibrillar ATPase

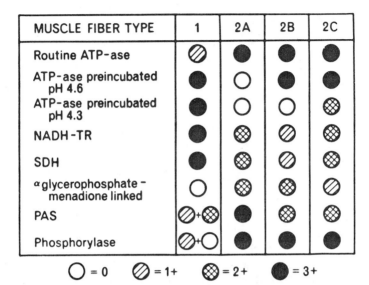

MUSCLE FIBER TYPE	1	2A	2B	2C
Routine ATP-ase	�/1+	●3+	●3+	●3+
ATP-ase preincubated pH 4.6	●3+	○0	●3+	●3+
ATP-ase preincubated pH 4.3	●3+	○0	○0	⊗2+
NADH-TR	●3+	⊗2+	◍1+	⊗2+
SDH	●3+	⊗2+	◍1+	⊗2+
α glycerophosphate – menadione linked	○0	⊗2+	⊗2+	◍1+
PAS	◍+⊗	●3+	⊗2+	⊗2+
Phosphorylase	◍+○	●3+	●3+	●3+

○ = 0   ◍ = 1+   ⊗ = 2+   ● = 3+

Fig. 5-1 Histochemical reactions in human muscle. (Reproduced with permission from Dubowitz V, Brooke MH, *Muscle Biopsy: A Modern Approach,* Saunders, Philadelphia, 1973.)

because muscle fibers demonstrate either a weak (type I) or strong (type II) reaction (Figure 5-1). The two-fiber type system can be determined by the activity of oxidative enzymes such as NADH-TR, succinic dehydrogenase, or with a standard ATPase reaction (pH 9.4).

Electrodiagnostic studies, an important part of the patient evaluation, consist of electromyography (EMG) and determination of nerve conduction velocities. EMG demonstrates electrical activity of muscle and enables the examiner to identify whether the lesion is limited to the nerve or muscle. EMG findings are never specifically diagnostic of a disease process, but are useful in corroborating a clinical diagnosis. If the neural segment of the motor unit is involved, it is often possible to determine if the lesion is in the anterior horn cell, the axon as it traverses a spinal root, peripheral nerve, or the myoneural junction.

Motor nerve conduction velocities are obtained by stimulating a peripheral nerve while recording the activity (compound muscle action potential) from the muscle innervated by that nerve. Sensory nerve conduction studies are obtained by stimulating and recording from a cutaneous nerve while stimulating a mixed nerve.

Conduction velocities of motor and sensory nerves vary with age because of nerve fiber size, the degree of myelination, and the internodal distance. There are significant changes of motor nerve conduction velocities with maturation (Table 5-2).

Table 5-2   Motor Conduction Velocities in Infants and Children
Expressed in meters/second

Age	Ulnar	Median	Peroneal
0-1 week	32(21-39)	29(21-38)	29(19-31)
1 week-4 months	42(27-53)	34(22-42)	36(23-53)
4 months-1 year	49(40-63)	40(26-58)	48(31-61)
1-3 years	59(47-73)	50(41-62)	54(44-74)
3-8 years	66(51-76)	58(47-72)	57(46-70)
8-16 years	68(58-78)	64(54-72)	57(47-63)
Adults	63(52-75)	63(51-75)	56(47-63)

Adapted from Gamstorp, I: Acta Paediat Suppl 1963, 146:68-76

DISORDERS OF THE ANTERIOR HORN CELL

The clinical features of anterior horn cell disorders are those of a lower
motor neuron lesion (Table 1-3).

CONGENITAL ABNORMALITIES

A variety of congenital malformations of the brain stem and spinal cord
may affect the large motor cells of some cranial nerve nuclei and the anterior horn cells of the spinal cord. Some major malformations include
diastematomyelia, syringomyelia, syringobulbia, and hydromyelia. Duane
and Mobius syndromes may affect the motor cells of cranial nerve nuclei
VI and VII, respectively.

PROGRESSIVE SPINAL MUSCULAR ATROPHY (PSMA)

PSMA is a degenerative disease of unknown etiology which affects the
anterior horn cells of the spinal cord and some motor cells of cranial nerve
nuclei. It is inherited as an autosomal recessive trait, although some have
suggested there are factors which modify gene expression. A variety of
classifications of the disease have been described, each of which is based
on the age at onset of symptoms and the length of survival of patients.
Generally, the earlier the onset, the shorter the survival. Some believe
PSMA is one genetic disease with variability of clinical expression; whereas
others believe in a genetic heterogeneity. It seems reasonable to view the
spectrum of this disease in the following manner: an acute type in which
symptoms begin before the age of 6 months and survival is generally 12-24
months; a chronic type in which the symptoms begin after 6 months of
age and the patient may survive to adolescence or young adulthood; a mild
type (juvenile; Kugelberg-Welander) in which symptoms are first apparent
from 5-15 years of age and patients live to adult life.

ACUTE INFANTILE PSMA (Werdnig-Hoffmann Disease)

The clinical presentation is rather typical although it is difficult to know when the weakness begins. About one third of mothers, when specifically questioned, experienced decreased fetal activity during the last few months of pregnancy. Unless symptoms are present at birth, mothers gradually become aware the infant is not normally active. The cry becomes feeble and the patient has difficulty with sucking and swallowing. As the disease progresses, motor milestones are not achieved and the infant may not be able to support his head, roll over, or sit up. Often the patient assumes a 'frog-like' or 'jug-handle' posture, lying supine with arms extended and internally rotated, and legs abducted and flexed at the knee. Extraocular motility remains intact and though unable to move the limbs, the patients are alert.

Fasciculations of the tongue are present in most patients. It may require several examinations to document this finding and they are best seen during periods of quiet. Flickering (small muscle twitches) of fingers and hands may be present; this is a valuable sign of anterior horn cell disease. There is generalized muscle wasting and weakness.

The thorax is commonly flattened, sometimes with pectus excavatum and intercostal muscle weakness. There may be a flaring of the lower rib cage and paradoxical respiration is often seen. Stretch reflexes are severely depressed to absent; the sensory examination is normal. There is no notable cardiac abnormality.

No specific treatment is available for this group of diseases but the clinician must pay meticulous attention to pulmonary function, potentially recurring pulmonary infection, and the patient's nutrition. In this acute form of disease, contractures are rarely a problem; physical therapy may be of some benefit. Usually the disease progresses relentlessly and patients have increasing difficulty handling oropharyngeal secretions. Patients expire within 12-24 months of age, usually from pneumonia and respiratory failure.

CHRONIC INFANTILE PSMA

The onset of symptoms is usually between 6 and 12 months of age and progression of weakness is insidious. Infants seem normal until onset of weakness, when a delay in achieving milestones becomes apparent. Patients may sit with support, but are often never able to sit alone. They are not able to stand or walk and are confined to a wheelchair in early life.

Extraocular motility remains intact, and weakness of oropharyngeal muscles is seldom a problem. Lingual fasciculations are common. There is muscle wasting and weakness, proximal muscles more than distal, and a fine tremulousness, or flickering of small muscles of the fingers and hands is commonly seen. Stretch reflexes are decreased to absent.

It is imprudent to predict the length of survival of children with the chronic form of disease for some may have a relatively benign course. The longer the survival, the greater is the likelihood of joint contractures of hips and knees. Other problems include kyphoscoliosis and equinovarus deformities. Recurring pulmonary infection is a potential problem and with increased patient longevity, particular attention must be directed to pulmonary function.

As in the case of acute PSMA, there is no specific treatment, except for supportive management including antibiotics when specifically indicated, and physical therapy. Parents can be instructed to carry out the physical therapy maneuvers at home, but patients should be reassessed periodically by physical therapists. In older, cooperative patients, breathing exercises and pulmonary drainage are important.

JUVENILE PSMA (KUGELBERG - WELANDER)

This variety of PSMA was thought earlier to be a form of muscular dystrophy. Symptom onset is usually from 5-15 years of age, although the initially reported age range of symptom onset was 2-17 years. Weakness progresses gradually. The pelvic girdle is first affected and patients have gait abnormalities and difficulty climbing steps. The arms and shoulders become weak, and the patient may be unaware of this until examined. Patients may walk on their toes and appear unusually lordotic.

There is loss of bulk of the thigh muscles, but calf musculature seems relatively normal. Progressive weakness appears insidiously and it may be some time until the child is seen by a physician. Only later are shoulder girdle and arm muscles affected. There is atrophy of forearm muscles with weakness of the flexor muscles greater than extensors. The hands and fingers are relatively unaffected until late in the disease course. Facial weakness may be apparent later and some patients have lingual fasciculations. Progressive ophthalmoplegia and bulbar symptoms and signs have been reported. Stretch reflexes are normal to depressed. There are no sensory abnormalities.

This type of PSMA is relatively mild and patients may have a full life for decades, remaining able to walk 20 years or more after the diagnosis. It is inherited as an autosomal recessive trait, but reports of autosomal dominant and x-linked inheritance have been recorded.

AMYOTROPHIC LATERAL SCLEROSIS

This is a progressive, degenerative disease with signs of corticospinal tract dysfunction and anterior horn cell loss. Although primarily affecting adults, there are reports of patients with onset of symptoms in the first or second decades. Both hereditary and sporadic cases are reported in childhood.

Initial symptoms vary, but there is usually an asymmetrical weakness of distal muscles; some patients may first have weakness of oropharyngeal muscles with dysphagia. There is progressive bulbar paralysis and patients complain of muscle spasms, cramps, or a 'dull-heavy feeling' in the legs.

Neurological findings are consistent with upper and lower motor nerve dysfunction. There is loss of muscle bulk, and fasciculations are seen in the tongue and limb muscles. Stretch reflexes are usually increased but may be decreased; plantar responses are extensor. No sensory abnormalities are detected; however, abnormalities of responses to quantified sensory stimuli have been reported with structural changes of peripheral nerves. There is continual progression of muscle wasting and weakness, and death comes within months to several years after onset of symptoms.

Autopsies have shown loss of motor neurons of the brain stem and spinal cord, demyelination of corticospinal tracts and anterior nerve roots. Motor nuclei of the medulla are generally severely affected. Neuronal inclusions derived from Nissl substance have been reported in sporadic juvenile cases, but not in adults with the sporadic type of ALS.

Treatment includes vigorous supportive measures and careful attention must be directed to pulmonary function and potential pulmonary infection.

PROGRESSIVE BULBAR PALSY (Fazio-Londe Syndrome)

This is a rare disease of childhood in which there is loss of motor neurons of some brain-stem nuclei particularly VII. Other nuclei which have been affected include III, IV, V, VI, X, and XII. The number of reported patients is few and onset of symptoms has ranged from 2-12 years. Most patients have facial weakness, dysphagia and/or dysarthria. There is progressive bulbar involvement and death occurs months to years after symptom onset. The etiology is unknown.

Few autopsy studies are available, but findings are generally consistent with neuronal loss in cranial nerve nuclei III, IV, V, VI, VII, X, and XII. Other abnormalities were found in the spinal cord with loss of anterior horn cells in upper cervical and thoracic regions. Loss of Purkinje cells and decreased cells of midline cerebellar nuclei have been noted.

SCAPULOPERONEAL/FACIOSCAPULOHUMERAL MUSCULAR ATROPHY

Several reports have been published describing children and adults with weakness and atrophy of the shoulder girdle, anterior tibial, and peroneal muscles. Facial and neck muscles are occasionally involved. There has been confusion regarding some reports and other diagnoses have been suggested. There is, nonetheless, a small number of patients with scapuloperoneal or facioscapuloperoneal syndromes whose clinical findings, muscle biopsy, and EMG features are all consistent with a neurogenic process.

TRANSVERSE MYELOPATHY

Although commonly known as transverse myelitis, it is more appropriate to use the term 'myelopathy,' for neuropathological studies are seldom available and one often cannot be certain of the etiology. It must be noted however, that one half to two thirds of patients have a preceding history of nonspecfic 'viral illness,' the relationship of which is usually unclear.

Patients usually complain of leg or back pain; there is acute or subacute onset of hypotonia, commonly progressing to flaccidity of legs and occasionally the arms. A sensory level is usually demonstrable in the thoracic region (67%) and less commonly in the cervical (22%), or lumbar regions (11%). There is a loss of bladder and anal sphincter tone. Some patients are febrile and may have nuchal rigidity. Signs and symptoms reach their nadir within hours to 1 or 2 days, and within days to several weeks, flaccidity disappears and the patient has increased tone, or spasticity, with hyperreflexia and extensor plantar responses.

It must quickly be determined if the patient has a space-occupying lesion which requires immediate neurosurgical intervention, and myelography must be performed early. Epidural abscesses, spinal cord tumors, and vascular malformations are generally identified by myelography. Both physician and neurosurgeon should follow the patient from the onset until the need for neurosurgical procedure is established. A minimal amount of CSF should be removed for examination at the time of myelography to minimize the risk of spinal cord compression. In transverse myelopathy, the CSF may be normal or have a mild pleocytosis. The CSF glucose and protein are normal. A variety of viruses have been implicated as causative agents, including mumps, rubella, rubeola, varicella, variola, and infectious mononucleosis.

The clinical course is chronic and patients require careful, supportive care and physical therapy; appropriate bowel and bladder care is essential. According to one study of children and adults with transverse myelopathy, one third had good recovery, one third had fair recovery and one third of patients had little or no return of function.

Neuropathological studies have demonstrated myelomalacia with focal lesions extending over many segments. Other pathological findings include demyelination and cyst formation.

NEUROMYELITIS OPTICA (Devic's Disease)

This is a rare disease characterized by optic neuritis and acute transverse myelopathy which may appear simultaneously or subsequently. Both eyes are almost always involved, either simultaneously or in sequence. Visual loss is rapid, occurring within hours to days and precedes the paraplegia in about 80% of cases. The interval between optic neuritis and onset of transverse myelopathy may be days, weeks, or months.

Prognosis for recovery of vision is good and vision usually returns to normal. The overall outlook for transverse myelopathy is less favorable. The etiology is unclear, although it is probably related to multiple sclerosis for neuropathological features are similar.

ARTHROGRYPOSIS

This syndrome is characterized by contractures of joints and is often associated with muscular atrophy. A number of pathophysiological processes can be involved. It may occur as a result of restricted in-utero activity with normal neuromuscular function. It is, however, most commonly associated with anterior horn cell loss and less frequently with myopathy, radiculopathy, and anomalies of brain and spinal cord. Arthrogryposis has also been linked to peripheral neuropathies and abnormalities of collagen. One unusual familial syndrome of arthrogryposis found in Eskimos, is Kuskokwim disease (named after a region in Alaska) characterized by multiple joint contractures primarily affecting the knees and ankles. Studies of muscle and nerve in this unusual condition are normal, but a periarticular fibrosis has been found.

Since arthrogryposis is caused by a number of different pathological processes, one should determine whether the joint contractures are on a neurogenic or myopathic basis, or if it represents a specific joint disease.

Treatment includes vigorous physical therapy, and orthopedic procedures may be of significant benefit to patients.

DISORDERS OF PERIPHERAL NERVES

The peripheral nervous system is composed of the neural elements external to the pial membrane which surrounds the brain stem and spinal cord. The neural bundles attached to the lateral brain stem and dorsal and ventral aspects of spinal cord within the spinal canal are the nerve roots. The dorsal root (comprised of sensory fibers) and the ventral root (comprised of motor and autonomic fibers) join to form the peripheral nerve (Figure 5-2). Axons of the dorsal root ganglia are sensory and terminate in specialized sensory nerve endings; whereas, the ventral root axons terminate in muscle fibers or in parasympathetic or sympathetic ganglia.

Diseases of the peripheral nerve have been classified in a variety of ways and there is not one classification which is universally acceptable. Mononeuropathy refers to involvement of one nerve and polyneuropathy when more than one nerve is affected. The etiology of polyneuropathies remains obscure in over one half of cases.

The entire nerve can be transected in traumatic lesions and other pathophysiological processes can affect the axon, the Schwann cell and myelin, or the nutrient neural vessels. Unless there is evidence of specific inflammation of the peripheral nerve, it is more appropriate to use the term neuropathy, rather than neuritis, to indicate abnormal nerve function without regard to specific etiology.

Symptoms of peripheral nerve disorders are motor and sensory; rarely patients have a neuropathic process with only sensory or motor findings. When autonomic nerves are affected, abnormalities of pupillary reaction, intestinal or bladder dysfunction, or impotence are found; anhidrosis or orthostatic hypotension may also occur.

The typical features of polyneuropathy are weakness of the feet and legs; the hands and arms are usually affected later and are often less severely involved. Stretch reflexes are reduced to absent. There may be a loss of muscle bulk, but fasciculations are not present. The disorder is often heralded by paresthesias and dysesthesias, and patients complain of being 'numb - tingling - hypersensitive - burning.' Objective findings are usually distal, legs more than arms, and most often all sensory modalities are impaired or lost. Vibration is usually affected more than position sense. The sensory loss roughly conforms to a 'stocking' or 'glove' distribution.

Pathological changes of a peripheral nerve include wallerian degeneration, segmental demyelination and axonal degeneration.

The changes of **wallerian degeneration** were initially considered in relation to a transected nerve; however, it now refers to the degenerative changes of the severed nerve from whatever process. There is irregular swelling of the axon which is followed by granular disintegration of neurofibrils, fragmentation of the axon, and longitudinal retraction of fragments. There is retraction of the myelin from the node Ranvier and the myelin tubes split. Fragments of myelin enclose the broken segments of axon, forming ovoids or 'digestion chambers.' The Schwann cell undergoes reactive changes and the cytoplasm ultimately engulfs the myelin debris. Recovery requires months to over a year.

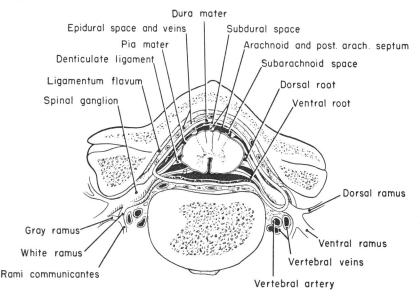

Fig. 5-2 Spinal cord and its meningeal coverings. (Reproduced with permission from Carpenter, *Human Neuroanatomy*, Baltimore, Williams & Wilkins, 1976.)

Segmental demyelination occurs in diseases primarily affecting the Schwann cell in which the axon remains intact. The cytoplasm swells and there is splitting of myelin lamellae. Concurrently, Schwann cells proliferate and cytoplasmic processes insert themselves around the myelin fragments making contact with the axon. When the new Schwann cell makes contact with the axon, remyelination begins by formation of a mesaxon and encircles the axon. Throughout the process, the basement membrane of nerve fibers remains intact. Recovery of function is relatively rapid. Examples of segmental demyelination are seen in Guillain-Barre syndrome and lead poisoning. It is also seen in diabetes mellitus in which there may also be axonal degeneration and involvement of the nutrient vessels of the nerve.

Axonal degeneration occurs when the distal aspect of the axon is first affected and there is commonly a 'dying-back' phenomenon. Examples of axonal degeneration include the toxic neuropathies, those associated with malnutrition and/or alcoholism, Fabry's disease, alphalipoproteinemia and abetalipoproteinemia. An unusual neuropathy which has its onset in childhood, giant axonal neuropathy is characterized by swollen segments which are filled with neurofilamentous masses.

THE HEREDITARY POLYNEUROPATHIES

The hereditary polyneuropathies have been divided into those with primarily sensory or sensorimotor findings (see Tables 5-3 and 5-4). There are

Table 5-3 The Hereditary Sensory Neuropathies (HSN)

HSN I   Onset of cellulitis, lymphangitis, and ulceration of feet is usually in the 2nd or 3rd decades but may occur in the 1st decade. Ulcers are usually painless but if associated with osteomyelitis may be present; upper limbs may be affected. Sensory loss of all modalities is greatest distally; usually the trunk is not involved. There may be moderate distal weakness and absent ankle jerks. In-vitro studies of sural nerves showed decreased amplitudes of A, AS, and C compound action potentials. Sphincters and sexual function are preserved. Patients usually have normal life expectancy but must be instructed in meticulous foot care. Inherited as autosomal dominant trait with variable severity.

HSN II Onset of mutilating ulcerative lesions of the hands and feet is in infancy or early childhood. Fractures may go unrecognized. There is loss of all sensory modalities, particularly distally, and the trunk can be involved. Decreased to absent stretch reflexes. Nerve action potentials of afferent fibers are not detectable. Natural history is not well known. Heritability is probably autosomal recessive trait.

HSN III **Familial dysautonomia. Riley-Day syndrome.** Onset in infancy characterized by poor feeding, vomiting, emotional lability, and pulmonary infections. Signs of autonomic dysfunction include decreased or absent tearing, abnormal temperature regulation with increased sweating, skin blotching and labile blood pressure. Patients have insensitivity to pain. Fungiform papillae of tongue are absent. Mental retardation has been reported. Stretch reflexes are decreased to absent. Abnormal local axonal reflex demonstrated by failure of skin scratch or intradermal injection of histamine to produce erythematous flair of triple response. Marked decrease in unmyelinated fibers of cutaneous nerves; decreased myelination in the dorsal root fibers and posterior columns. Motor nerve conduction velocities have been reported as decreased compared with controls. Autosomal recessive inheritance, primarily in patients of Jewish ancestry.

HSN IV HSN with anhidrosis; probably autosomal recessive inheritance. Present from birth and characterized by insensitivity to pain, anhidrosis, and mild mental retardation. Patients may have significant injuries without evidence of pain. Autopsy of one patient demonstrated absence of small neurons in spinal ganglia, decreased small fibers in dorsal roots, and absence of Lissauer's tract.

Table 5-4 The Hereditary Sensorimotor Neuropathies (HSMN)

HSMN I	**Peroneal muscular atrophy** Onset in childhood with foot deformity (pes cavus and/or hammer toe) or disorder of gait. Progressive weakness and atrophy beginning in the intrinsic hand muscles, anterolateral calf muscles, and later affecting intrinsic hand muscles. Stretch reflexes are decreased to absent. Sensory function normal to slightly impaired. Peripheral nerves may be hypertrophic. Reduced motor nerve conduction velocities are a hallmark of this disease. Inherited as autosomal dominant trait.
HSMN II	Similar clinical findings to those in HSMN I although symptoms begin later. Weakness of hand muscles less severe; there is greater weakness in foot plantar flexor muscles. Gait abnormality is prominent and sensory loss apparent in most patients affecting distal aspects of lower limbs. Motor nerve conduction velocities are only slightly decreased. Inherited as autosomal dominant trait.
HSMN III	**Hypertrophic interstitial neuropathy; Dejerine-Sottas** Onset in infancy with delayed motor development. Walking is impaired because of distal weakness, increasing in severity during the 2nd decade. Stretch reflexes are absent; some patients are ataxic. Impaired sensation in all modalities without affecting pain and temperature discrimination. Peripheral nerves are hypertrophic. Meiosis and decreased pupillary responses are present. Deafness may occur. Some have kyphoscoliosis and foot deformities. CSF protein is increased. Reduced motor nerve conduction velocities. Inherited as autosomal recessive trait.
HSMN IV	**Refsum's disease** The onset is insidious and varies from early childhood to the 2nd or 3rd decades. Characterized by night blindness, retinitis pigmentosa, ichthyosis, deafness, anosmia, and polyneuropathy. Pes cavus and hammer toes are frequently reported. Distal symmetrical muscle wasting, weakness, and areflexia. Increased CSF protein. Pathophysiological basis of disease is the inability to oxidize phytanic acid. Inherited as an autosomal recessive trait.
HSMN V	**Familial spastic paraplegia** The onset is usually in the 2nd decade or later. Progressive spasticity with hyperreflexia and adductor tightness with extensor plantar responses. There is no sensory impairment. Motor nerve conduction velocities are usually normal or reduced in legs. There may be a progressive decrease in numbers of myelinated peripheral sensory neurons with increasing age of patient.

reports of individual patients with sensory neuropathies that are not readily classified, an example of which is **congenital indifference to pain.** In this rare condition, patients do not withdraw from painful stimuli. They have no analgesia and no concomitant acceleration of pulse or increased blood pressure when exposed to pain. They are, rather, 'indifferent' to pain. Sensory modalities are intact and muscle bulk, power, and stretch reflexes are normal. Earlier studies have demonstrated no abnormality in cutaneous nerves, spinal cord, or thalamus. Sweat glands were present in the skin but were not innervated. (See also Tables 5-5, 5-6, and 5-7.)

BELL'S PALSY

An idiopathic neuropathy, Bell's palsy is a paralysis of the facial nerve, presumably secondary to edema and inflammation, as the nerve traverses the facial canal or the stylomastoid foramen. Patients often have symptoms of a mild respiratory infection or complain of pain about or behind the ear for 1 or 2 days before the paralysis. Onset of facial weakness can be acute or subacute, but most patients reach the nadir of facial weakness within 2 days. In child patients it is often difficult, though not impossible, to determine the site of the lesion along the facial nerve, and one should attempt to determine if there are abnormalities of taste (chorda tympani), sound perception (stapedius nerve), or decreased lacrimation (petrosal nerve). The diagnosis of Bell's palsy is one of exclusion. Other diagnostic possibilities include congenital facial palsies, infection (mastoiditis, meningitis, osteomyelitis, otitis media, parotitis, and Ramsay-Hunt syndrome). Trauma and tumors may also cause facial palsy. Less common diagnostic possibilities include varicella and mumps.

Treatment has included a variety of methods but more than 60% of patients recover completely without any treatment. Electromyography may be of prognostic value for if there is evidence of denervation after 10 days, there will probably be a prolonged recovery period which may be incomplete.

Prednisone, given within 72 hours of symptom onset may decrease the incidence of facial denervation. Children over 10 years should receive 40 mg daily in divided doses for 4 days with gradual reduction of dosage to 5 mg daily to discontinue at 8 days. Younger children should receive 20 mg daily for 4 days with gradual dosage reduction to 5 mg to be discontinued at 8 days.

There is no evidence that surgical decompression is effective. If the eye does not close, it should be protected with an eye patch, and ophthalmic solutions of methyl cellulose are beneficial to keep the cornea moist. There is no evidence that electrical stimulation of facial muscles is of valu.e Generally, the younger the patient the better is the prognosis.

MELKERSSON SYNDROME

An unusual idiopathic neuropathy characterized by recurrent facial palsy, facial swelling, and a lingual corrugation (lingua plicata). Eventually, after repeated episodes, there may be permanent swelling of the face and lips, with cheilitis and lingua plicata. There is no treatment of significant benefit. The etiology remains unknown.

GUILLAIN - BARRE SYNDROME (Idiopathic Polyneuritis)

Idiopathic polyneuritis may occur from infancy throughout adulthood. About 75% of children have nonspecific respiratory or gastrointestinal symptoms during the preceding several weeks. It has been reported to follow infectious mononucleosis, mumps, rubella, and rubeola.

Paresthesias or dysesthesias may precede or accompany weakness which usually begins in the legs and ascends to affect the hands and arms. A small number of cases have proximal weakness greater than distal. About one half of patients have cranial nerves involved and facial diplegia is most commonly seen. Papilledema is present in a small number of patients, and may be related to impaired CSF resorption. The degree of muscle weakness varies; it is symmetrical and primarily distal. The stretch reflexes are decreased to absent. Rarely, plantar responses are extensor.

Sensory deficits are minimal, but impairment of position sense may be present. Less commonly there is impairment of vibration, touch, pain, and temperature. Patients often complain of muscle pain or tenderness.

Autonomic dysfunction may occur and is manifested by facial flushing, labile blood pressures, and cardiac arrhythmias. Rarely, patients have urinary retention but, if present, lasts only for a few days. Inappropriate ADH has been reported. The **Fisher variant** of Guillain-Barre syndrome is characterized by ataxia, external ophthalmoplegia, and areflexia.

Elevation of CSF protein is typically present reaching its peak within several weeks and then gradually decreasing. The cell count is usually normal, but 5% or less of patients will have pleocytosis. About 80% of patients will have nerve conduction slowing at some time during the illness. Distal latencies may be increased as much as three times normal.

Treatment is supportive and particular attention should be directed to pulmonary function. Appropriate ventilatory equipment and trained personnel must be readily available if tracheostomy is required. If the patient has any respiratory impairment, ventilatory assistance is needed at that time rather than waiting for potentially calamitous respiratory problems to occur. Because of labile blood pressures, careful monitoring is essential. Physical therapy should be started as soon as the patient is clinically stable.

There is controversy regarding the administration of corticosteroids to these patients, but at this time there is no evidence they are of benefit. Plasmapheresis has also been recommended as another treatment method; however, this requires further clinical documentation. It is not possible to state what therapeutic role plasmapheresis has in this disease.

A small number of children have relapses over the course of months to years and others have fluctuating courses without complete recovery between exacerbations. These patients appear to respond favorably to administration of corticosteroids.

INFECTIOUS CAUSES OF NEUROPATHY

Ramsay-Hunt syndrome, characterized by facial paralysis and a vesicular eruption within the external auditory canal, is secondary to herpes zoster infection of the geniculate ganglion. The eighth cranial nerve may sometimes be affected.

Table 5-5 Polyneuropathy in Heritable Metabolic Diseases

Ataxia-telangiectasia	Clinical and pathological evidence of mild neuropathy found in some older patients. Delayed sensory and motor nerve conduction velocities have been reported (see Chapter 9).
Abetalipoproteinemia (Bassen-Kornzweig)	A rare disorder of autosomal recessive inheritance. Characterized by early steatorrhea and poor growth; ataxia and weakness with decreased to absent stretch reflexes. Retinal pigmentary degeneration is present and sensory examination demonstrates loss of position sense and vibration. Demyelination of peripheral nerves; loss of neurons in spinal cord (posterior columns) and cerebellum.
Adrenoleuko-dystrophy	Leukodystrophy and adrenal insufficiency of x-linked recessive inheritance. Onset from 4-16 years with cerebral degeneration and ultimately death. Adrenomyeloneuropathy described in older patients with spastic paraparesis and mild polyneuropathy. Long chain fatty acids in cholesterol esters isolated from brain and adrenal glands.
Alphalipoprotein deficiency (Tangier disease)	Motor and/or sensory impairment with muscle weakness, wasting and absent stretch reflexes, paresthesias, dysesthesias, and increased sweating. Notable for recurrent neuropathic episodes. Motor nerve conduction velocities generally slowed. Autosomal recessive inheritance probable.
Chediak-Higashi syndrome	Oculocutaneous albinism, mental retardation, fits and muscle weakness. Giant peroxidase positive lysosome granules in leukocytes and Schwann cells. No sensory impairment detected; motor nerve conduction progressively reduced. Giant C-H granules in Schwann cells. Patients have marked sensitivity to infection. Those who survive this period frequently die from lymphoreticular malignancy.
Fabry's disease (angiokeratoma corporis diffusum)	Onset in childhood or adolescence with recurrent episodes of severe leg pains, cutaneous vascular lesions, angiokeratoma, hypohidrosis, and corneal dystrophy. Vascular involvement prominent in central and peripheral nervous system. Loss of small myelinated and unmyelinated fibers as well as small cell bodies of spinal ganglion. There is an absence of alpha-galactosidase-A. X-linked recessive inheritance.

Diabetes mellitus	Neuropathy uncommon in childhood; occurs usually in poorly controlled disease of long duration. Some have mild distal weakness of small muscles of feet and sensory loss of stocking-glove distribution. Others have only electrophysiological evidence of neuropathy.
Krabbe's disease (globoid cell leukodystrophy)	Acute infantile leukodystrophy of autosomal recessive inheritance. Progressive spasticity and hyper-reflexia; optic atrophy and ultimately decorticate posturing. Reduced motor nerve conduction velocity demonstrated. Infant may become hypotonic with decreased reflexes. Nerve biopsy shows reduced number of myelinated fibers.
Leigh disease	Onset in infancy or childhood, but may occur at any age. Typically oculomotor and bulbar dysfunction with weakness, ataxia, dysphagia, and abnormalities of respiration. Polyneuropathy present. Evidence of disorder of brain pyruvate metabolism; autosomal recessive trait.
Metachromatic leukodystrophy	Cerebral degenerative disease of autosomal recessive inheritance. Hypotonia with progressive weakness; decreased to absent reflexes and marked reduction of peripheral nerve conduction velocity. Nerve biopsy characterized by metachromasia, decreased myelinated fibers, and evidence of segmental demyelination. Metabolic abnormality defined as deficiency of arylsulfatase A.
Porphyria	Neuropathy found in acute intermittent type of disease. Back and limb pains followed by weakness; arms affected more than legs and proximal muscles more than distal. Usually symmetrical. Occasional dysesthesias and paresthesias in proximal limbs and/or buttock that precede motor symptoms. Autonomic nervous system can be involved. Stretch reflexes decreased to absent.
Refsum's disease	See Table 5-4 (HSMN IV).

Table 5-6 Adverse Effects of Drugs

Amitriptyline	Numbness, paresthesias and tingling with mild sensory impairment; reduced to absent ankle and knee stretch reflexes. May occur after chronic administration. Patients who have sensory abnormalities in lower limbs also have optic neuritis. Symptoms disappear when the drug is discontinued.
Carbon disulfide	Usually after moderately heavy exposure. Initially paresthesias, muscle pain, decreased strength, and sensory loss. Stretch reflexes decreased to absent. Usually worse in legs; in severe cases difficulty in walking. Motor nerve conduction velocities decreased. No specific treatment, although vitamin B_6 has been recommended.
Chloramphenicol	Most often occurs in patients receiving prolonged treatment. Numbness of feet progressing to pain and tenderness. There are few objective signs, and loss of reflexes uncommon. Optic neuritis has been reported. Recommended treatment is discontinuation of drug. Vitamin B_6 has been suggested, but rationale equivocal.
Clioquinol	Restricted to use as oral intestinal amebicide in the USA since 1961. Not marketed in USA since 1972; used frequently in Asia and Southern hemisphere. Thought to be responsible for subacute myelo-optico neuropathy in Japan with symmetrical sensory disturbance in lower limbs from feet to thorax. Some patients have weakness with increased reflexes and bladder dysfunction. Motor and sensory nerve conduction velocities delayed.
Dapsone	An unusual complication of drug therapy where motor loss is predominant; mechanism thought to be an axonal degeneration.
Disulfiram	Neuropathy can occur at standard therapeutic doses. Symptoms begin several months after treatment and reverse several months after discontinuation of drug. Paresthesias followed by weakness; gradually all sensory modalities and stretch reflexes are impaired distally to proximally. Optic neuritis reported. Disulfiram catabolized to carbon disulfide (see above).
Glutethimide	Predominantly sensory neuropathy with paresthesias of feet and legs, cramping, and tenderness. All sensory modalities are lost and ankle reflexes absent. Symptoms appear after months of exposure and disappear within several months following drug withdrawal.

Hydralazine	Distal numbness and paresthesias; mild distal weakness may occur. Findings may be asymmetrical and gradually resolve following discontinuation of drug or following administration of pyridoxine. Proposed mechanism of action: hydralazine reacts with pyridoxine to form inactive, readily excreted compounds, resulting in pyridoxine deficiency.
Isoniazid	Numbness and paresthesias in feet and legs; some complain of burning or aching. There is weakness of distal muscles and loss of stretch reflexes. Interferes with vitamin B_6-dependent enzymes. Prevented by administration of pyridoxine which does not interfere with antibacterial effect of the drug (isoniazid).
Nitrofurantoin	Neuropathy appears after using medication for weeks to months. Symptoms include numbness and pain; sensory findings include impaired distal vibration and position sense. Pain and temperature are less affected. Distal weakness and decreased to absent stretch reflexes.
Phenytoin	Reported to occur in some patients on long-term drug administration and characterized by mild distal symmetrical impairment of sensation, reduced to absent ankle and knee reflexes. No unequivocal relationship established.
Stilbamidine	May produce sensory neuropathy in distribution of trigeminal nerve.
Trichlorethylene	Used as inhalant anesthetic as well as organic solvent. May result in trigeminal neuropathy with loss of sensory modalities over entire distribution of the nerve. May have weakness of muscles of mastication. Optic and facial nerves may be involved. Recovery occurs within several months. Pathophysiology unknown.
Vincristine	Sensorimotor neuropathy after several months of treatment; numbness, paresthesias and dysesthesias in all distal limbs. Weakness seen first in distal extensor muscles of arms and legs; loss of ankle jerks. Symptoms reduced when dosage decreased or drug discontinued.

Table 5-7 Polyneuropathy Secondary to Toxic Agents

Acrylamide	Distal motor and sensory fibers are affected, resulting in clumsiness of hand movements and walking difficulty. Stretch reflexes are lost early. Sensory symptoms include numbness in feet and fingers; decreased vibration in hands and feet are also commonly reported and position sense is impaired in distal joints. Motor symptoms greater than sensory. Excessive sweating is universally found.
Arsenic	Symptoms appear insidiously in low-level environmental contamination, or subacutely in unsuccessful murder or suicidal attempts. Numbness and paresthesias of distal limbs, followed by distal weakness. Sensory involvement often severe. All sensory modalities, particularly position sense, are affected. Recovery is gradual; there is complete recovery in mild cases.
n-Hexane (normal hexane)	Motor and sensory dysfunction develop slowly, except in cases of 'glue sniffers' where onset is subacute, predominantly with motor findings. History of weight loss, distal paresthesias and weakness of hands and feet. Ankle jerks decreased to absent. Severe cases have progressive distal weakness and atrophy of hands and legs. Proximal muscles may be involved. Moderate loss of touch, pain, vibration, and temperature. Other systemic manifestations include hyperkeratosis, brown skin with pitting edema, and lesions of the mucous membranes.
Lead	Children usually have encephalopathy; however, there may be an initial polyneuropathy. It is primarily a motor neuropathy which affects legs before arms in children and the reverse in adults. Stretch reflexes are absent. Sensory loss usually minor. There is commonly history of pica and a confirmatory test is lead blood level greater than 60 μg/dl. (See Chapter 17.)
Methyl-m-butyl ketone	An organic solvent thought to be metabolized similarly to n-hexane (see above).

Methyl bromide	Colorless gas at room temperature used as fire extinguisher, fumigant, insecticide, and refrigerant. After chronic exposure, paresthesias of limbs, usually legs, with distal weakness and sensory loss. Stretch reflexes decreased to absent. Thought to cause axonal degeneration.
Organophosphorous compounds	Most cases caused by triortho-tolyl phosphate. Shortly following ingestion, GI distress with nausea, vomiting, and diarrhea. After 8-18 days, patients complain of numbness and tingling in feet and hands with cramping in calves, followed by weakness of lower limbs. Hip girdle and proximal muscles can be involved; decreased to absent stretch reflexes. Sensory loss may conform to weakness. Recovery may be poor.
Mercury (organic)	Earliest complaints are tingling and paresthesias of fingers followed by numbness which can affect tongue. Generalized weakness of limbs and progressive ataxia; tremor occurs in about 70% of patients. Constriction of visual fields; ultimately results in blindness.
(inorganic)	Fine tremor of hands and fingers followed by eyelids, tongue, cheeks, head, and legs. Extreme irritability, muscle weakness and brisk stretch reflexes. Personality changes occur. Occasional patients have deposition of brown pigment in the anterior lenticular capsule.
Thallium	Most common sign is alopecia. Several days following ingestion, paresthesias of feet and legs. May complain of joint pain with numbness of fingers and toes. Impaired sensation in all modalities. Distal weakness, but stretch reflexes generally preserved. Other findings include psychosis, ataxia, choreoathetosis, tremor, cranial nerve palsies, convulsions, and death.

Herpes zoster can affect other peripheral nerves resulting in pain and weakness in the distribution of the involved nerves. This neuropathy results from activation of a latent virus and has been seen following spinal cord injury, lymphomas, or leukemia.

Herpes simplex has also been shown to cause peripheral nerve impairment in some patients with recurrent herpes infection. Pain always precedes the eruption. Usually, the pain begins 24 hours before the cutaneous rash and disappears soon thereafter. On occasion, pain occurs earlier and persists longer until the vesicles begin to break. The distribution of pain may not conform to dermatomes or myotomes, but there is a general correlation. It is important to distinguish whether the neuropathy is secondary to herpes zoster or herpes simplex. In herpes zoster infections the neuropathy is not recurrent and is almost always unilateral. Manifestations of herpes simplex infection are recurrent and usually bilateral. There is no universally accepted treatment, although a variety of analgesics have been used empirically.

Transient paralyses of other cranial nerves occurring as an isolated finding have been described in children following nonspecific infections. The abducens, glossopharyngeal, and vagus nerves have been reported with symptoms persisting weeks to months and gradually resolving. This diagnosis is one of exclusion and one must be particularly cautious that some other specific pathologic lesion is not overlooked.

TRAUMATIC NEUROPATHY

Congenital brachial plexus palsy About 80% of patients have lesions involving the C5-C6 roots which usually result from traction on the shoulder during the delivery of the head in a difficult cephalic or breech presentation. Commonly the infant birth-weight is high. About 90% of congenital brachial plexus injuries are unilateral in which the right side is affected more often than left.

The problem is usually apparent at birth for the arm is adducted and internally rotated at the shoulder, with extension and pronation at the elbow. If muscles innervated by C7 root are affected, the ulnar wrist extensors, thumb, and finger extensors are weak. If the entire brachial plexus is involved, the arm hangs limply to the side without movement and the hand is dry. Sensory loss does not correspond to the extent of motor involvement. If the C4 root is injured, there is paralysis of the diaphragm and the infant may have respiratory distress, tachypnea, cyanosis, and decreased movement of that hemithorax.

Only a small percentage of all patients have the lower plexus root affected with weakness of intrinsic muscles of hands, and flexors of the wrist and fingers. A unilateral Horner's syndrome may be present resulting from injury to cervical sympathetic nerves. This may cause delay, or failure, of pigmentation of iris.

The Moro reflex is asymmetrical and there is an absence of reflex and voluntary movement of the involved limb. Fractures of the clavicle and humerus should be ruled out by radiography.

In severe avulsion injuries the CSF is bloody. Myelography may be of assistance in demonstrating the root avulsion. EMG can be performed after several weeks to document the extent of denervation. The affected limb and shoulder should be carefully handled. The arm should be placed in its natural position by pinning the sleeve of the night shirt; the wrist should be supported with a splint. Gentle physical therapy can be started about 1 week after birth. About 30% of patients recover by 6 months with minimal residual weakness, 55% have fair recovery by 12 months and 15% have severe residual weakness.

NEUROPATHIES ASSOCIATED WITH TUMORS

Neoplasia in childhood may have an associated neuropathy, the most notable of which is neurofibromatosis. Leukemia (lymphomas) are also exemplary, for as the mortality of these diseases has decreased, morbidity has increased, and signs of CNS involvement are more common including meningeal leukemia, focal infiltration of leukemic cells throughout the CNS, and leukemic infiltration of cranial and peripheral nerves. Patients may have sensory and/or motor findings with weakness and loss of stretch reflexes. It is important to separate the neurological complications of anti-leukemic drugs from the signs of leukemic infiltration of both central and peripheral nervous systems.

Hodgkin's disease also affects the central and peripheral nervous systems and can be associated with polyneuropathy similar to that of Guillain-Barre syndrome. The presence of neurologic findings often indicates the disease may undergo rapid progression.

NEUROPATHY ASSOCIATED WITH VASCULAR DISEASE

The connective tissue (vascular) diseases are sometimes accompanied by a polyneuropathy which is usually asymmetrical and sensorimotor. Diseases included in this category are dermatomyositis, lupus erythematosus, polyarteritis nodosa, rheumatoid arthritis, and scleroderma. The lesions are caused by abnormalities (angiitis) of small nutrient vessels of the peripheral nerve.

DISORDERS OF THE MYONEURAL JUNCTION

Myasthenia gravis is a chronic disease characterized by fluctuating weakness of skeletal muscles. It occurs at any age and affects both sexes, although it is more common in females. It has occurred in several family members and has been reported in twins. Children comprise about 1% of all patients. There are three clinical forms of myasthenia gravis in chilhood: neonatal, congenital, and juvenile.

NEONATAL MYASTHENIA GRAVIS

About 10-15% of mothers with this disease have offspring similarly, though transiently, affected. There is no relationship between the severity of the mother's illness and the severity of her myasthenic infant. Symptoms include ptosis, feeble cry and a faltering suck, and occur at any time during the first several days of life. Infants are generally weak and their movements are reduced. There is usually no impairment of pulmonary function.

Attention must be directed to the efficiency of the patient's suck; swallow, and pulmonary function should be carefully observed. Usually anticholinesterase drugs are not required; however, there is good symptom response to these drugs if needed. Symptoms subside within 3-5 weeks.

CONGENITAL MYASTHENIA GRAVIS

The congenital form is uncommon, occurring in infants of mothers who do not have the disease. There is a tendency for familial occurrence in other siblings. Symptoms may occur on the first day of life and are similar, though less marked, to those of the neonatal form; with ptosis, faltering suck, feeble cry, and generalized weakness.

Because the symptoms are usually mild, the diagnosis may not be made for 1 or 2 years. Mothers often note spontaneously, though in retrospect, that the child had decreased in-utero activity and a weak suck compared to her other children. A small number of these patients will have spontaneous remission, but most will have the disease throughout their lives.

JUVENILE MYASTHENIA GRAVIS

Signs and symptoms of this form of disease are similar to the adult variety; however, females are affected up to six times more frequently than males. The adult female is affected three times more often than male until the fifth decade when the sex incidence is about the same. Onset of symptoms is insidious or subacute and may follow a febrile illness.

Ptosis and external ophthalmoplegia are the most common signs, but other bulbar symptoms can occur and generalized weakness is common. Though generally worse at day's end, muscle weakness fluctuates unpredictably. The patient may have unilateral ptosis on one occasion, only to return with ptosis of the other lid or both lids. The ptosis may clear and other muscles can be involved. There is a wide spectrum of symptoms, ranging from those with mild ptosis to others with severe weakness requiring ventilatory assistance. Partial or complete remission occurs in about 25% of patients, usually within the first 2 years after onset. Muscle atrophy is seen rarely and only in severe cases. Despite the unpredictably fluctuating weakness and hypotonia, stretch reflexes are normal. If muscle tendons are repeatedly percussed, the reflexes will dampen and finally disappear.

About 5% of patients have evidence of hyperthyroidism at some time during the course of their illness. Symptoms may occur, however, when patients are hypothyroid or euthyroid. The explanation for this association is obscure.

MYASTHENIC SYNDROME

The myasthenic syndrome is associated with a congenital syndrome of end-plate acetylcholinesterase deficiency, small nerve terminals and reduced acetylcholine release, lupus erythematosus, rheumatoid arthritis, acute leukemia, administration of trimethadione and a variety of antibiotics including neomycin, streptomycin, kanamycin, polymyxin, bacitracin dihydrostreptomycin, colistin and with combinations thereof. The myasthenic syndrome has also been reported following a bee sting.

DIAGNOSIS OF MYASTHENIA GRAVIS

It is important to distinguish myasthenia gravis from the myasthenic syndrome secondary to a variety of etiologies. This should not be a major problem if the typical clinical features are present and the patient has no history or evidence of preceding or concomitant illness known to be associated with myasthenia gravis, and has received none of the medications known to be associated with the myasthenic syndrome. Some patients with dermatomyositis or polymyositis have had symptomatic improvement following administration of anticholinesterase drugs.

The **diagnostic test** for this disease is the administration of a short-acting anticholinesterase; namely, edrophonium chloride (Tensilon). Appropriate personnel and equipment must be available before the test is carried out. Dosage for infants is 0.15 mg/kg, IV; and for children 0.2 mg/kg, IV. Subcutaneous or IM administration of edrophonium chloride is generally not as satisfactory.

After the IV administration of edrophonium chloride, muscle weakness decreases within several minutes and the beneficial effect of the drug persists about 5 minutes. The administration of neostigmine is occasionally used with less pleasant effects. Curare testing is not recommended unless experienced personnel and equipment are readily available.

Electrophysiological abnormalities typical of this disease are obttained by stimulating a motor nerve, recording the evoked potentials from the contracting muscle. The amplitude provides an indication of the number of fibers activated. There is a variable decrement, depending upon the technique used, to repetitive supramaximal stimulation. A decrease of 7% is usually considered abnormal.

The **muscle biopsy** of these patients is not particularly notable. Fibers are generally small and there appears to be focal atrophy of type II fibers; atrophy of type I fibers is occasionally seen. In some cases, there is necrosis of muscle fibers and lymphorrhages are seen. Thymomas occur in 10% of the adult population, but not in childhood.

BOTULISM

The heat-labile neurotoxin of *Clostridium botulinum*, a gram-negative spore-bearing anaerobic bacillus, produces symptoms either by ingestion of inadequately canned or prepared foods, or wound infection by the organism which then elaborates the toxin. Symptoms appear within several hours to a few days following the introduction of the toxin, usually beginning with nausea, vomiting, or diarrhea. Neurologic symptoms include cranial nerve dysfunction and generalized weakness manifested by blurred or double vision, vertigo, dysphagia and/or dysphonia. Swallowing may be significantly impaired, dyspnea may occur and some patients have associated generalized weakness.

Patients are often alert but may seem lethargic. Pupils are dilated and are either fixed or react sluggishly to light. Other cranial nerves may be impaired. Generalized weakness becomes apparent with stretch reflexes that are initially normal but later in the course of the disease become depressed. The sensory system is normal.

A syndrome of **infant botulism,** first identified in 1976, apparently results from in-vivo germination of *C botulinum* spores within the infant gut, producing botulinum toxin. Over a period of hours to several days, infant patients become remarkably hypotonic, have a poor suck, swallow, and a feeble cry. They may have ptosis, external ophthalmoplegia, and facial weakness; most patients are somewhat listless.

Electrophysiologic studies greatly assist in establishing the diagnosis. The motor nerve conduction velocities are normal; however, needle electrode examination demonstrates abundant, low-amplitude, brief action potentials. Repetitive nerve stimulation, in moderate to severely affected patients, shows a decremental response at low-frequency stimulation.

Both types A and B toxin have been implicated. In adult patients, toxin may be demonstrable from the patient's blood; toxin may also be isolated from the suspected contaminated food source or from the infected wound. In cases of infant botulism, the toxin is best identified in stool specimens.

Treatment is directed to general supportive measures and particularly to meticulous respiratory support. Ventilatory support may be required for several months. There is no specific therapy known to be of value at this time.

PRIMARY DISEASES OF MUSCLE

A **myopathy** is any primary disease of muscle, whether the abnormality is structural, electrophysiological, or biochemical and in which there is no related neurological abnormality. A **muscular dystrophy** is a genetically determined primary disease of muscle characterized by muscle fiber degeneration. The hallmark of muscle disease is weakness.

DUCHENNE'S MUSCULAR DYSTROPHY

This malignant form of muscular dystrophy is inherited as an x-linked recessive trait and is expressed almost entirely in males, and occurs sporadically in about one third of patients. Rarely, females who have chromosomal abnormalities have been reported with typical clinical findings of this disease.

The patient appears normal until he begins to walk or run; there may be a delay in walking unaided. Parents become aware the child is clumsy, falls easily, and has a waddling gait. He has difficulty rising from the floor and ultimately 'climbs up' his legs (Gower's sign); he is inordinately lordotic, often walks on his toes, and has difficulty climbing stairs. Commonly, at day's end, the child complains of leg or calf pain. Symptoms are usually apparent by the age of 3 or 4 years. If a second child of the same parents is similarly affected, the parents identify muscle weakness earlier.

There is often an enlargement of the posterior compartment of the calf; less commonly other muscles are enlarged, including the quadriceps, deltoid, or infraspinatus. Muscles feel 'doughey' or 'rubbery' on palpation. Early in the course of the disease, weakness of upper limbs is usually mild. Weakness is generally symmetrical and proximal muscles are more severely affected than distal. Stretch reflexes are decreased to absent, except for the ankle jerks which may persist until the disease is well advanced.

There is progressive loss of muscle power and most patients are confined to wheelchair by early adolescence. Periods of immobilization seem to hasten the patient's inability to walk, and when confined to a wheelchair, the hips, knees, and particularly the heel cords are vulnerable to contracture. Shoulders and elbows are sometimes affected by contractures and kyphoscoliosis may become apparent.

With further progression of weakness, there is decreased facial movement and poor head control. Chest deformities impair pulmonary function and patients are subject to recurring pulmonary infection. Many children become obese but a small number remains rather thin. An inordinate number of patients are mentally dull, and chronic depression is common. Most patients do not survive beyond the age of 20 years, although some have survived to the third decade.

Rarely does one find such marked elevation of serum CPK as in Duchenne's dystrophy. The enzyme may be significantly elevated in early life before there is clinical evidence of weakness. Serum levels of the enzyme appear to parallel the loss of muscle bulk and as the disease progresses there is a decline in the level of CPK. Other enzymes, including aldolase, lactic dehydrogenase, glutamic oxaloacetic transaminase, and glutamic pyruvate transaminase are also increased, but to a lesser degree. Cardiac muscle is abnormal in about 80% of patients and arrhythmias are sometimes noted. The most consistent ECG findings include tall, right precordial R waves and deep Q waves in the limb and precordial leads.

There is no specific **treatment** for Duchenne's dystrophy and one must provide vigorous supportive care with particular attention directed to pulmonary function. **Physical therapy** is most important and early in the disease should be directed to prevention of heel cord contractures. When it is apparent that heel cord stretching is no longer of value, surgical lengthening of the Achilles tendon can be done, preferably under local anesthesia. Following surgery the patient should be ambulatory as quickly as possible, at least within several days. Surgical release of hip contractures should also be considered and long leg braces may prolong the patient's ambulation for several years. As always, one cannot separate the child from the family; it is of great usefulness to have the family involved in some common sense counseling program.

Because of the known x-linked recessive inheritance of Duchenne's muscular dystrophy, questions regarding carrier detection must be explained carefully to the family. It is important to screen the female members of the family to identify carriers.

Determination of serum CPK is the most reliable **screening test** available. Determinations of serum CPK should be done at weekly intervals for 3 or 4 weeks, and if any one value is abnormally high, it is presumed that person is a carrier. If all enzyme levels are normal, however, there is still a 20% chance that person may yet be a carrier. There is no enzyme assay of value in prenatal detection of this disease; however, prenatal sex determination can be carried out if parents desire abortion of a male fetus.

BECKER TYPE MUSCULAR DYSTROPHY

This type of muscular dystrophy is relatively benign, although similar in clinical presentation to Duchenne's dystrophy. Symptoms of muscle weakness are usually apparent by the second decade, but progression of weakness is slower.

Patients develop similar weakness of the hips and later the shoulder girdle, and may have a tendency to walk on their toes. Some have muscle compartment enlargement as in Duchenne's dystrophy. The time of onset, as well as the time course, is delayed and patients remain ambulatory for several decades, and commonly survive until mid-adult life.

There is less likelihood of developing joint contractures or kyphoscoliosis and the incidence of mental subnormality is less. Serum CPK may be moderately increased and the ECG is often similar to patients with Duchenne's dystrophy.

Carrier detection of this type of muscular dystrophy is less reliable than in Duchenne's dystrophy for only about one half of carriers will have abnormal elevations of serum CPK. There is sufficient genetic evidence to separate this benign type (Becker) from the malignant variety of the disease (Duchenne's).

FACIOSCAPULOHUMERAL MUSCULAR DYSTROPHY

This disease is inherited as an autosomal dominant trait. Onset of symptoms is insidious, commonly beginning in the second decade, though signs and symptoms are sometimes present in the first. Patients realize they have difficulty in whistling, inflating a balloon, or sipping a straw, but think little about the matter until attention is directed to their scapular winging. When initially evaluated, there is wasting and weakness of facial muscles, shoulder girdle, and proximal muscles of the arms. Progression of signs and symptoms is usually slow. Ultimately there is weakness of the anterolateral compartment of the lower limbs and foot drop; the pelvic girdle is often weak.

The spectrum of clinical findings ranges from mild facial weakness which may be unrecognized, to those with severe muscle wasting and weakness. Some patients compensate so well for their decreased strength, they are surprised when it is discovered on examination. This is important to acknowledge when obtaining a family history of others who may have muscle weakness.

There is decreased bulk of facial muscles and a paucity of facial movement. The orbicularis oris and zygomaticus are weak and often there is pursing of the lips referred to as 'tapir mouth' or 'bouche de tapir.' Neck muscles, shoulder girdle, and proximal arms are wasted and weak and the shoulders may droop. The deltoid muscles, surprisingly, retain good power.

Muscle pseudohypertrophy is uncommon, but may occur in the deltoid or calf muscles. Some patients have a remarkable asymmetry of limbs. The scapulae are not stabilized by normal musculature and attempts to abduct the arm result in scapular winging. Weakness of the pelvic girdle may pass unnoticed until the patient is examined. Commonly, patients are quite lordotic; the posterior calf muscles remain more powerful than the antero-lateral muscles and the patient may have a footdrop. Stretch reflexes are reduced to absent.

If symptoms are present in early childhood, the clinical course is usually more severe. Facial weakness may be so marked the child is unable to close the eyelids or mouth. Muscle wasting and weakness of the limbs and trunk is also marked and the child may be confined to a bed or a wheelchair during the first decade. Often these children have severe lordo-sis or a 'poker' back appearance.

Serum CPK may be normal or mildly elevated. Cardiac abnormali-ties are not typically seen in this disease, and intelligence is generally within the normal range.

Most patients have a relatively benign course, but they should be carefully followed on a long-term basis. Those few patients with marked difficulty in elevation of arms, but in whom the disease course is relatively static may benefit from orthopedic procedures which fixate the scapulae. These patients must be carefully selected.

SCAPULOPERONEAL MUSCULAR DYSTROPHY

There are reports of patients with muscle wasting and weakness primarily affecting the scapular and anterolateral calf muscles. Less commonly, other muscles are affected. Symptoms are mild and become apparent be-tween the second and fourth decades. Reports are controversial and pa-tients have been described with physical findings, muscle biopsy, and EMG characteristics consistent with a myopathic process; whereas, other pa-tients have findings consistent with neurogenic disease. One must use care when attaching this diagnostic label. There has been no consistent pattern of inheritance identified although more patients are reported as autosomal recessive trait.

MYOTONIC DYSTROPHY

This disease, inherited as an autosomal dominant trait, affects patients of all ages and is characterized by muscle wasting, weakness, and myotonia. It is common for the diagnosis to be unrecognized for decades with patients knowing they have 'a little stiffness,' but making no complaint, often be-cause other family members are similarly affected.

The disease affects other tissues including the optic lens, testes and other endocrine tissues, and bone. The muscles involved include the leva-tor palpebrae, facial, temporalis, masseter, and sternocleidomastoid. There is often 'hollowing' of the temporal fossae, ptosis, and patients have a 'swan neck' appearance. Muscles of the forearm, hand, and anterolateral muscles of the lower limbs are commonly affected. Distal weakness is greater than proximal. As the disease progresses there is a generalized weakness and palatal/pharyngeal weakness results in a nasal voice. There is often a narrow high-arched palate. There may be extraocular involvement as manifested by tightly closing the eyelids followed by lid relaxation. The eyes remain in upward deviation for several seconds after the eyes are opened.

The physical appearance of patients is striking and mental subnormality is common. Cataracts are frequent and examination by slit lamp will best demonstrate the irridescent lenticular subcapsular dots (both anterior and posterior) in most affected children and virtually all adults. Cardiac abnormalities may be present including conduction abnormalities and arrhythmias; the ECG may show prolongation of the PR interval. Characteristically, the male has progressive frontal balding and testicular atrophy, and though he may be impotent is not necessarily infertile. Females often have menstrual irregularities, but fertility is only slightly diminished. The prevalence of clinical diabetes is only slightly increased, but increased insulin response to glucose load is common. Skull abnormalities include hyperostosis of the cranial vault, small sella turcica, and enlarged paranasal sinuses.

There is no known specific treatment for the muscle wasting and weakness. Some patients have noted a lessening of myotonia following administration of procainamide, quinine, or phenytoin, but there is no universally recognized improvement with these drugs. Weakness and dementia are more serious problems than myotonia.

CONGENITAL MYOTONIC DYSTROPHY

This condition occurs when one parent, almost invariably the mother (89%) is affected. There is often a maternal history of hydramnios. The infant is usually hypotonic at birth, has facial diplegia, impaired sucking and swallowing. Most, if not all patients, have contractures of one or more joints; some have diaphragmatic hypoplasia. The lack of facial movement, poor suck and swallow, and feeble cry may erroneously lead one to consider diagnoses such as Mobius syndrome, spinal muscular atrophy, congenital myopathies, or severe myasthenia gravis.

If airway and nutritional problems can be managed satisfactorily during the first several months of life, there is usually significant improvement in swallowing and pulmonary function. As the child grows, the commonly recognized features of myotonic dystrophy become apparent with expressionless face, open mouth and 'tenting' of the upper lip. Myotonia may first be apparent in the latter part of the first decade.

Serum CPK is of little diagnostic value and may be normal or only mildly elevated.

LIMB - GIRDLE MUSCULAR DYSTROPHY

This form of muscular dystrophy is uncommon. Weakness is apparent during the second or third decades and either pelvic or shoulder girdle is first affected. Usually, however, the hip flexors and extensors are the first to become weak and mildly atrophic; muscles of the posterior compartment of the calves are enlarged. Gradually, the anterolateral leg muscles become weak.

The shoulder girdle is affected any time during the next 10-15 years with sagging of shoulders and weakness of neck flexors and extensors. Proximal arm muscles are also weak, but there is no sparing of the deltoids as seen in facioscapulohumeral muscular dystrophy. Localized areas of muscular wasting are noted in the biceps or quadriceps resulting in a 'scalloped effect.' Facial weakness, if present is mild. The stretch reflexes are decreased. There is no notable intellectual impairment.

Because of the lack of specificity of this disease category, one must be particularly careful not to overlook some other myopathic process. Limb-girdle muscular dystrophy is an autosomal recessive trait in about 60% of cases; the remainder are sporadic.

OCULAR MUSCULAR DYSTROPHY

An uncommon condition characterized by ptosis that is usually apparent in the second or third decades, but may appear earlier. It is slowly progressive, and extraocular muscles are often involved; pupils remain unaffected. Patients usually do not complain of diplopia, but often tilt their head backwards or wrinkle their forehead to compensate for the ptosis. Ultimately other muscles may be involved, particularly those of the face, and some patients have weakness of the limbs. Reflexes are often depressed to absent.

Some patients have an unusual sensitivity to curare which in small doses may produce marked ptosis or external ophthalmoplegia, as well as increased weakness of the neck and limb muscles. This disease is inherited as an autosomal dominant trait.

Treatment is individualized. Some patients have found it useful to wear superior eyelid crutches attached to their spectacles; others have preferred surgical correction of the ptosis. The unusual response to curare must be emphasized in those patients who have a surgical procedure with anesthesia.

OCULOPHARYNGEAL MUSCULAR DYSTROPHY

This condition is inherited as an autosomal dominant trait, although sporadic cases occur. It is primarily seen in the adult population with symptoms starting in the third or fourth decade. Most patients are of French-Canadian stock, but an increased incidence of the disease has been found in the southwestern part of the USA. There is progressive ocular ptosis and dysphagia; some patients have weakness of external eye muscles, as well as facial and masseter muscles. Occasionally, there is decreased strength in proximal limb muscles. The combination of these neurological findings and a similar family history should present no problem in making the appropriate diagnosis. One should be cautious in attaching this diagnostic label to child patients.

DISTAL MUSCULAR DYSTROPHY

This very rare form of dystrophy is inherited as an autosomal dominant trait. Weakness of distal muscles can be present by 2 years of age and bilateral foot drop and weakness of hands and forearms are evident during early childhood. There appears to be no progression of symptoms after 18 years of age.

Serum CPK levels are normal; EMG and muscle biopsy are characteristic of a myopathic process. This disease is different from other muscular

Table 5-8 Congenital Myopathies

Disease	Clinical features	Muscle biopsy
Central core disease	Hypotonia noted at birth or shortly thereafter; motor development delayed. Diffuse weakness, primarily proximal; stretch reflexes normal to reduced. Skeletal abnormalities may occur (hip dislocation, kyphoscoliosis, lordosis, pes cavus). Inherited as autosomal dominant trait, but sporadic cases occur. Serum CPK usually normal; EMG findings nonspecific. Malignant hyperthermia known to occur.	Variability of fiber diameter, often with predominance of type I fibers. Within the fiber, centrally or peripherally, are cores devoid of oxidative enzyme activity. Myofibrillary ATPase activity of cores normal to decreased.
Myotubular myopathy (centronuclear)	Hypotonic at birth with ptosis, external ophthalmoplegia and occasionally facial weakness. Decreased muscle power throughout, greater distally than proximally. Neonatal type described with profound weakness at birth (may die in infancy). Inheritance reported as usually x-linked recessive, but autosomal dominant and recessive traits reported. Serum CPK normal to moderately increased. EMG nonspecific.	Predominance of type I fibers with central nuclei surrounded by clear area. Type I atrophy has been recorded. Increased central staining with oxidative enzymes and pale central area with ATPase reactions.
Congenital fiber type disproportion	Hypotonia and generalized weakness present at birth. Muscle contractures are often present with skeletal abnormalities (high arched palate, congenital hip dislocation, kyphoscoliosis, varus or valgus foot deformities). Rarely, external ophthalmoplegia occurs. Commonly, clinical status remains static or improves.	Type I fibers are more numerous and smaller than type II fibers.
Mitochondrial myopathies	Heterogeneous group of diseases with normal as well as abnormally shaped and enlarged mitochondria within muscle fibers. Symptoms usually begin in childhood but may appear at any time. External ocular muscle weakness a frequent finding. Excessive muscular fatigue following exercise is common. Inheritance is variable. Structural changes of muscle are nonspecific and have been reported in a variety of disorders (hypothyroidism, polymyositis, thyrotoxic myopathy, and spinal muscular atrophy).	Mitochondrial abnormalities suspected on light microscopy by accumulation of subsarcolemmal or intramyofibrillary granules which are irregular and stain red with modified trichrome stain — 'ragged red fibers.'

117

Multicore disease	Several patients described with nonprogressive generalized hypotonia and weakness of trunk and limb muscles, proximal greater than distal. Stretch reflexes are decreased. Serum CPK is normal; EMG demonstrates short duration motor unit potentials or normal findings.	Predominance of type I fibers and numerous small randomly distributed areas of types I and II, with focal decreased oxidative enzyme activity and focal myofibrillary degeneration.
Nemaline myopathy	Hypotonia at birth; some mothers indicate decreased fetal movement. Poor suck, swallow, and respiratory embarrassment; delay in achieving milestones. Elongated face with narrow high arched palate, prognathism, dental malocclusion and pigeon chest. Stretch reflexes reduced to absent. Inherited as autosomal recessive or dominant traits; sporadic cases known to occur. Serum CPK normal to mildly increased. EMG demonstrates brief low amplitude abundant polyphasic motor potentials.	Usually a predominance of type I fibers; about half of type I fibers are small. Subsarcolemmal collection of ('nemaline') rods seen with vesicular nuclei and prominent nucleoli.
Trilaminar neuromuscular disease	Very rare congenital neuromuscular disease with muscular rigidity at birth. Muscles are hard on palpation. Stretch reflexes are normal. CPK in early infancy reported as markedly increased, but decreases near end of 1st year. EMG has been normal.	About 15% of fibers demonstrate 3 concentric zones of differential staining (trilaminar fibers).. At EM, a sharp delineation is demonstrated between the outer and middle zones, but junction is not defined by membrane.
Reducing body myopathy	Profound hypotonia with decreased muscle bulk, generalized weakness, and stretch reflexes depressed to absent. Milestones delayed. Serum CPK normal to mildly elevated. EMG demonstrated myopathic potentials.	Variability of fiber size with predominance of type I fibers. Large numbers of fibers contain 'reducing bodies' rich in sulphydryl groups and RNA.
Fingerprint body myopathy	Hypotonia and generalized weakness, usually with sparing of external ocular and bulbar muscles. Stretch reflexes reduced to absent. Muscle bulk reduced. Serum CPK normal to mildly elevated and EMG studies have varied from normal to 'consistent with myopathy.'	Small type I fibers and hypertrophied type II fibers. EM demonstrates inclusions composed of concentric lamellae resembling fingerprints. Similar structures also found in dermatomyositis, myotonic dystrophy, and oculopharyngeal muscular dystrophy.
Sarcotubular myopathy	One case report of two brothers whose parents were 3rd cousins. Patients were clumsy and had mild weakness of proximal limb muscles and neck flexors. Stretch reflexes were normal to mildly decreased. Serum CPK normal to mildly elevated.	Vacuolar changes seen selectively affecting type II fibers. A 'myriad' of small spaces were seen on cross-section in affected muscles and in longitudinal section; vacuolization was segmental.

dystrophies because of the distal distribution of weakness and wasting compared to the usual proximal involvement.

CONGENITAL MUSCULAR DYSTROPHY

This diagnostic label has been applied to infant patients who are hypotonic at birth and have weakness of limbs, trunk, and facial muscles and in whom muscle biopsies demonstrate changes consistent with muscular dystrophy. A wide spectrum of clinical reports has been included under this heading and one must be cautious in making the diagnosis.

Often patients have difficulty sucking and swallowing. Contractures affecting different muscles are common and may be progressive. The decrease in muscle power tends to be static; the stretch reflexes are decreased to absent. Sensation is normal. Developmental milestones are delayed and mental function is probably normal.

Serum CPK is normal to moderately increased. EMG usually has findings consistent with a myopathic process. The muscle biopsy is usually striking, with typical features of muscular dystrophy. Since the course is relatively mild, vigorous physical therapy should be adopted and the use of orthopedic appliances, such as night splints or plaster casts considered.

CONGENITAL MYOPATHIES

These conditions are apparent at birth or soon after, and are characterized by weakness and usually hypotonia. There is no evidence of recognized central or peripheral nervous system abnormality. Microscopic structural changes of muscle are demonstrated, after which the diseases have been named (see Table 5-8). It is unclear whether the pathological changes reflect a primary muscle disease or some other pathological process. Associated skeletal abnormalities are sometimes seen, including an elongation of facial features, narrow high palate, hip dislocation, lordosis, kyphoscoliosis, and pes cavus.

Muscle weakness is usually more marked proximally than distally; there may be a paucity of muscle bulk and stretch reflexes are normal to decreased. The serum CPK is commonly normal to mildly increased. EMG studies may be normal, but often demonstrate short duration, low amplitude polyphasic motor unit potentials.

THE MYOTONIC DISORDERS

Myotonia is the prolonged contraction of skeletal muscles following stimulation, either electrically or by percussion, and the delay in relaxation after voluntary muscular contraction.

MYOTONIA CONGENITA

Although this disease is characterized by myotonia, patients usually complain of muscle 'stiffness' or that they 'can't get going.' There are two recognized disease types; one is inherited as an autosomal dominant trait, and the other an autosomal recessive trait. The **dominant type, or Thomsen's disease,** is less common. Symptoms are usually mild and may be identified only in retrospect. Some children have feeding difficulties and delayed development, but show no progression in severity of myotonia. Often they have difficulty relaxing muscle contraction, but with repetiion of movement there is less difficulty as if they 'loosen up.' Both sexes are equally involved.

In the **recessive (Becker) type,** males are affected more frequently than females. Patients are aware of muscle stiffness at 5 or 6 years of age. They may appear clumsy during initiation of movement, but with continued movement appear normal and may even run.

All skeletal muscles are affected by myotonia, but this is most notable in limbs. The face and tongue may also be affected. Myotonia is exaggerated after exposure to cold or emotional stress. The stretch reflexes are normal. Muscles often appear hypertrophic and, indeed, some patients have such muscular development they have been called 'infant Hercules.' These patients should be distinguished from the rare form of hypothyroidism associated with muscle hypertrophy (Debre-Semelaigne syndrome).

Serum CPK is normal. Electrodiagnostic studies demonstrate typical myotonic discharges which are evoked by electrode movement, by percussion, or voluntary contraction of those muscles being examined.

There is no uniformly beneficial treatment for myotonia congenita. Phenytoin, procainamide, and quinine have been used and some patients have experienced improvement for short periods of time.

PARAMYOTONIA CONGENITA

This disease, inherited as an autosomal dominant trait, is characterized by myotonia following exposure to cold. Patients may also have episodic weakness following exposure to low temperature or after muscle exercise. Symptoms begin in childhood and are believed not to be progressive. Aside from percussion myotonia, the neurological examination is normal between attacks. If examined while weak, stretch reflexes may be decreased. There is no muscle atrophy and no sensory defects have been discerned.

Serum CPK is normal and electrodiagnostic studies demonstrate findings of myotonia. It has been suggested that paramyotonia congenita and familial hyperkalemic periodic paralysis are the same disease; this view has not been confirmed.

MYOTONIC CHONDRODYSTROPHY (Schwartz-Jampel Syndrome)

This rare disease is characterized by severe generalized myotonia, muscular hypertrophy, dwarfism, and unusual facies with blepharospasm and pursed lips. Bone and joint abnormalities are present, including kyphoscoliosis and deformities of the ribs and sternum.

There is some progression with restriction of joint mobility. EMG demonstrates continuous muscle high-frequency potentials and no electrical silence at rest, general anesthesia, or following administration of curare. Malignant hyperthermia has been associated with this syndrome. It is inherited as an autosomal recessive trait.

INFLAMMATORY DISEASES OF MUSCLE

Muscle is no less a victim of infection than other tissues. Inflammation of muscle is generally considered as those conditions in which the etiology is known compared with those of unknown etiology. Commonly recognized infectious agents including bacterial, viral, fungal, and parasitic may cause myositis.

MYOSITIS OF KNOWN ETIOLOGY

Bacterial infections of muscle are usually the result of extension of a local infectious process but may result from direct contamination of a traumatic wound. Infections caused by hematogenous spread are relatively uncommon.

Fungal infections usually follow a traumatic wound and include actinomyces sp. blastomycosis, or nocardia. Parasitic infections are uncommon in the USA but may be caused by a variety of tapeworms including *Trichinella spiralis*, *Taenia solium*, echinococcosis, and toxoplasmosis.

Viral agents as a cause of myositis are less readily identified. The syndrome of acute myositis, secondary to influenza types A and B, is characterized in children by an acute or subacute tenderness and pain in the gastrocnemius and soleus muscles. Serum CPK is generally moderately elevated. The process may last for days to several months. There is no specific treatment aside from rest.

MYOSITIS OF UNKNOWN ETIOLOGY

Polymyositis is an inflammation and degeneration of skeletal muscle and in the presence of 'typical' skin rash is called dermatomyositis. The combination of acute or subacute muscle weakness associated with the skin rash makes the diagnosis of dermatomyositis highly probable. Polymyositis is less common than dermatomyositis in childhood.

The disease may occur at any time from infancy to adulthood. The onset of weakness is usually subacute but often may continue unrecognized for weeks to months. The hallmark of the disease is weakness, usually with proximal muscles affected more than distal, and there is often a predilection for involving anterior neck muscles. Facial weakness is relatively uncommon but dysphagia is often a prominent symptom.

The skin rash of dermatomyositis is characterized by a violaceous hue (heliotrope) of the eyelids, commonly associated with lid edema. The typical skin rash is erythematous and scaly, found particularly over the extensor surfaces of the metacarpophalangeal and interphalangeal joints. The same kind of rash may be present on the elbows, knees, and sometimes the malleoli.

Subcutaneous calcification may be palpable and sometimes extends through the skin's surface; some calcifications must be removed surgically. Presence of calcification usually suggests the acute inflammatory process is waning. Other findings often include lymphadenopathy, splenomegally, and Raynaud's phenomenon.

Diagnosis The presence of this kind of muscle weakness, particularly when associated with the described skin rash, generally makes the diagnosis highly probable. The serum CPK is significantly elevated and the most useful enzyme to follow the cause of the disease's activity. Other enzymes including aldolase, SGOT, SGPT, and LDH are commonly elevated but are usually of less value in following the patient.

The EMG is useful in establishing the diagnosis, and is characterized by low amplitude polyphasic potentials sometimes associated with repetitive discharges.

The muscle biopsy is notable for abnormal variability of fiber diameter, central nuclei that are commonly vesicular, and the presence of basophilic fibers. Necrosis is commonly seen with typical inflammatory changes. It must be remembered that the biopsy of at least one-third of patients demonstrate no inflammatory changes.

Treatment Patients should receive prednisone at a dose of 1-2 mg/kg/day and continued until the patient has symptomatic improvement and the serum enzymes have returned to normal or nearly normal. There is some evidence to suggest that the sooner the medication is started after symptom onset, the better is the outlook.

Steroids should be only gradually reduced to the lowest dosage level which enables the patient to have a functional life. Exacerbations and remissions are known to occur. Some patients have little response to steroid administration and methotrexate, an immunosuppressive agent, has been administered. No conclusions can be made regarding its efficacy at this time because clinical experience with the drug in these circumstances is limited.

Active physical therapy throughout the course of the disease is required.

REFERENCES

Brooke MH: *A Clinician's View of Neuromuscular Disorders.* Williams and Wilkins, Baltimore, 1977.

Dubowitz V, Brooke MH: *Muscle Biopsy: A Modern Approach.* Saunders, Philadelphia, 1973

Dyck PJ, Thomas PK, Lambert EH: *Peripheral Neuropathy.* Saunders, Philadelphia, 1975.

Swaiman KF, Wright FS: *Pediatric Neuromuscular Diseases.* Mosby, St. Louis, 1979.

Walton JN (Ed.): *Disorders of Voluntary Muscle,* 4th Ed. Little-Brown, Boston, 1981

6

Infections of the Nervous System

James F. Schwartz, MD

BACTERIAL MENINGITIS

Despite advances in antimicrobial therapy, an increased incidence of bacterial meningitis, the most common serious CNS infection in childhood, has been documented over the past three decades. *Haemophilus influenzae* type b, *Streptococcus pneumoniae*, and *Neisseria meningitidis* are the etiologic organisms in approximately 95% of cases of bacterial meningitis in children. The Center for Disease Control, in 1972, estimated that there were approximately 29,000 cases of meningitis due to *H influenzae* type b, 4800 cases of pneumococcal meningitis, and 4600 cases of meningococcal meningitis. Ninety percent of the cases occur between 1 month and 5 years of age, with the age of greatest risk being 6-12 months. Unlike meningococcal and pneumococcal meningitis, *H influenzae* infection primarily occurs in children under 3 years of age.

Meningitis in the first month of life, most commonly caused by group B streptococci, followed by coliform bacilli, poses a particular problem with a high morbidity and mortality. The clinical signs are frequently subtle, the infections are often fulminating, and with gram-negative organisms in particular, it is difficult to achieve and maintain therapeutic levels of antibiotics within the subarachnoid space and ventricular system, so that bacteriologic relapse is not infrequent (see Table 6-1).

CLINICAL DIAGNOSIS

The diagnosis of bacterial meningitis in children over 1 year of age rarely presents any problems, except when prior antibiotic therapy has masked the clinical findings. Typical manifestations include fever, headache, vomiting, irritability, confusion and lethargy, and signs of meningeal inflammation including nuchal rigidity, and positive Kernig and Brudzinski signs. Increased intracranial pressure may be reflected by headache in older children or bulging fontanelle in infants. Focal or generalized convulsions may occur early in the course of illness, and occasionally the onset of illness may be signalled by a seizure. Since convulsions with fever may be the most prominent early manifestations of meningitis, even the experienced clinician may be unable to distinguish on the basis of physical findings between a simple febrile seizure in a child under 1 year of age and a convulsion associated with bacterial meningitis, because the young child (under 1 year) may lack the usual common clinical signs of meningeal infection, particularly early in the course of illness.

Table 6-1   Most Common Causes of Bacterial Meningitis
Related to Age

Age	Organism
Birth to 4 weeks	Group B *Streptococcus*
	Escherichia coli, other coliforms
4 to 12 weeks	Group B *Streptococcus*
	Streptococcus pneumoniae
	Salmonella species
	Listeria monocytogenes
	Hemophilus influenzae
3 months to 3 years	*H influenzae*
	Streptococcus pneumoniae
	Neisseria meningitidis
3 years to 16 years	*Streptococcus pneumoniae*
	N meningitidis
	Other rare organisms
Birth to 3 months	*Proteus mirabilis*
	Paracolon bacillus
	Pseudomonas aeruginosa
	Klebsiella - aerobacteria
	Vibrio fetus
	Serratia marscescens
3 months to 16 years	*Staphylococcus aureus*
	P mirabilis
	Herellea vaginicola
	Mima polymorphea
	Bacteroides

Diagnosis may be more difficult in the neonate, in whom the only signs of overwhelming bacterial meningitis may be sudden onset of decreased activity, decreased feeding, and hypotonia. The affected newborn may be afebrile or hypothermic; bulging fontanelle occurs in less than one-third of newborns with meningitis, and nuchal rigidity is extremely unusual in this age group. Seizures occur in approximately 40% of cases of neonatal meningitis. If the newborn or older infant or child has received antibiotic treatment early in the course of illness prior to diagnosis, the clinical picture may be confused since the classical manifestations may be modified or absent.

Laboratory diagnosis   Lumbar puncture should be performed immediately on any child with suspected meningitis. The benefits to be gained far outweigh the potential harm of the procedure; only under unusual circumstances, i.e., the presence of papilledema, a third nerve palsy, possibly decerebrate or decorticate posture which might be evidence of impending herniation, should lumbar puncture be withheld. Cerebrospinal fluid (CSF) that appears turbid or frankly purulent clearly suggests the presence of bacterial infection. If CSF pleocytosis exceeds 1000 cells/mm³ and polymorphonuclear leukocytes predominate, suspicion of bacterial meningitis is increased. CSF examination must include a count of the total number of white blood cells in a counting chamber, a differential cell count performed on a Wright's stained smear of centrifuged sediment of CSF, gram stained smears, and aerobic and anerobic cultures. Gram stained smears provide an etiologic diagnosis in up to 80% of cases, negative gram stains but positive cultures of CSF occur in 10-15% of cases of bacterial meningitis. **CSF glucose and protein determinations** are also essential. If CSF glucose is less than 40 mg/dl, or less than two-thirds of a simultaneously obtained blood glucose, and CSF protein is increased, antibiotic therapy should be started immediately, even if the cell count is low. Rarely, there may be a polymorphonuclear leukocytosis in CSF, but gram stained smear is negative and CSF glucose is normal or only slightly reduced, so that the diagnosis is uncertain. Another test of CSF which may then be indicated, especially if prior antibiotic treatment has been given, is **counter immunoelectrophoresis (CIE)**. CIE, which depends on the migration of capsular polysaccharide antigens of *H influenzae* b, meningococcus, and pneumococcus in an electrical field in the presence of specific antisera, appears to be extremely accurate in providing a rapid, etiologic diagnosis and can detect nonviable bacteria.

A repeat lumbar puncture within 8 hours after the initial tap may be of great value in permitting a clear distinction between nonbacterial and bacterial meningitis in most cases. A reduced CSF glucose concentration may also occur in nonbacterial infections including tuberculous and cryptococcal meningitis, meningitis due to mumps virus, herpes simplex virus, and meningeal neoplasm. Determination of enzymes including SGOT, LDH, and CPK has not proved to be a useful means of distinguishing bacterial and nonbacterial meningitis nor are enzyme levels useful in predicting response to treatment.

NEUROPATHOLOGY

Although bacterial meningitis is frequently thought of in simplistic terms as a disease involving only the subarachnoid space, characterized by bacteria in the CSF with reduced glucose, elevated protein, and a positive culture, the morbid process is not limited to the leptomeninges. Bacterial multiplication within the subarachnoid space can result in dissemination of bacteria over the surface of the brain and cerebellum, and into the ventricular system. Inflammatory change around leptomeningeal vessels may produce vasculitis and secondary thrombosis of small veins, sinuses, and small arteries. The result may be impaired cerebral perfusion, infarction, and necrosis. Hypoxia, shock, and impaired respiratory and cardiovascular function may cause additional cerebral parenchymal injury and brain edema. The development of abscesses within brain parenchyma as an extension of infection from the leptomeninges is uncommon with most types of bacterial meningitis. The extensive inflammatory process in the subarachnoid space may also involve cranial nerves and spinal nerve roots. Thick inflammatory exudate at the exits of the fourth ventricle, in the subarachnoid cisterns, or in the aqueduct of Sylvius may interfere with CSF circulation, producing acute or slowly progressive hydrocephalus. Mild degrees of brain swelling may merely complicate the effects of the primary inflammation, but severe brain swelling may result in caudal shift of midline structures, with resultant transtentorial or foramen magnum herniation.

NEUROLOGICAL SIGNS AND SYMPTOMS

In addition to the common signs of meningeal inflammation, alterations in level of consciousness are common, with variable degrees of **stupor or coma**. The coma may be related to the inflammatory changes in meninges and vessels, but accompanying fever, brain swelling, increased intracranial pressure, and impaired cerebral perfusion also play a role. Fluid and electrolyte disequilibrium, caused by the syndrome of inappropriate secretion of antidiuretic hormone, which commonly occurs in patients with bacterial meningitis, may also be partially responsible for altered states of consciousness as well as causing seizures.

Seizures occur in 20-30% of all cases of meningitis in childhood. They are most frequent in neonatal meningitis and are not uncommon in pneumococcal or *H influenzae* meningitis. The seizures most commonly occur in the first 48 hours of illness; they may be brief or continuous, focal or generalized, and they are clearly an indication for anticonvulsant therapy.

Focal signs including hemiparesis, asymmetrical reflexes or asymmetrical changes in muscle tone may reflect either vascular or parenchymal disturbance or may be transient postictal phenomena. Ataxia may occur as an early manifestation, especially with *H influenzae* infection, although it is more commonly noted as a sequelae. Cranial nerves III, VI, VII, and VIII may be affected in the course of illness. Blindness which may also occur is usually related to occipital cortex involvement rather than to disease of the optic nerves. Involvement of the third cranial nerve with a dilated pupil, ptosis, and impaired adduction may be secondary to medial temporal lobe swelling and herniation. Transient unilateral or bilateral sixth nerve palsy may be indicative of increased intracranial pressure and not be of any localizing significance. Deafness, a not infrequent sequelae of bacterial meningitis, is rarely noted early in the course of illness, perhaps because of difficulty in assessing hearing in the critically ill child; it may be a permanent disability. Increased intracranial pressure, manifested by a bulging fontanelle, headache, reduced level of consciousness, or abducens palsy is rarely associated with papilledema. If papilledema occurs, this finding should suggest the presence of some other intracranial process such as localized suppuration, i.e., brain abscess, subdural empyema, etc.

NEUROLOGICAL COMPLICATIONS AND SEQUELAE

Persisting seizures may occur and are an indication for prolonged anticonvulsant therapy. **Hydrocephalus** which may complicate bacterial meningitis at any age is more common following neonatal meningitis. It is rarely an acute problem requiring emergency treatment, but if there is progressive head enlargement, a fontanelle remains tense, or there are other signs of increased intracranial pressure, a CT scan may be indicated. Shunting may be necessary. Early and late hydrocephalus is especially common with meningitis caused by gram-negative organisms in the neonate and with tuberculous meningitis. Serial daily head circumference measurements should be recorded during the acute illness for any child under 2 years of age.

Subdural effusions, although common, are rarely clinically significant. In the past, fever which persisted after the first several days of antibiotic therapy or recurrence of fever was an indication for the performance of subdural taps. When subdural taps were routinely done on every infant with meningitis with an open fontanelle, effusions almost invariably sterile, were found in 34% of the infants. These effusions are, however, usually very small, and they should not be considered the cause of seizures, impaired consciousness, or persistent fever; these findings are more likely related to the severity of the meningeal inflammation. Diagnostic subdural taps are rarely indicated in the absence of signs of increased intracranial pressure, such as a persistently bulging fontanelle after the first 4-5 days of therapy, progressive increase in head circumference or other signs suggestive of increased pressure. Therapeutic subdural taps are not recommended for small fluid collections noted on CT scan. Only in instances of large volumes of subdural fluid and evidence of significant cerebrocranial disproportion on CT scan or angiogram should further intervention (i.e., repeated taps or shunting) be considered. Subdural empyema is a very rare complication of meningitis and is associated with persisting fever, lethargy, and lack of clinical improvement with adequate antibiotic therapy. Brain abscess is an extremely rare complication of bacterial meningitis except in the neonate with gram-negative organisms, particularly *Citrobacter*, or in meningitis occurring in association with open head injury.

Long-term sequelae may include mental retardation, seizure disorders, motor deficits of varying magnitude, deafness, blindness, learning disabilities or attention deficit disorder with poor impulse control. As many as 50% of the survivors of *H influenzae* meningitis may have some sequelae, including subtle defects in school performance or behavior. The prognosis for ultimate outcome is dependent on many factors including the age of the patient, duration of illness prior to treatment, the severity and duration of seizures, degree and persistence of coma, as well as laboratory findings including the concentrations of bacterial antigen and of bacteria in CSF.

TREATMENT

For the child over 2 months of age, unless there is evidence suggesting an unusual organism is causing the meningitis, combined therapy with ampicillin and chloramphenicol is recommended, pending laboratory identification of the etiologic organism. Current recommended dosage of ampicillin is 200 mg/kg/day, in 4-6 divided doses, each dose to be given by rapid IV infusion in less than ½ hour. Following 7 days of IV therapy, ampicillin may be administered by IM injections. Because of the widespread appearance of ampicillin-resistant *H influenzae*, choramphenicol, 100 mg/kg/day, should be administered concurrently. If the bacteria are found to be beta lactamase negative (i.e., sensitive to ampicillin) the chloramphenicol may subsequently be discontinued. Treatment with either ampicillin or chloramphenicol should be given for 10 days. If pneumococcus or meningococcus are identified as the etiologic organisms, penicillin G, in a dose of 250,000 units/kg/24 hours, in 6 divided doses, should be substituted for the ampicillin and chloramphenicol and continued for 10 days.

There are no rigid criteria uniformly applicable to all patients beyond the neonatal period regarding need for repeat LP, or CSF cell counts, protein or glucose at time of terminating antibiotics. With the common organisms and satisfactory clinical course, a repeat LP is unnecessary. If clinical improvement is unsatisfactory or delayed, LP can be repeated at any time. If LP is done at the end of 10-14 days of parenteral antibiotic therapy, 60 cells/mm^3 or more may still be present in CSF. Persistent pleocytosis occurs more often in patients with prolonged fever, but it does not appear to be an indication for continuing antibiotics. CSF glucose levels may still be quite low, with CSF to blood ratios still below 0.66 in many instances.

Neonatal meningitis therapy requires monitoring with repeated lumbar punctures both because of difficulty of clinical assessment of response to treatment and because of prolonged persistence of positive bacterial cultures, especially with gram-negative infections. Initial antibiotic treatment of neonatal meningitis consists of ampicillin and an aminoglycoside, either kanamycin or gentamicin. The particular aminoglycoside chosen depends on the sensitivity of gram-negative bacteria in the specific geographic locale or nursery population. Ampicillin is administered IV, aminoglycosides are administered IM or IV and dosages are determined on basis of both weight and age of the newborn infant.

Antibiotic dosages, route of administration, are as indicated in Table 6-2.

Neither lumbar intrathecal nor intraventricular injections of gentamicin are beneficial or required in the usual case of neonatal meningitis caused by coliform bacteria. However, in cases with persistent positive CSF cultures, despite IV therapy, daily instillations of gentamicin into the ventricles, either by direct needle puncture or by an indwelling Rickham reservoir, may be advantageous. Cefamandole may also be administered in cases of neonatal meningitis caused by coliform bacteria.

Recommended antibiotic treatment for various types of bacterial meningitis are shown in Table 6-3.

Duration of antibiotic treatment for neonatal meningitis is for approximately 2 weeks after bacteriologic cure, and this must be documented with repeat lumbar puncture. For the gram-negative organisms, antibiotics should be administered for at least 14 days after CSF cultures are negative or for 21 days, whichever is longer. All infants with meningitis should have a repeat CSF examination and culture at 24-36 hours after initiation of therapy as well as repeat LP at the conclusion of therapy, and at any other time during the course of treatment if the clinical response is less than satisfactory.

Table 6-2   Antibiotic Dosages and Routes of Administration

Antibiotic route	Dosage Age 1 week	Dosage Age 1-4 weeks
Ampicillin, IV	100 mg/kg/day (2 divided doses)	200 mg/kg/day (3 divided doses)
Gentamicin, IM or IV	5 mg/kg/day (2 divided doses)	7.5 mg/kg/day (3 divided doses)
*Kanamycin, IM Weight< 2000 gm	15 mg/kg/day (2 divided doses)	20 mg/kg/day (2 divided doses)
Weight> 2000 gm	20 mg/kg/day (2 divided doses)	30 mg/kg/day (3 divided doses)
Penicillin G, IV	150,000 units/kg/day (2 divided doses)	250,000 units/kg/day (3 or 4 divided doses)
Carbenicillin, IV Weight <2000 gm	100 mg/kg = initial 225 mg/kg/day (3 divided doses)	100 mg/kg = initial 400 mg/kg/day (4 divided doses)
Weight> 2000 gm	300 mg/kg/day (4 divided doses)	400 mg/kg/day (4 divided doses)
Ticarcillin	150-225 mg/kg/day (3 divided doses)	300 mg/kg/day (4 divided doses)
Methicillin, IV	50 mg/kg/day (2 divided doses)	100-150 mg/kg/day (3 divided doses)

* Total kanamycin dosage should not exceed 500 mg/kg during the course of treatment.

Table 6-3   Antibiotics for bacterial meningitis

Organism	Antibiotic
Group B *Streptococcus*	Penicillin G
Group D *Streptococcus* (enterococcal)	Ampicillin + gentamicin
Listeria monocytogenes	Ampicillin + gentamicin
Escherichia coli, other coliforms	Ampicillin + gentamicin, or kanamycin
Pseudomonas aeruginosa	Carbenicillin + gentamicin, or ticarcillin + gentamicin
Staphylococcus aureus	Methicillin (vancomycin for methicillin-resistant strains)

VIRAL MENINGITIS AND ENCEPHALITIS

Viral infections of the nervous system may primarily involve meninges, brain, spinal cord, or a combination of these areas, producing meningitis, encephalitis, myelitis, meningoencephalitis, etc. Multiple sites within the nervous system may be simultaneously affected. Although such viral illnesses may be mild, and without serious sequelae, there may be dramatic clinical manifestations, with high morbidity and mortality. The clinical course of the usual case of viral meningitis is mild, and most patients recover completely; whereas encephalitis caused by one of the arboviruses or the herpesviruses may be devastating, with profound sequelae or death.

The viruses associated with these illnesses include the agents listed in Table 6-4.

CLINICAL MANIFESTATIONS

The viruses most commonly identified as causes of **viral meningitis** are the echo, coxsackie, and mumps viruses. Prior to polio immunization, poliovirus was also a commonly recognized cause of viral meningitis. Clinical manifestations of viral meningitis include headache, fever, irritability, vomiting, photophobia, stiff neck, and mild alterations of consciousness. Associated symptoms and signs may be a result of systemic viral infection; i.e., gastrointestinal symptoms including vomiting, diarrhea, abdominal pain; various exanthems or petechial rashes are noted with some of the echoviruses; pharyngeal vesicles, sore throat, or chest pain may occur with some coxsackievirus infections. The systemic manifestations may be the clinical clue to the specific viral etiology of the neurological disease.

If seizures, paralysis, cranial nerve palsies, and ataxia occur, these clinical manifestations are evidence that the infection involves other parts of the nervous system in addition to the meninges, and the illness should therefore be correctly referred to as a meningoencephalitis, meningomyelitis, and so on.

Enteroviral infections occur most commonly in epidemics in summer months, are frequent in infants as well as in school-aged children or adults. Neonatal CNS infection with enteroviruses may also occur.

Mumps meningitis and **meningoencephalitis** are also common. The clue to the etiology may be the associated parotitis, or less commonly, orchitis or pancreatitis, although mumps meningitis may occur without clinical evidence of parotitis or other organ involvement in as high as 50% of the cases. Although usually a benign illness with complete recovery anticipated, mumps virus infection of the nervous system may be severe, with coma, convulsions, and serious neurological sequelae including mental retardation and chronic seizure disorders. Much less common than either mumps or enteroviral meningitis is **lymphocytic choriomeningitis**. This is usually a relatively mild illness, affecting older children or adults, with systemic symptoms of malaise, arthralgia, or myalgia, which may be more prominent than the symptoms of CNS infection. Other viruses which may also cause viral meningitis include influenza viruses, adenoviruses, Epstein-Barr viruses, and the herpesviruses.

Table 6-4   Viruses Associated with CNS Infections

Viral meningitis

Enteroviruses:
>   Polioviruses (3 types)
>   Coxsackieviruses, groups A and B
>   Echoviruses

Mumps virus
Lymphocytic choriomeningitis virus
Epstein-Barr viruses
Adenoviruses
Influenza viruses

Viral encephalitis

Any of the above viruses that cause viral meningitis

Arboviruses:
>   California encephalitis virus
>   St. Louis encephalitis virus
>   Western equine encephalitis virus
>   Eastern equine encephalitis virus
>   Japanese B encephalitis virus
>   Venezuelan equine encephalitis virus
>   Colorado tick fever virus

Herpesviruses:
>   Herpes hominis types 1, 2
>   Varicella-zoster viruses
>   Cytomegaloviruses

Postinfectious encephalitis viruses:
>   Varicella virus
>   Rubeola virus
>   Rubella virus
>   Mumps virus

Nonviral (nonbacterial) meningitis/encephalitis:
>   Mycoplasma
>   Leptospirosis
>   Toxoplasma
>   Rocky Mountain spotted fever
>   Cat scratch disease
>   Syphilis
>   Funguses: *Cryptococcus, Coccidioides, Candida,*
>   *Mucormycosis, Aspergilla*

Encephalitis is highly variable in severity. Typical manifestations include the abrupt onset of fever, headache, dizziness, irritability, and lethargy, with progressive confusion, disorientation including hallucinations, and declining level of consciousness. Tremors, convulsions, and coma may develop within a period of several days. Focal or generalized seizures may be prominent and may be relatively resistant to anticonvulsant therapy. Focal motor deficits, with weakness of one or more extremities, spasticity, and reflex changes, including extensor plantar responses are not uncommon. Brain stem involvement, although uncommon, may develop with multiple cranial nerve palsies and ataxia. The illness may be fulminating over a matter of hours or days, with rapidly developing coma, seizures, and increased intracranial pressure. Papilledema may occur but is uncommon, and if present, the accuracy of the diagnosis should be in serious question. Along with increased intracranial pressure, progressive deterioration may occur, with decorticate or decerebrate posturing. As with viral meningitis, systemic signs of illness may be clues to the underlying etiology. Also of diagnostic aid may be information regarding disease outbreaks in the community or school, the seasonal incidence of specific viral infections, and other epidemiologic data. Of the various viruses causing encephalitis, St. Louis encephalitis is the most frequently diagnosed arboviral encephalitis in the USA, although it is much more common in adults than children. California encephalitis occurs predominantly in children and especially infants. Most of these arboviral infections occur in the spring and summer months; mumps is more common in winter and spring months. Although it has been stated that in the winter months encephalitis is most likely due to the herpesvirus, the majority of winter encephalitides go undiagnosed despite adequate attempts made at viral identification in the laboratory.

Postinfectious encephalitis or **encephalomyelitis,** related to infection with the viruses causing the common childhood illnesses rubeola, rubella, varicella, and mumps were once considered the most common viral encephalitides in childhood. Viral invasion of the brain has been well documented with varicella, rubella and mumps, and even measles virus has been isolated from the brain of fatal cases of measles encephalitis. However, in measles encephalitis and in many cases of encephalitis related to mumps and varicella, the pathologic changes differ from those considered distinctive for a viral encephalitis. The microscopic changes show a striking similarity to the lesions of experimental allergic encephalomyelitis, which is presumably related to some form of allergic or immunologic reaction of the host to the virus. Whether these illnesses are truly viral encephalitides or postviral illnesses, remains a very complicated question which is still not completely answered. Measles encephalitis occurs in about one of 1000 cases of measles; when measles was a common illness, measles encephalitis was a relatively common and often serious disease. Immunization has produced a dramatic reduction in the occurrence of measles and therefore of measles encephalitis. The control of measles by immunization has also resulted in a marked reduction in the incidence of subacute sclerosing panencephalitis.

Encephalitis after varicella resembles other types of acute viral encephalitis but is relatively rare. Acute cerebellar ataxia associated with varicella is a special form of neurologic complication of varicella, but it is not clear whether it is caused by direct virus invasion or is similar to the postinfectious encephalitis of measles. Of greater importance in relation to varicella is the association between varicella infection and Reye's syndrome. Varicella is probably second only to influenza virus infection as the viral illness predisposing to the development of Reye's syndrome. Varicella-zoster virus may cause a meningoencephalitis, but zoster involvement of nerve roots is much less common in childhood than in adults.

Herpes hominis virus encephalitis is currently considered one of the most frequent severe and often fatal nonseasonal encephalitides. It can occur at any time of the year and affect all age groups. Type I virus is most common after the neonatal period. Identification of the etiologic agent is particularly important since an effective drug, adenine arabinoside (Ara-A) is available. The treatment is effective, provided diagnosis is established early in the course of illness. The level of consciousness and age of the patient appear to be major variables influencing the outcome; younger patients and particularly those who are not comatose have a better outcome. At present, diagnosis requires brain biopsy and viral isolation of the herpesvirus from brain tissue, or specific virus identification by fluorescent antibody tests or by special electron microscopy on brain tissue. Herpes infection is likely to occur in the immunocompromised host, as are CNS infections with the cytomegaloviruses and toxoplasma, but herpes CNS infection is being increasingly recognized in previously healthy children.

LABORATORY DIAGNOSIS

Cerebrospinal fluid examination in cases of viral meningitis and encephalitis generally reveals a lymphocytic pleocytosis, varying from as few as 10 cells to over 1000 cells/mm^3. In the first days of illness, polymorphonuclear leukocytes may predominate, but then lymphocytes become the predominant cell type. Protein content may be normal or only slightly elevated; in the more severe and necrotizing forms of encephalitis caused by some of the arboviruses and herpesvirus, protein levels may become elevated to several hundred mg/dl. CSF glucose is usually normal, although slight reductions of glucose are occasionally found with mumps or lymphocytic choriomeningitis virus infection.

The frequency of virus isolation or identification in cases of viral meningitis and encephalitis varies considerably.

Laboratory confirmation of **specific viral etiology** requires either virus isolation from an appropriate tissue or fluid, or diagnostic serological results showing at least a 4-fold rise in antibody titer between acute and convalescent serum specimens. This usually requires the facilities of a highly specialized laboratory, either in a university medical center or a state health department laboratory. Presumptive identification includes cases with compatible virus isolation from non-CNS sites (throat, stool) without supporting serologic evidence. When adequate specimens of CSF, throat washings, feces, and paired sera are available, in laboratories with appropriate facilities for viral identification, etiologic determination is possible in no greater than 50% of cases. With the availability of antiviral agents, such as adenine arabinoside, there is increasing need for identification of etiologic agents, and particularly with herpes simplex encephalitis, brain biopsy, viral isolation, and specific fluorescent antibody tests may be essential.

The role for other diagnostic tests in the evaluation of a patient with presumptive diagnosis of viral meningitis or encephalitis is not always clear. The **differential diagnosis** not uncommonly includes primary bacterial or fungal infection, and tuberculous CNS infection. Diagnostic difficulties particularly arise if patients have been given antibiotics prior to diagnostic evaluation. Changes in CSF cell type, from polymorphonuclear leukocytes to lymphocytes on repeat lumbar puncture may be helpful in ruling out the likelihood of bacterial disease, as is the absence of organisms on CSF smear and negative counterimmunoelectrophoresis. At times the diagnosis of partially treated bacterial meningitis cannot be excluded, and a full course of antibiotic treatment may be obligatory. Tuberculous and crypto-coccal meningitis also commonly enter into the differential diagnosis. Chest x-rays, tuberculin skin testing, history of possible exposure, determination of cryptococcal antigen on repeated CSF specimens, and cultures may be helpful. Brain abscess may also be considered in the differential diagnosis of viral meningitis and encephalitis. Localized cranial tenderness on percussion, underlying cyanotic congenital heart disease, chronic sino-pulmonary infection or other pericranial infection may be clues to the likelihood of brain abscess. CSF findings may be very similar in patients with brain abscess and encephalitis.

Electroencephalography may be helpful. Generalized slowing of variable degree is common with meningitis or encephalitis. Localized delta activity occurs with brain abscess, or localized frontal, temporal or even bilateral frontotemporal spike discharge may be found in cases of herpes encephalitis. CT scanning may be indicated, particularly in an effort to exclude brain abscess, epidural empyema, or to identify localized frontotemporal involvement in herpes simplex encephalitis.

CT scan The CT changes in herpes encephalitis are primarily areas of decreased attenuation in temporal lobes, at times extending to insular cortex and often to frontal or even parietal lobes. These changes may be extremely subtle and may not develop until the 10th to 11th day of illness; furthermore, the changes may be bilateral rather than being restricted to one temporal lobe.

Other disorders which must be considered in the differential diagnosis of viral meningitis or encephalitis include Reye's syndrome and a variety of other toxic and metabolic encephalopathies. Determination of serum ammonia, aminotransferases, blood glucose, serum electrolytes, osmolality, as well as toxicological analysis of blood and urine may be required.

TREATMENT

The treatment of infants and children with viral meningitis is supportive. The only viral encephalitis for which specific treatment is presently available is herpes hominis. Supportive care may include fluid restriction, especially if there is inappropriate secretion of antidiuretic hormone. Anticonvulsants are indicated for the control of seizures. Mannitol or other osmotic agents may be used in case of progressive increases in intracranial pressure although the role of intracranial pressure monitoring in such cases is not clearly established at the present.

SEQUELAE

The prognosis in most viral meningitis illness is extremely good, and the overwhelming majority of patients recover completely. In viral encephalitis, the prognosis is highly variable. The arboviral encephalitides and herpes encephalitis have perhaps the worst prognosis, with varying degrees of mental retardation, seizure disorders, and motor handicaps persisting. The sequelae are more common in those patients with the most severe and recurring seizures and the longest duration of coma during the acute illness.

REFERENCES

Bell WE, McCormick WF: *Neurologic Infections in Children,* 2nd Ed. Saunders, Philadelphia, 1981.

Feigin RD, Cherry JD: *Textbook of Pediatric Infectious Diseases.* Saunders, Philadelphia, 1981.

Nelson JD: *Pocketbook of Pediatric Antimicrobial Therapy,* 4th Ed. Jodone Publishing, Dallas, 1981.

Smith DH, et al: Bacterial meningitis, a symposium. Pediatrics 52:586-600, 1973.

Swartz MN, Dodge PR: Bacterial meningitis — a review of selected aspects. N Engl J Med 272:725-731, 842-848, 898-902, 954-960, 1003-1010, 1965.

7

Trauma of the Brain & Spinal Cord

Michael S. B. Edwards, MD and Lawrence H. Pitts, MD

Accidents account for more childhood deaths than do the four most common fatal diseases of childhood combined, and approximately 30% of the accidental deaths are associated with a head injury. It is estimated that nearly 5 million children sustain head trauma each year; the majority of these injuries are associated with automotive accidents. In approximately 200,000, the injury is severe enough to require hospitalization, and in nearly 4000 children, it results in death.

EPIDEMIOLOGY

Approximately 10% of these fatal head injuries occur before age 10 years. Boys are injured two times more often than girls, although this sex difference is less prominent in children under the age of 5 years. Skull fractures accompany 26% of all pediatric head injuries. The incidence of fracture rises to 60% of fatal head injury in children younger than 10, and 75% in children older than 10 years. The peak incidence of fracture is in children under 1 year of age, and 50% of these fractures are due to 'birth trauma.' There is a smaller secondary peak between 3 and 4 years of age. Precautions such as closing open windows, using car seats and restraints, and not allowing children to play with dangerous toys or guns, can prevent these injuries.

MECHANISMS

Children, especially infants, are particularly susceptible to head trauma because of the large mass of their head in relation to their weight and length, and because they lack full dexterity and have little fear. The majority of pediatric head injuries result in temporary loss of consciousness (concussion) associated with a variable period of retrograde amnesia. The mechanism is thought to be a temporary alteration in the function of the reticular activating system at the brain stem level.

Blunt trauma to the skull may result in a cerebral contusion directly beneath the site of impact (coup injuries) or at the opposite side of the brain (contrecoup injuries). Contrecoup injury (injury 180° from the site of direct trauma) usually occurs when the head in motion suddenly comes to an abrupt stop, such as may happen in a fall. Most commonly, contrecoup injuries involve the frontal and/or temporal poles; less frequently, they involve the occipital tips. Contrecoup injury occurs in 10% of children less than 3 years old, in 25% of children from 3-4 years old, and in 70% of children over the age of 4 years.

Cerebral contusion is usually accompanied by at least an initial loss of consciousness. Focal neurologic deficits may be seen and are related to the anatomic site of cerebral injury.

Interestingly, cerebral contusion is relatively rare in young children. In children under 5 months of age, stress to the head more commonly results in tears of white matter rather than contusion and/or hemorrhage, probably because of poor myelinization at this stage of development. In older children, severe head injuries may result in cerebral lacerations that involve the cortex primarily, and white matter secondarily.

EVALUATION

The child with a mild head injury is usually awake and irritable when first seen by the physician. The child with a severe head injury, however, is unable to obey commands, may not speak or cry, and is not capable of spontaneous and pain-elicited eye opening. The first priority, before obtaining a history or performing a detailed neurologic examination, is to assure that the airway is adequate and that circulation is maintained. In establishing an airway, care must be taken to prevent spinal cord injury in the child who has an unstable cervical spine. In all cases, until proven otherwise, one should assume that a child with severe head injury has an associated spinal injury.

Once an airway has been established and any hypotension reversed, the level of consciousness and neurologic status can be assessed. A standardized method for neurologic assessment, such as the Glasgow Coma Score (Table 7-1), helps to categorize the patient and allows subsequent examinations to be compared to the initial findings. In young children without language skills, the verbal response must be modified. The usual sequence is to evaluate verbal responses, brain stem reflexes, and motor function. After the initial evaluation, frequent neurologic reassessments are made. (See Chapter 19.)

Children who are in coma or who exhibit focal neurologic findings should undergo immediate CT scanning to exclude a lesion that requires surgical removal. More frequently, a diffuse cerebral injury will be diagnosed by CT scan (see p. 142). Children who show rapid deterioration should have bilateral exploratory trephination immediately. If no lesion is identified during the operation, a postoperative CT scan should be performed to rule out an intracerebral or posterior fossa hematoma. In infants with open fontanelles, ultrasonography may prove useful in screening and in making a rapid diagnosis of intracerebral mass lesions.

Table 7-1   Glasgow Coma Score

Best motor response		Verbal response		Eye opening	
Obeys	6	Oriented	5	Spontaneous	4
Localizes	5	Confused conversation	4	To speech	3
Withdraws	4	Inappropriate words	3	To pain	2
Abnormal flexion	3	Incomprehensible sounds	2	Nil	1
Extensor response	2	nil	1		
Nil	1				

Coma score (M + V + E) = 3-15

CEPHALOHEMATOMA

Cephalohematoma (hemorrhage beneath the periosteum of the skull) occurs in 2.5% of live births. The hematoma is usually unilateral and, as opposed to subgaleal hematomas, does not cross suture lines. Cephalohematomas most frequently involve the parietal region, and up to 25% are associated with an underlying linear skull fracture. On palpation, a distinct circular edge is felt that is often confused with a depressed skull fracture.

In general, these are benign lesions and resolve in a few weeks. Large lesions may cause anemia, and hyperbilirubinemia may occur as the lesion reabsorbs. These hematomas occasionally become infected in children with sepsis. Needle drainage is contraindicated because of the risk of introducing an infection. Long-standing lesions sometimes calcify.

SKULL FRACTURE

Skull fractures are a frequent complication of head trauma. Linear fractures are usually of little consequence. However, linear fractures that cross major dural sinuses or meningeal arteries may be associated with significant epidural hematomas. Even if awake and neurologically intact, children with such fractures should always be admitted to the hospital for observation.

Basilar skull fractures are visible on plain x-rays in only 20% of patients; the diagnosis is made on the basis of the physical examination. The presence of a hemotympanum or a CSF leak from the nose, mouth, or ears is diagnostic of basilar fracture. Also diagnostic is Battle's sign (ecchymosis overlying the mastoid) or raccoons' eyes (periorbital ecchymosis), which tends to develop a few hours following the initial trauma.

Depressed skull fractures, in which fractured bone is displaced below the normal skull contour, are of greater potential clinical significance. The spectrum of depressed fractures is wide; it ranges from a simple depression of the outer table, which generally is of little consequence, to a severe compound depressed fracture with underlying contusion or laceration.

The clinical examination usually demonstrates an area of scalp swelling, but identification of the depression by palpation is unreliable. If a depressed skull fracture is suspected, routine skull x-rays should be obtained. Suspicious areas should be further evaluated with tangential x-ray views. CT scanning with bone windows is a very sensitive technique for defining skull fractures, both linear and depressed.

In the older child, the decision to elevate a simple depressed fracture depends on: whether the depth of depression is greater than the skull thickness or about 0.5 cm; the location of the fracture and its correlation with the underlying neurologic deficit; the presence of active hemorrhage; and the possibility of cosmetic disfigurement, as occurs with frontally placed fractures. Compound depressed fractures and those associated with a penetrating foreign body require emergency repair. In younger children and neonates, simple depressed fractures, especially of the parietal bone, may on occasion spontaneously spring back into their anatomic position without treatment ('ping-pong' fracture). In the infant, we recommend the elevation of fractures that are depressed more than 5 mm.

Skull fractures in the neonate may occur in utero, during labor, or during delivery, as a consequence of physical trauma to the mother's abdomen or pelvis, or they may occur in the early neonatal period. The recommendations for treatment are the same as those for all children.

COMPLICATIONS OF SKULL FRACTURES

SUBGALEAL HYGROMA

An accumulation of CSF beneath the galea can occur in association with skull fracture. Examination demonstrates a soft, fluctuant swelling that resembles diffuse edema beneath the scalp. Hygromas are best treated conservatively and usually resolve over a few weeks' time; they should not be aspirated because of the risk of introducing an infection. Children under 3 years of age should be followed for possible development of a leptomeningeal cyst.

LEPTOMENINGEAL CYST ('Growing Fracture of Childhood')

This entity is seen primarily in infants and children who sustain skull fracture before 3 years of age. The initial injury typically is a parietal or parieto-occipital skull fracture with a diastasis greater than 4 mm and with an underlying dural tear; these combine to allow the arachnoid to be trapped within the fracture site.

The clinical manifestations may include seizures, hemiparesis, headache, and local discomfort. Plain x-rays of the skull demonstrate an elongated area of lucency with scalloped, irregular margins at the original fracture site; the inner table is more involved than the outer table.

Treatment consists of surgical correction of the skull defect with a watertight dural repair. Early detection facilitates repair; therefore, to detect such leptomeningeal cysts, children younger than 3 years old who sustain skull fractures should be followed at intervals of 3-6 months for several years.

PNEUMOCEPHALUS

Leakage of air into the intracranial fossa is associated with basilar fractures or linear skull fractures involving the air-containing sinuses. Air may leak into the epidural, subdural, or subarachnoid spaces. Intracranial air generally produces significant headache and/or irritability and may cause symptoms and signs of meningeal irritation. The major risk is the development of bacterial meningitis.

CEREBROSPINAL FLUID FISTULA

Fractures involving the skull base or paranasal sinuses may result in CSF rhinorrhea or otorrhea. The leak usually occurs immediately, but can be delayed days or weeks following trauma. Most of these fistulae will close spontaneously. **Treatment** consists of head elevation, together with multiple lumbar punctures or continuous lumbar drainage. Diamox (3-5 mg/kg daily) may be beneficial in decreasing CSF production. If the leak persists for longer than 2-3 weeks, surgical repair may be necessary.

The major risk of CSF leakage is meningitis, which occurs in up to 25% of cases. The usual organism is pneumococcus, which is more common with frontal than temporal bone fractures. The use of prophylactic antibiotics (penicillin, 50,000 units/kg daily) for basilar skull fractures is controversial, but we recommend this treatment when an active CSF leak is present.

VENOUS SINUS THROMBOSIS

Venous sinus thrombosis is a disastrous complication of depressed skull fracture. The most common site of this fracture is the vertex; thus, the thrombosis involves the sagittal sinus. This complication has been described following traumatic delivery in the neonate and after a fall or automobile accident in older children. **Therapy** consists of treatment for seizures and of raised intracranial pressure; despite appropriate therapy, significant brain injury often occurs.

SUBDURAL HEMATOMA

Bleeding into the subdural space may occur from various forms of trauma. The blood may originate from tearing of veins that bridge the space from the brain to dural or calvarial sinuses — or from tearing of venous sinuses or cortical vessels when there is a cerebral laceration.

An **acute subdural hematoma (SDH)** is defined as one that presents within 1 day of injury. It is usually the result of significant head trauma and frequently is associated with an underlying cerebral contusion and edema. Acute SDH can occur at birth; in this case, it always is associated with a difficult delivery and rapid neurologic deterioration postpartum.

Localizing neurologic findings, such as an ipsilateral dilated pupil and contralateral hemiparesis in association with an altered state of conciousness, are often present. On occasion, the paralysis may be ipsilateral to the mass lesion (Wolkman-Kernohan notch phenomenon), due to pressure of the tentorial edge on the cerebral peduncle contralateral to the mass lesion. The mass lesion is virtually always on the side of the pupillary abnormality. Rapid diagnosis is imperative and is best accomplished by CT scanning, which will demonstrate a hyperdense subdural collection.

Depending on the patient's clinical condition, a CT scan may be obtained first, before surgical evacuation. However, if the patient deteriorates rapidly, then immediate intubation, hyperventilation, and emergency surgery may be necessary without benefit of a CT scan. The outcome will depend on the patient's age, neurologic status at time of evacuation, and the severity and nature of cerebral and associated systemic injuries.

Subacute SDH (presenting between 1 day and 3 weeks following injury) and **chronic SDH** (presenting after 3 weeks) may occur at any age, but the peak incidence is between 2 months and 8 months after birth. The incidence decreases after age 2, and is infrequent between the ages of 5 and 16. In one-half of the cases, there is no history of head trauma, and the SDH may be a result of deformation of the skull at birth, an accidental fall, or child abuse.

In infants, 80-85% of SDHs are bilateral. The clinical presentation includes an increasing head circumference, irritability, decreased appetite and recurrent vomiting. However, the clinical course may be protracted and subtle. Focal or grand mal seizures occur in approximately 50% of cases, and children older than 6 months may show retardation of developmental skills.

Examination usually reveals a tense fontanelle and increased tone, especially in the lower extremities; there is a concomitant increase in the deep tendon reflexes. In more severe cases, a hemiparesis or alteration in the level of consciousness may be noted. Papilledema is rarely seen; however, retinal or subhyaloid hemorrhages may be observed. Anemia may be found as a result of blood loss into the subdural space. The diagnosis is confirmed by sonogram or CT scan. On CT scans made without contrast material, subacute SDH appears isodense and chronic SDH appears hypodense in relation to cerebral tissue.

Treatment consists of daily subdural taps, and the vast majority of these hematomas resolve within 2 weeks. Subdural hematoma in an older child with closed sutures requires the placement of a burr hole for drainage and irrigation. If reaccumulation persists after 2 weeks or the head progressively enlarges, subdural to peritoneal shunts may be necessary. Stripping of subdural membranes is of no benefit.

Chronic untreated subdural hematomas may calcify. In this case, they are usually associated with seizures and mental retardation. Surgery does not benefit these symptoms. Rarely, subdural hematoma in the posterior fossa may occur as the result of a tear of the tentorium during a difficult delivery. Surgical evacuation may be life-saving. The prognosis following SDH is not related to the method of treatment, but rather to the severity of the initial brain injury.

Subdural hygromas are the result of arachnoidal tears with resultant leakage of CSF into the subdural spaces. They may occur days or weeks following head trauma and usually resolve spontaneously.

EPIDURAL HEMATOMA

Epidural hematoma is rare in infants and young children; the reasons are that sharp-edged skull fractures are unusual, branches of the middle meningeal artery are not as yet grooved within the inner table, and the dura is still tightly adherent at the suture lines. These hematomas occur more commonly in boys, and almost always are unilateral. Classically, they develop in the temporal region and are associated with a skull fracture. Approximately 4% occur in the posterior fossa; this location is more common in children than adults. Epidural hematomas may follow relatively minor head trauma in which there is no skull fracture or loss of consciousness.

Classically, there is an initial loss of consciousness followed by a lucid interval. The onset of symptoms may occur as early as 15 minutes or as long as days or weeks after the initial incident. Progression may be very rapid. Plain x-rays of the skull usually reveal a skull fracture crossing the middle meningeal artery or a major dural venous sinus, but a normal x-ray does not exclude the possibility of epidural hematoma. A CT scan is the diagnostic procedure of choice. However, if the child rapidly becomes comatose, an immediate craniotomy and evacuation should be performed.

As in SDH, the outcome relates to the neurologic state at the time of surgical decompression, rapidity of deterioration, and accompanying brain injuries. Subjacent brain is injured less frequently with an epidural than with a subdural hematoma, and the outcome in a child with epidural hematoma is usually excellent.

INTRACEREBRAL HEMATOMA

The majority of intracerebral hematomas occur in the frontal and/or temporal lobes and are usually contralateral to the site of skull impact; traumatic subdural hematoma commonly coexists. A CT scan is critical for precise localization.

In general, surgical removal is advocated if the hematoma is accessible and is causing neurologic symptoms or a shift of the midline structures. Deep-seated lesions are best observed, but evacuation should be considered when there is progressive neurologic dysfunction. If the CT scan demonstrates a hemorrhagic contusion rather than an intracerebral hematoma, aggressive nonsurgical management is indicated.

In the newborn, intracerebral hematoma is associated with prematurity (28-33 weeks), low birth-weight (less than 1500 gm), hypoxia, and acidosis. These hemorrhages classically occur in the germinal matrix of the frontal horn of the lateral ventricle. **Treatment** consists of multiple lumbar punctures to control increased ICP; Lasix (furosemide, 1-2 mg/kg) and/or Diamox (acetazolamide, 5-30 mg/kg) may be useful. Progressive increase in ventricular size and head circumference despite these measures are indications for external ventricular drainage or ventriculoperitoneal shunting.

In large-term infants, head distortion during delivery, especially with breech presentations, may cause a laceration of the tentorium, posteriorly situated bridging veins, or choroid plexus. A subdural hematoma is the usual consequence of these tears; however, they may be associated with intracerebral hemorrhages in the supratentorial and/or infratentorial compartment. Depending on the infant's neurologic condition, emergency surgical evacuation may be necessary.

DIFFUSE HEAD INJURY

The vast majority of children who die from head injury exhibit diffuse cerebral swelling with obliteration of the CSF spaces and venous congestion, rather than a mass lesion. The syndrome of diffuse cerebral swelling has been attributed to progressive cerebral edema, but recent evidence suggests that the swelling results from cerebral hyperemia and increased cerebral blood volume.

Criteria for establishing the diagnosis of diffuse cerebral swelling on the basis of CT scan are the presence of small ventricles and cisterns with compression or absence of the perimesencephalic cisterns. These CT patterns may be present in up to 40% of children with Glasgow Coma Scores of 8 or less. With aggressive management of raised ICP, as many as 94% of children with diffuse brain swelling exhibit a good to excellent recovery. The management of this pathologic process is the control of raised ICP (see p. 282).

POSTCONCUSSION SYNDROME

The postconcussion syndrome has various manifestations in children. After mild head trauma, prolonged nausea and vomiting is not unusual. Somnolence and irritability may persist for days. Uncommon sequelae are transient blindness, hemiparesis, and the onset of migraine attacks. In general, all of these symptoms are short-lived. However, trouble with concentration and poor performance in school may persist for weeks or months. (See Chapter 15.)

BATTERED CHILD SYNDROME

The term 'battered child syndrome' was introduced by Kempe in 1962 in referring to infants and children who sustain physical injury from purposeful abuse by others. A variety of cranial lesions, including skull and facial fractures, acute and chronic subdural hematomas, cerebral infarction, and hydrocephalus, may be seen in these children.

Any child with head injury arising from unknown or unusual circumstances should be considered as a possibly abused child. The physician must be alert to this entity, which crosses all racial and social boundaries and can only be investigated and corrected when recognized by an astute health care system.

Kempe noted that 25% of all fractures in children under age 2 appear in these battered children. Radiographs of the skull, ribs, and long bones should be taken in all suspected cases. The radiologic hallmark is multiple traumatic skeletal lesions of different ages.

SPINAL CORD INJURY

Injuries to the bony spine and spinal cord are not uncommon in the pediatric population. Spinal injuries in children may result from an automobile or motorcycle accident, a fall on the head, or an athletic mishap such as a dive into shallow water or severe neck flexion while skiing or playing contact sports. The majority of injuries result in closed trauma, which may produce a varying degree of neurologic injury ranging from concussion to complete anatomic transection.

Common sites for childhood spinal cord injuries are the C1-C2, C5-C6, and T12-L1 spinal segments. Fracture dislocations of the vertebral column are the most frequent cause of injury; however, a child may have major spinal cord injury, including complete anatomic cord transection, without showing radiologic evidence of fracture dislocation on plain and/or dynamic spine x-rays.

Spinal cord concussion (transient loss of spinal cord function without anatomic injury) usually occurs as the result of severe trauma, such as a long-distance fall or a blow from a flying blunt object. There is temporary and reversible loss of all spinal cord function below the level of injury. All precautions should be taken to rule out spine instability. Recovery usually begins within hours and generally proceeds to complete recovery.

In neonates, birth trauma as a result of a difficult delivery requiring extension of the neck (e.g., a breech extraction) may result in cord transsection or diffuse intraparenchymal hemorrhage with no evidence of bone injury. This can occur because the laxity of the supporting ligamentous spine structures allows traction of the less elastic neural elements. Operative intervention is not recommended and treatment is generally limited to supportive measures. High cervical cord injuries resulting in quadriplegia and loss of ventilatory mechanisms carry a grave prognosis.

In very young children, the following anatomical and developmental factors predispose the upper cervical spine to injury:
    (1)   A relatively large head and a small body, which results in high loading forces during acceleration and deceleration injuries.
    (2)   Laxity of the ligaments and joint capsules in this region.

(3) Horizontal position of the facet joints.
(4) General laxity of the immature uncovertebral joints at C2-3-4.

As a general rule, vertebral fractures in children occur through the cartilaginous growth plate of the vertebrae at the junction of bone and joint, rather than through the vertebral body, as occurs in adults. For example, the majority of odontoid fractures in children occur through the subdental synchrondrosis (below the superior facets), rather than through the odontoid waist (above the superior facets), as in most adults.

In younger children, cervical spine fractures tend to heal spontaneously with appropriate external immobilization, and surgical intervention for fusion is necessary only in cases of gross instability.

In older children, the pattern of injury is similar to that in adults. The entire cervical spine is at risk and skeletal injuries are increasingly severe, tending to involve the vertebral body.

Compression fracture of a vertebral body usually occurs in older children and adolescents following forceful flexion of the spine or following abrupt axial loading, as in a fall from height in which the child lands directly on the feet or buttocks. Compressive fractures most commonly involve the mid-cervical to low-cervical region and thoracolumbar junction. Spinal cord injury may result from angulation of the bony spine or from posterior displacement of bone or disk tissue into the spinal canal.

Fracture dislocation, in which vertebral displacement is anteroposterior, lateral, or rotational, usually results from a flexion or flexion-rotation type of injury. The clinical picture depends on the severity and level of spinal cord injury. Often the clinical picture may be dominated by spinal shock. This represents a transient loss of synaptic excitability below the level of the injury. During spinal shock, the extent of injury cannot be fully determined. Return of spinal segmental reflexes, such as bulbocavernous and deep tendon reflexes, represents the termination of spinal shock. If total loss of voluntary motor function and sensory function persists, the injury is termed complete. In incomplete spinal cord lesions, return of motor, sensory, and reflex function will be variable, depending on the severity of injury.

Evidence of trauma is usually present or a history of trauma can be elicited. It may be difficult to establish the spinal level and extent of injury, particularly in infants and small children. The level of injury to the spine may be determined by assessing the motor response to pain and the reflex function. Another method is to demonstrate the level of impairment of autonomic dysfunction by determining the level of sweating. The dermatomes below the level of injury will be dry and exhibit loss of vasomotor tone.

Plain x-rays of the spine should be obtained, but sometimes they are difficult to interpret. In all suspected spinal injuries, the spine should be immobilized (preferably with sandbags) until its stability can be determined. When the spine appears normal on the x-ray, focal swelling may help localize the site of injury; therefore, the prevertebral space should be examined carefully for swelling. Most recently, spinal CT scanning has been useful in determining the extent of injury to bone and in localizing compromise of the spinal canal by bone fragments.

In a patient with evidence of an **anterior cord syndrome** (loss of motor function and pain sensation with preservation of dorsal column function) or progression of incomplete lesion, myelography should be performed to rule out a surgical lesion, such as disk material that has ruptured into the spinal canal.

In a patient with a fracture dislocation, the first goal is realignment of the bony spine. This is generally done by skeletal traction (halo, halo-tibial, or halo-pelvic). Stable or improving neurologic deficits are treated conservatively. However, if there is neurologic progression despite good alignment of the spine, myelography and/or spinal CT scanning should be performed. If evidence of a subarachnoid block or bony fragments within the spinal canal is identified, then surgical decompression is warranted. In children, most fracture dislocations will fuse spontaneously if correct alignment is maintained. On occasion, if a spontaneous fusion does not develop or if the injury to the bony spine is felt to be unusually unstable, then spinal fusion with internal stabilization (Harrington rods) may be necessary.

Hyperextension injuries of the cervical cord may produce a **central cord syndrome**. This syndrome is manifest by lower motor neuron findings at the level of injury; these affect the distal portion of the upper extremities and there is relatively greater preservation of function in the lower extremities. Conservative management usually is appropriate, but on occasion, decompression of the cervical cord may be of benefit.

The ultimate outlook for recovery following spinal cord injury depends on the severity and site of cord injury. In general, improvement may be seen for up to 1 year following the initial injury.

Transient apparent atlantoaxial subluxation is an unusual clinical picture that occurs exclusively in children. It often follows an upper respiratory infection, and is sometimes mistaken for a spinal injury. The child usually presents with head tilt to the affected side, and there is often tenderness to palpation over the C1 and C2 spinous process. This syndrome is rarely associated with root or cord signs and resolves spontaneously with cervical traction.

REFERENCES

Bell WE, McCormick WMF: *Increased Intracranial Pressure in Children*, 2nd Ed. Saunders, Philadelphia, 1978.

Bruce DA, et al: Outcome following severe head injuries in children. J Neurosurg 48: 679-688, 1978.

Bruce DA, et al: Diffuse cerebral swelling following head injuries in children: the syndrome of 'malignant brain edema.' J Neurosurg 54:170-178, 1981.

Matson DD: *Neurosurgery of Infancy and Childhood*, 2nd Ed. Charles C Thomas, Springfield, 1969, pp 271-281.

McLaurin RL, McLennan JE: Diagnosis and treatment of head injury in children. *In* Youmans JR (Ed): *Neurological Surgery*, 2nd Ed. Saunders, Philadelphia, 1982, pp 2084-2136.

Raphaely RC, et al: Management of severe pediatric head trauma. Pediatr Clin NA, 27:715-727, 1980.

Teasdale G, Jennett B: Assessment of coma and impaired consciousness. A practical scale. Lancet 2:81-84, 1974.

8

Craniospinal Neoplasms

Michael S. B. Edwards, MD

INCIDENCE

Primary intracranial tumors are the second most frequent cause of cancer-related deaths in children. At least 60% of tumors in children of age 2 years and older are located below the tentorium cerebelli. In infants, as in adults, supratentorial tumors predominate. Approximately 70% of brain tumors in children are glial in origin (Table 8-1). In most series, the most common tumor is cerebellar astrocytoma, followed in order of frequency by medulloblastoma, ependymoma, brain stem glioma, and craniopharyngioma.

Although some intracranial tumors are present at birth and an increasing number are discovered during infancy, the overall incidence of intracranial neoplasms in the pediatric population reaches a peak during the second half of the first decade of life. The incidence declines during the period of puberty, then increases gradually until late adolescence, when it reaches a second peak.

CLINICAL MANIFESTATIONS

Pediatric brain tumors manifest themselves either by signs and symptoms of increased intracranial pressure (ICP) due to obstruction of the cerebrospinal fluid (CSF) pathway or by focal findings correlated with the site at which the central nervous system (CNS) is involved by tumor (Table 8-2).

The possibility of a brain tumor should be suspected in any child who has unexplained vomiting. The vomiting characteristically occurs soon after the child awakens from sleep, either early in the morning hours or after a nap. It is frequently described as projectile, and, in general, is not preceded by nausea. In the infant, irritability, a full fontanelle, or an increasing head circumference may be the earliest manifestations of increased ICP. The child who complains of a headache that is severe, recurrent, or increasing in frequency should be referred for a neurologic evaluation. Such headaches are often localized to the suboccipital area, reflecting the high incidence of posterior fossa tumors. In infants and young children headaches due to increased ICP are often manifested in irritable behavior, restlessness, and a dislike of being touched. Irritation of the lower cranial nerves and upper cervical nerve roots resulting from incipient herniation of the cerebellar tonsils produces neck stiffness which may be confused with meningitis.

The presence of papilledema, an unequivocal sign of increased ICP, may be difficult to determine in the irritable, uncooperative child or infant.

Table 8-1 Types of Brain Tumors Arising in Children

Tumor type	Incidence (%)
Glial origin	
Astrocytoma	
Cystic/solid cerebellar astrocytoma	20-30
Brain stem glioma	10-20
Optic nerve, chiasm, hypothalamic glioma	5
Cerebral hemisphere astrocytoma	8
Medulloblastoma	18
Ependymoma	8
Nonglial origin	
Craniopharyngioma	5
Choroid plexus papilloma	less than 0.5
Pineal region tumors	1
Meningioma	1
Metastatic tumors	—*

* Incidence unknown

Sedation may be necessary before a funduscopic examination can be performed. The sedation must be done carefully to prevent hypoventilation and hypercarbia, which could cause a sudden rise in ICP. On occasion, mydriasis may also be required. Only short-acting agents should be used, and the child's chart should be labeled as to the time they were administered, in order to prevent confusion about the clinical significance of a dilated pupil.

Cranial nerve dysfunction may result from direct involvement by tumor or as a secondary manifestation of increased ICP. When it is a consequence of increased ICP, it often involves the sixth nerve (abducens) and results in a strabismus — although any cranial nerve may be involved. The presence of a new strabismus in a child should always raise the suspicion of a tumor.

Certain tumors have a propensity to arise in distinctive locations and produce focal neurologic findings. In this chapter, the characteristic focal neurologic findings associated with specific locations within the CNS are discussed in conjunction with the specific tumor types.

NEURODIAGNOSTIC TESTS

Whenever there is clinical suspicion of a brain tumor, the physician should always be alert to the subtle signs of increased ICP. In the child who has persistent vomiting, a funduscopic examination is mandatory before embarking on a gastrointestinal evaluation.

Radiographic examination (plain x-rays) of the skull should be the initial diagnostic step. Elevated ICP in infancy and early childhood causes

Table 8-2   Clinical Manifestations of Pediatric Brain Tumors

Increased intracranial pressure
Headache, stiff neck
Vomiting
Impaired vision
Papilledema
Cranial nerve dysfunction
Enlargement of the head (infants)

Focal CNS involvement
Cranial nerve dysfunction (e.g., brain-stem glioma)
Long tract signs (e.g., brain-stem glioma)
Cerebellar dysfunction (e.g., cerebellar astrocytoma)
Endocrine dysfunction (hypothalamic glioma, craniopharyngioma)
Visual loss (optic glioma, craniopharyngioma)
Seizures (cerebral hemisphere tumors)

splitting of the cranial sutures. During late childhood and adolescence, suture separation may be less obvious; however, there may be demineralization of the dorsum sella. Abnormal intracranial calcification is observed in cases of craniopharyngioma, tumors of the pineal region, and cerebral glioma. Focal thinning of the skull, bone erosion, and abnormalities of the skull may be evident.

Ultrasonography is a very useful diagnostic tool for evaluating the infant with an open fontanelle. It can rapidly confirm a diagnosis of hydrocephalus, and may reveal brain shifts in cases of cerebral hemispheric tumors. In children and adolescents with surgically created calvarial defects, it is useful in following cystic lesions, such as craniopharyngioma.

Radionuclide brain scans are more accurate in the diagnosis of supratentorial tumors than they are for those that arise beneath the tentorium. The possibility of tumor cannot be excluded if the scan shows no abnormalities, however, because low grade tumors with an intact blood-brain barrier may not be detectable with presently available techniques.

Angiography usually must be performed with the patient under general anesthesia. Modern angiography employing magnification and subtraction techniques is useful in the diagnosis of vascular disease and in the precise localization of the tumor's position and vascular supply.

Computerized tomography has supplanted pneumoencephalography in the diagnosis of brain tumors. It is the single most important diagnostic test available. The new generation of scanners (GE 8800) is capable of delineating tumors both below and above the tentorium with a resolution of 0.5 cm. Coronal scans and a computer-reconstructed image help to delineate the tumor in more than one plane, and afford a better evaluation of the suprasellar and parasellar regions. Scans should always be performed both without and with the intravenous administration of contrast material. Noncontrast studies are used to determine the presence of calcification or hemorrhage within the tumor. Contrast-enhanced scans reveal the vascularity and blood-brain barrier defect associated with the tumor. Small, extra-axial masses situated at the base of the brain or foramen magnum may be more clearly demonstrated by combining metrizamide cisternography with CT scanning. Scans made immediately postoperatively can aid in determining the extent of tumor removal. Sequential scans are useful in determining the tumor's response to therapeutic intervention such as irradiation, chemotherapy, or combined therapy with both of these modalities.

Lumbar puncture is mentioned only to condemn it. It should be used *only* when there is a serious possibility of either bacterial or fungal meningitis or subarachnoid spread of tumor. Before lumbar puncture is performed, a CT scan should be made to rule out a mass lesion.

PRIMARY TUMORS

CEREBELLAR ASTROCYTOMA

Cerebellar astrocytomas are the most common childhood brain tumors, constituting from 20-30% of tumors in most large series. They may arise at any age, including infancy, but they are most prevalent among children between 5 and 9 years of age. Children of both sexes are affected equally. These tumors are characteristically slow-growing and noninvasive, and they only rarely metastasize within the CNS. They usually arise in the vermis and tend to expand laterally into the cerebellar hemispheres. They may be cystic or solid, and they have the most favorable prognosis of all intracranial tumors of childhood.

The duration of symptoms is quite variable, averaging 6-12 months. The patient usually presents with signs and symptoms of increased ICP. When the tumor is laterally placed, cerebellar appendicular dysfunction (dysmetria, disdiadokineses, hyporeflexia, hypotonia) and nystagmus are evident.

Cerebellar astrocytomas are generally divided into two histologic types: (1) juvenile astrocytoma, constituting 70% of cases, and (2) diffuse astrocytoma comprising the other 30% of cases. It has been the opinion of most neurosurgeons that the macrocystic cerebellar astrocytoma is surgically curable by excision of the mural nodule. However, some investigators have found a 15% recurrence rate over the course of 10 years in children with this tumor. It appeared that cure depended more on the microscopic features of the tumor and on the attainment of total surgical excision than it did on the presence of macrocyst formation. In this series of 132 tumors the 10-year survival rate was 94% for patients with glioma A, which is characterized histologically by: (1) microcyst formation, (2) Rosenthal fibers, (3) leptomeningeal deposits, and (4) foci of oligodendroglia. Of this group, total excision had been achieved in 80% of patients, and 69.6% of tumors showed macrocyst formation. In contrast, the 10-year survival rate was only 29% for patients with tumors designated glioma B, which is characterized histologically by either (1) perivascular pseudorosette formation, (2) necrosis, high cell density, or mitosis, or (3) calcification in the absence of any glioma A features. Total surgical excision of glioma B was possible in only 27.7% of patients, and 23.3% of tumors showed macrocyst formation. Thus, it can be expected that somewhere between 20 and 30% of cerebellar astrocytomas will recur within a 10-year period and require some form of subsequent treatment.

The effectiveness of radiation therapy against these tumors is clear. However, its use initially should be considered only for subtotally resected tumors, especially those with glioma B features, and for tumors of all histologic types at the time of recurrence.

MEDULLOBLASTOMA

Medulloblastomas account for approximately 18% of childhood brain tumors, occurring 2-3 times more frequently in males than females. They are highly malignant tumors, and have a propensity to seed along the CSF pathways and, on rare occasions, outside the CNS.

It is postulated that these embryonic tumors arise from remnants of the fetal external granular layer of the cerebellum. In young children, they arise from the vermis and occupy the midline. In older children and young adults, however, they tend to develop laterally in the cerebellar hemispheres. The vast majority of patients with these tumors develop them during the first decade of life, most frequently between the ages of 3 and 7 years.

Medulloblastoma is a highly cellular tumor composed of clearly staining cells with hyperchromatic nuclei, ill-defined cytoplasmic borders, and frequently with mitotic figures. Pseudorosettes, originally described by Homer Wright, are seen in approximately one-third of tumors.

Children usually present with a short history of increased ICP and signs of midline cerebellar dysfunction (truncal ataxia). On occasion, the presenting complaint may be related to CSF metastasis (such as spinal and/ or cranial nerve dysfunction) rather than the primary tumor.

Total resection of localized lesions, if it is feasible, is advocated. Surgical diagnosis should be followed by aggressive neuroaxis irradiation of the posterior fossa (5500 rads), whole brain (3500-4500 rads), and spinal cord (4000-4500 rads). If there are no signs of increased ICP, then myelography and CSF cytology should precede irradiation, as they are helpful in the diagnosis of silent metastatic lesions.

A 5-year survival of 35%, and 10-year survival of 25%, of patients treated with aggressive craniospinal irradiation has been reported. Approximately 75-80% of recurrences occur during the first 3 years after treatment. The vast majority of tumors recur at the primary site in the posterior fossa. Sequential evaluations of CSF polyamine levels have been useful in predicting recurrence before a clinical change or CT evidence of tumor regrowth is seen.

The use of adjunctive chemotherapy (cis-chloronitrosourea [CCNU], vincristine, prednisone) against medulloblastoma has been investigated by the Children's Cancer Study Group. They were not able to document an increase in the survival of patients in the chemotherapy arm of their study. However, females in both arms of the study appeared to have a better prognosis than males. Chemotherapy at recurrence has been very effective in prolonging survival, but cure has not as yet been obtainable.

EPENDYMOMA

Ependymoma of the fourth ventricle constitutes 8% of the intracranial gliomas in children. These tumors occur most frequently in the young child, 2-3 years of age. There is a slight predilection of the tumor for males.

The majority of ependymomas arise from the floor of the fourth ventricle and grow to fill the fourth ventricle, producing obstructive hydrocephalus. These tumors may grow through the foramen of Magendie and extend to fill the cisterna magna and upper cervical canal. They tend to enlarge slowly and usually remain circumscribed. They are modestly cellular and classically form ependymal (true) rosettes. They have a tendency to calcify, and approximately 23% are cystic.

At the initial presentation, the patient has increased ICP secondary to fourth ventricle obstruction and hydrocephalus. Papilledema is usually present, and ataxia of gait and limb or diplopia may be noted in a careful neurologic examination.

Surgery, with the goal of total resection, followed by radiation therapy is the treatment of choice. Investigators have found that local radiation doses greater than 4500 rads significantly decreased the recurrence rate. Despite radiation therapy, the 5-year survival is only 13.7%. Chemotherapy with 1,3-bis (2-chloroethyl)-1-nitrosourea (BCNU) at recurrence has shown some effectiveness against this tumor.

Less frequently, ependymomas may occur in the cerebral hemispheres. These constitute 5-6% of childhood brain tumors, and tend to occur at a later age (median 5-7 years). They arise from the ependyma of the lateral ventricles and may grow to fill them. They are more often cystic than are infratentorial ependymomas, and they frequently calcify. The presentation is usually that of increased ICP, although there may be focal hemispheric symptoms. Surgery followed by radiation therapy offers the best chance for a long-term survival, although the reported 5-year survival rate is only 10%.

In general, local irradiation is recommended for both the supratentorial and infratentorial lesions. However, some ependymomas (ependymoblastoma) may show histologic signs of malignancy, are often invasive, and have the capability to seed along the CSF pathways. Extraneural metastases have also been reported. To determine appropriate therapy, CSF cytology and myelography are recommended. If the results are positive, craniospinal radiation therapy should be given.

BRAIN STEM GLIOMA

These neoplasms constitute from 10-20% of pediatric brain tumors. They usually arise in the pons and grow cephalad and caudal, to involve the midbrain and medulla, respectively. They occur during the first decade of life, reaching a peak incidence around age 6 years. They may be diffusely invasive, infiltrating between normal neural structures, or they may grow as a localized or exophytic brain-stem mass lesion. The histologic picture is quite variable, ranging from that of a low grade pilocytic astrocytoma to that of a highly anaplastic glioblastoma multiforme.

Because of this tumor's tendency to infiltrate the brain stem, presenting complaints are related to the tumor's location rather than to increased ICP due to CSF obstruction. Most commonly, the child presents with progressive multiple cranial nerve palsy (usually involving cranial nerves VI and VII) with long tract findings, and ataxia without increased ICP.

Occasionally, the tumor may grow with an exophytic portion in the fourth ventricle, causing a presenting complaint related to increased ICP, or with an exophytic component into the cerebellopontine angle, involving cranial nerves V, VII, and VIII.

In general, the prognosis for patients with this lesion is poor. Untreated children live for 6-18 months from the time of diagnosis. Surgery is indicated in cases of exophytic and cystic lesions or when the diagnosis is in question. Local irradiation with doses of 4000-5500 rads directed to the tumor prolongs survival and reverses signs and symptoms in 75% of children. Recurrences are inevitable, and most children die within the first 3-5 years after treatment. However, up to 30% may survive for more than 5 years.

A benign form of brain-stem tumor that presents as an enhancing exophytic fourth ventricular mass in young children (usually those under 2 years of age) has been described. Long-term survival, after treatment with surgical decompression alone, was reported to have been achieved in this group.

Chemotherapy as an adjunct to radiation therapy has not, as yet, been shown to be of benefit against these tumors; however, when it is used at recurrence, survival may be enhanced.

TUMORS OF THE PINEAL REGION

Primary pineal tumors constitute approximately 1% of primary brain neoplasms in the USA and Europe, but the incidence is higher in Japan. These tumors are of various histologic types. The most common of them are of germ cell origin (germinoma, embryonal carcinoma, choriocarcinoma, teratoma) or originate in primary pineal tissues (pineocytoma, pineoblastoma). However, tumors of glial origin also occur in this region. Although the vast majority are histologically malignant, up to 25% may be encapsulated or benign (meningioma, epidermoid, dermoid, benign teratoma). Males are more frequently affected than females.

Regardless of the histology, the clinical features of the various pineal tumors are similar. Because of their location, they produce obstructive hydrocephalus due to involvement of the posterior third ventricle and blockage of the aqueduct of Sylvius. Pressure on the tectum of the brain stem causes a Parinaud's syndrome with loss of upward gaze, convergence nystagmus, and pupillary dilatation. Germinomas may spread to involve the anterior third ventricle, hypothalamus, and suprasellar region, producing either precocious or delayed puberty. Many of the germinal tumors produce CSF markers, such as alpha-fetoprotein and beta-human chorionic gonadotropin, which are useful for making a diagnosis and for evaluation after therapy.

The tumor type can occasionally be delineated with the aid of CT scanning, but in general there is no preoperative test that can be used to accurately differentiate the benign from the malignant neoplasm. For many years, treatment consisted of shunting procedures to control hydrocephalus followed by the administration of local irradiation. If definite evidence of malignancy can be determined preoperatively by CSF cytology, CSF markers, or CSF dissemination (or if a germinoma is considered the most likely diagnosis) then the reasonable course is to waive surgical histologic confirmation and institute radiation therapy. In general, germinomas are highly radiosensitive; the 5-year survival of patients so treated is approximately 80%.

The prognosis for other germ cell tumors is quite poor. The majority recur within 2 years after the completion of radiation therapy. Careful staging of tumor spread with myelography and CSF cytology is essential because these tumors have a high propensity for CSF dissemination.

The Japanese reports suggest that irradiation be used as a diagnostic modality. They suggest that radiation therapy (approximately 1500 rads) will result in the disappearance of germinoma, as documented on a CT scan. If CT scan evidence of tumor persists after irradiation with 1500 rads then they advocate surgical exploration to document tumor histology. Other reports suggest that, unless the diagnosis of germinoma is certain, surgical confirmation of tumor should be performed before irradiation is applied, because of the 25% incidence of benign lesions that can be surgically extirpated. The latter alternative is feasible because of modern microsurgical techniques that allow an approach to the pineal region with a very low risk of morbidity and mortality.

MISCELLANEOUS INFRATENTORIAL TUMORS

Choroid plexus papillomas occasionally develop from the choroid plexus within the roof of the fourth ventricle. In children, they more commonly develop in the lateral ventricles. Except for rare variants, they are histologically benign. The clinical signs and symptoms are those of increased ICP. In rare instances, these tumors develop from the choroid plexus within the foramina of Luschka and present as a mass in the cerebellopontine region. Total surgical excision is the treatment of choice.

Dermoid tumors account for approximately 2% of infratentorial tumors in childhood. Recurrent bouts of meningitis, usually from *Staphylococcus aureus*, should alert the physician to the possible presence of this entity. Dermoid tumors arise in the midline and are always connected via a sinus tract with a cutaneous dimple over the external occipital protuberance. X-rays of the skull may reveal a small defect in the occipital bone in the region of the inion. The CT scan generally reveals a well circumscribed, low-density midline mass in the posterior fossa. Total surgical removal is curative.

Epidermoid tumors, although congenital in origin, usually do not become manifest until adulthood. In contradistinction to the dermoid tumors, they usually occur off the midline, in the cerebellopontine angle, or anterior to the pons. The symptomatology may mimic that of brain-stem glioma; metrizamide CT scanning may help to differentiate these two entities. Surgical excision is the treatment of choice.

Cerebellar hemangioblastoma is predominantly a tumor of adulthood, but it may present during adolescence. The tumors are usually situated in the cerebellar hemispheres, and they may be solid or associated with a large cyst. This tumor is histologically benign. It may not be possible to differentiate it from a cystic cerebellar astrocytoma on a CT scan; however, a cerebral angiogram reveals a characteristic tumor blush. Hemangioblastoma is occasionally associated with von Hippel-Lindau disease, and may produce polycythemia. Total surgical removal is curative.

Acoustic neuromas, when encountered in children, are always associated with von Recklinghausen's disease. They often arise bilaterally. Surgical removal is the treatment of choice.

HEMISPHERIC ASTROCYTOMA

Astrocytomas constitute approximately 8% of the tumors of childhood. They may occur anywhere in the cerebral hemispheres. They arise in white matter and are locally infiltrative. They may be cystic or solid, and microscopic examination reveals fine calcification in approximately 25% of them. Histologically, they range from low-grade astrocytoma (34%) to malignant astrocytoma and glioblastoma multiforme (35%). The other 20% are ependymomas (see p. 151). Males are more commonly affected than females. There appears to be a greater incidence of this entity in children with neurofibromatosis, tuberous sclerosis, and familial polyposis.

Symptoms of this tumor are headache, seizures, behavioral changes, nausea, vomiting, and loss of recent memory. In young children, seizures, motor and speech delay, and an increasing head circumference are suggestive of supratentorial tumors. Papilledema is present in 75% of the cases at the time of diagnosis. Signs are specific for the area of brain involved, but may include hemiparesis, hemisensory loss, hemianopsia, and dysphasia.

Treatment consists of surgery with the goal of total removal, followed by local irradiation for tumors of a higher grade. Reoperation for recurrent low-grade lesions may improve survival. Complete removal is rarely possible. With current therapy, survival ranges from 1-5 years; however, histologically benign lesions (pilocytic cystic astrocytoma) may be associated with survival in excess of 10 years.

OPTIC NERVE AND CHIASMATIC GLIOMA

These tumors account for approximately 5% of intracranial tumors that arise during childhood. They may be situated entirely within the intraorbital portion of the optic nerve, or they may involve the nerve on either side of the optic foramen. Alternatively, they may originate in the optic chiasm and remain localized, or extend diffusely within both optic nerves as well as the chiasm. They may grow as exophytic masses from the chiasm and compress the anterior third ventricle, causing obstructive hydrocephalus.

Their microscopic configuration is quite variable, ranging from low-grade pilocytic astrocytoma with Rosenthal fibers (usually tumors within the optic nerve alone) to anaplastic astrocytomas (more commonly chiasmatic lesions). Some authors classify the most benign of these lesions as hamartomas. Children with von Recklinghausen's disease have an increased incidence of optic pathway gliomas. (See Chapter 9.)

The **clinical presentation** depends on the portion of the anterior optic pathways involved by tumor. Tumors involving primarily the optic nerve usually present with nonpulsatile exophthalmos and visual loss.

Gliomas arising in the optic chiasm produce bilateral visual loss. Extension that involves the anterior third ventricle may produce hypothalamic dysfunction (diabetes insipidus, obesity, precocious puberty) or symptoms of increased ICP resulting from obstructive hydrocephalus. Plain x-rays of the skull with views of the optic foramina are diagnostic if the tumor involves the nerve as it passes through the optic foramen. High-resolution CT scanning with orbital views is the diagnostic procedure of choice.

Treatment is controversial. Some authors contend that these are benign lesions with little or no growth potential, and should be left alone. Others recommend that tumors involving the anterior optic nerve be excised, in an attempt to prevent posterior extension and involvement of the optic chiasm. Large tumors involving the chiasm are unresectable — but as these lesions may be confused with craniopharyngioma, surgical biopsy is a reasonable course to follow when the diagnosis is uncertain. Tumors causing third ventricular obstruction are best treated with CSF shunting procedures. In most instances, these lesions may be managed expectantly to observe their growth potential, as the history is quite variable. Tumors causing progressive visual loss should be treated with radiation therapy.

HYPOTHALAMIC GLIOMA

It is often difficult to differentiate the hypothalamic glioma from the chiasmatic glioma. Over 75% of these tumors occur in children under the age of 12 years, and children of both sexes are affected equally. Histologically, these tumors vary from benign hamartoma to frank glioblastoma multiforme; however, the majority are low-grade astrocytomas. Two distinct presenting syndromes are recognized. The diencephalic syndrome of Russell occurs most frequently in children less than 1 year old, although it has been reported in children up to the age of 4 years. It is characterized by progressive and profound emaciation (in spite of the child's having a good appetite and adequate caloric intake), accelerated skeletal growth, hyperactivity, hypotension, and hypoglycemia. Tumor progression may cause visual loss, optic atrophy, diabetes insipidus, and seizures. Older children present with precocious puberty associated with visual loss, obesity, diabetes insipidus, extrapyramidal movement disorders, and fluid and electrolyte imbalance.

CT scanning is the diagnostic procedure of choice. Endocrinologic evaluation may reveal elevations of plasma leutinizing hormone (LH), follicle-stimulating hormone (FSH), and testosterone in children presenting with precocious puberty. Surgery is indicated to confirm the diagnosis and to exclude the possibility of a tumor with a more favorable prognosis, such as craniopharyngioma, teratoma, or hamartoma. Over one-half of children with hypothalamic glioma die within 1 year of presentation, although a few children treated with local irradiation have a more prolonged survival.

CRANIOPHARYNGIOMA

Craniopharyngiomas constitute 5% of intracranial neoplasms that occur in children. This tumor arises from the hypophyseal stalk (the remnant of Rathke's pouch). The majority are situated above the diaphragma sellae.

They may grow as dumbbell-shaped tumors (in any direction). Rarely, they are totally intrasellar. They are well encapsulated, slow-growing tumors that frequently have a cystic component. Plain x-rays of the skull demonstrate abnormalities of the sella turcica and/or suprasellar calcification in over 94% of patients. On the CT scan, a cystic, calcified lesion with a slightly enhancing solid component is frequently seen.

In the young child, the usual presenting complaints are related to increased ICP resulting from obstruction of the CSF pathways. Older children usually present with the triad of growth failure, progressive visual loss, and raised ICP.

Some surgeons advocate operating for total removal whenever feasible. Despite successful radical excision, the rate of recurrence within 10 years is still between 23 and 50%. The 5-year and 10-year survival rates are 88% and 75% respectively. Subtotal excision and postoperative irradiation produces similar results and is usually associated with less severe postoperative endocrine dysfunction. Children in whom total removal of tumor is confirmed by CT scan should not receive postoperative irradiation unless tumor recurrence is documented.

PRIMARY CEREBRAL NEUROBLASTOMA

Cerebral neuroblastomas, also known as primitive neuroectodermal tumors, may occur anywhere in the cerebral hemispheres. The majority present during the first 5 years of life. They are highly cellular, poorly differentiated tumors that resemble medulloblastoma.

Cerebral neuroblastomas appear to be well demarcated from brain tissue, but usually have invasive regions in the periphery. They appear as densely enhancing lesions on the contrast-enhanced CT scan. Treatment should consist of total surgical removal, whenever feasible, followed by localized irradiation. Some authors suggest that this tumor has a propensity to spread within the subarachnoid space and that, for this reason irradiation of the craniospinal axis should be given postoperatively. However, we have seen no evidence of such a propensity.

The reported survival rate for patients with this tumor is less than 10% at 1 year. In our experience, however, over 80% of patients treated with surgery and local irradiation were alive at 1 year, the best results being in older children with a cystic tumor that was totally resected.

MENINGIOMA

Meningiomas account for approximately 1% of intracranial tumors in childhood. Sixty-six percent of these tumors are located in the supratentorial compartment, 19% are infratentorial, and 17% are intraventricular tumors. The mean age of patients at diagnosis is 10.9 years. Males and females are affected equally. The most common presenting complaints are increased ICP, visual disturbance, cranial nerve palsies (excluding the optic nerve), and seizures. Calcification is commonly found in children older than 5 years of age. The tumor has a frequent association with neurofibromatosis. Total resection, when possible, may be curative.

MISCELLANEOUS SUPRATENTORIAL TUMORS

Tuberous sclerosis is a familial phakomatosis characterized by adenoma sebaceum, tumors of the heart and kidneys, and neuroglial nodules (tubers) in the brain. The usual clinical presentation is mental deficiency, epilepsy, and adenoma sebaceum. The tubers are found at the crests of the cerebral gyri and in the subependymal area surrounding the lateral ventricles.

Characteristically, these neoplastic lesions are composed of giant-cell astrocytes. They are slow growing and benign, but may enlarge to obstruct the foramen of Monro, causing hydrocephalus. They are usually densely calcified and nodular. Surgical exploration confirms the tissue diagnosis and may be useful in unblocking the foramen of Monro. Radiation therapy has not been effective against these tumors. (See Chapter 9.)

Epidermoid and dermoid tumors usually occur along the dorsal or ventral midline, but can occasionally arise within the cerebral hemispheres. Their most frequent sites include the sylvian fissure, lateral ventricles, and the third ventricle.

Pituitary tumors occur rarely among the pediatric population, although endocrine-active tumors causing Cushing's disease have been reported. CT scans performed with coronal and sagittal reformations are helpful for diagnosis and evaluation, especially in determining suprasellar and lateral extension of tumor. Transsphenoidal resection is feasible for microadenomas and for pituitary tumors with mild suprasellar extension. Tumors with major suprasellar extension should be approached by the subfrontal route. Radiation therapy is indicated in cases of subtotally resected tumors.

Suprasellar germinomas may occur as isolated lesions, but the vast majority occur in association with a pineal germinoma. The most common presentation is diabetes insipidus. This tumor is exquisitely radiosensitive, and the 10-year survival rate is in excess of 60%.

Hamartomas of the hypothalamus most commonly occur in males. The usual presentation is precocious puberty. Endocrine studies reveal normal adult levels of LH and FSH. Serum prolactin also may be elevated. CT scanning usually reveals a small mass attached to the tuber cinereum; this mass may show contrast enhancement. Methods for the chemical suppression of LH and FSH to reverse the signs and symptoms of precocious puberty are under investigation.

Suprasellar and parasellar teratomas, epidermoids, and lipomas have been reported. These lesions resemble those previously discussed. Surgical extirpation is the treatment of choice.

EPIDERMOID AND DERMOID TUMORS

These two tumors constitute the most frequent skull tumors occurring in childhood. Epidermoid cysts are lined solely by stratified squamous epithelium, and dermoid cysts include skin appendages, such as hair follicles and sebaceous glands or sweat glands. Collectively, these lesions are often called 'pearly tumors.' Both types are thought to result from inclusion of epithelial elements within the scalp or skull. Most of these tumors involve only the outer table of the skull and diploic space. Rarely, they may involve the dura and grow as a dumbbell tumor.

Dermoid tumors tend to occur in the midline, in the region of the anterior fontanelle. Epidermoid tumors are most frequently found in the frontal bone, placed laterally between the supraorbital rim and coronal suture, but they may arise anywhere in the skull. In-driven skin elements from prior scalp and skull trauma may be responsible for the development of either of these lesions. Their histopathology is similar to that described earlier in this chapter.

These lesions are typically nontender, immobile, and firm to palpation. They may become secondarily infected and produce tenderness and erythema. Rarely, osteomyelitis may develop.

Plain x-rays of the skull reveal a characteristic radiolucency with a well-circumscribed, sclerotic border. CT scanning with bone windows demonstrate erosion through the inner table. Surgical excision is indicated not only for cosmetic reasons, but also to prevent infection. The entire lesion must be removed or recurrence is inevitable. In older children, or if the lesion is large, a cranioplasty may be necessary to repair the skull defect.

HISTIOCYTOSIS

Histiocytosis constitutes a spectrum of diseases comprising both granulomatosis lesions with histiocytic proliferation confined to bone and widely disseminated lesions involving the liver and spleen. The etiology of the disease process is undetermined. There is no evidence of hereditary or familial transmission, and an infectious etiology has never been documented.

Eosinophilic granuloma is the most benign form of this disease. In 50% of patients, the lesions are confined to bone. The lesions may be either solitary or multiple, and they occur most commonnly in the skull, long bones, pelvis, and spine. Plain x-rays reveal a punched-out, radiolucent area without sclerotic margins. It is impossible to differentiate this tumor from a malignant bone tumor radiographically.

Eosinophilic granulomas are exquisitely sensitive to radiation. If the diagnosis is in question, a small biopsy or simple curettage is sufficient to establish the tumor type. Small doses of local irradiation (approximately 500 rads) are curative. The long-term prognosis is excellent in cases of a solitary lesion.

Hand-Schuller-Christian disease is characterized by the triad of osseous lesions, chronic otitis media, and diabetes insipidus. The skull lesions tend to be large, irregular, and multiple. They may involve the orbit resulting in proptosis, or the mastoid portion of the temporal bone, with resultant infection. Involvement of the hypothalamus (infundibular region) may result in obesity, hypogonadism, and diabetes insipidus. Biopsy to confirm the diagnosis, followed by local irradiation is the treatment of choice.

The most severe form of histiocytosis is termed **Letterer-Siwe disease.** This disorder usually appears in a child of 1-3 years of age, who presents with multiple areas of cerebral involvement. Disseminated lesions in bone, liver, and spleen are identified. Systemic chemotherapy and/or local irradiation is occasionally beneficial. The prognosis depends on the extent of visceral involvement. Death is usually the result of either organ failure or infection.

FIBROUS DYSPLASIA

This entity is characterized histologically by an accumulation of fibrous connective tissue within one or more bones. It is most likely a mesenchymal development defect. It affects females more often than males. There is a tendency for the osseous lesions to progress in parallel to normal skeletal growth. After the child reaches puberty, the lesions usually become densely ossified.

These lesions usually become symptomatic when the child is between 5 and 10 years of age. The most common site of involvement is the skull base — especially the frontal fossa, the wings of the splenoid bone, and the orbit. Characteristically, the lesion causes a mild cranial deformity usually seen as prominence of the forehead and narrowing of the palpebral fissure. Involvement of the maxilla and mandible is common. The complication of greatest concern is involvement of the orbit and optic nerve foramen, which causes progrsssive proptosis, decreased ocular mobility, and visual loss. The base of the skull may be involved, causing hearing loss or other deficits attributable to cranial nerve involvement.

Plain x-rays reveal diffuse sclerosis of bone and thickening of the skull. CT scanning is helpful in defining involvement of cranial nerve foramina. The differential diagnosis must take into consideration meningioma in bone, osteoma, hemangioma, osteomyelitis, and metastatic tumor. When the diagnosis is uncertain, biopsy is indicated.

Orbital involvement causing visual loss is an indication for optic nerve decompression. Severe proptosis responds to orbital decompression. Radiation therapy is of no benefit against this disease entity. The process usually arrests or regresses in late adolescence or early adulthood.

HEMANGIOMA

This tumor is common in adults, and is occasionally identified in children. It produces a firm, nontender skull mass that expands the diploic space and grows inward as an endosteoma. It does not invade dura. Plain x-rays of the skull are diagnostic, and reveal a well-circumscribed, honeycombed defect involving the diploic space. Surgical excision, with cranioplasty if the lesion is large, is the treatment of choice.

PRIMARY SARCOMAS

Osteogenic sarcomas, fibrosarcomas, and angiosarcomas have been reported to occur occasionally in children. Plain x-rays of the skull reveal irregular lesions with poorly defined margins. The lesions may be lytic, blastic, or both. Surgical excision followed by local irradiation and/or chemotherapy may be beneficial. In general, the prognosis is poor.

OSTEOMA

This is a benign, slow-growing exostosis which may arise from the inner or outer table of the skull. Osteomas are identified when a mass beneath the scalp becomes visible or when they are noted as an incidental finding on plain x-rays of the skull. On the x-rays, they appear as well-defined, radio-dense lesions. Surgery is indicated for cosmetic reasons and in the remote instance of endostosis causing neurologic findings related to compression.

SPINAL CORD TUMORS

Intraspinal tumors in children are relatively rare, occurring one-sixth as frequently as intracranial tumors. Males are more frequently affected than females. They most often present between the ages of 3 and 5 years. The prevalence of these tumors in early childhood is best explained by the high incidence of congenital neoplasms in the pediatric population.

Spinal tumors are divided into two main groups: **intradural tumors,** with intramedullary, extramedullary, and subarachnoid subdivisions, and **extradural tumors.** Among children, in contrast to adults, there is a high incidence of intradural intramedullary tumors (such as gliomas), and a much lower incidence of intradural extramedullary tumors (such as meningioma and neurofibroma). Intramedullary tumors constitute 35% of spinal tumors reported; intradural extramedullary tumors, 30%; extradural tumors, 30%; and subarachnoid tumors, 5%. Approximately 30% of spinal tumors occur in each of the major regions of the spinal cord (cervical, thoracic, and lumbar), and 10% arise in the sacral region.

At least 70% of intraspinal tumors in children are histologically benign (Table 8-3). Anaplastic tumors are almost always extradural in origin. Because the majority of pediatric spinal tumors are slow-growing, the early symptoms are apt to be missed. A high index of suspicion should be maintained in evaluating a child with a recently acquired gait dysfunction, back or radicular pain, progressive spinal deformity, segmental sensory complaints, progressive muscle weakness, or spastic sphincter disturbances (Table 8-4). In general, the course of the illness is shorter with extradural tumors than with intradural lesions.

Two unique syndromes must be considered. Firstly, in rare instances an intraspinal tumor may present with signs and symptoms of increased ICP resembling benign intracranial hypertension. There may be mild hydrocephalus, and papilledema may be noted during the physical examination. This syndrome may be associated with intradural tumors arising at any level of the spine, but it appears to occur more frequently in cases of lesions situated in the cervical area. The exact mechanism producing this syndrome has not been defined, but two alternatives have been proposed. The majority of these patients have a significant increase in CSF protein, which may be the causal factor in producing communicating hydrocephalus. The other proposed mechanism is the presence of small, recurrent subarachnoid hemorrhages. Secondly, recurrent bouts of meningitis, usually due to *Escherichia coli* or *Staphylococcus aureus*, should raise the suspicion of a dermal sinus tract associated with an intraspinal dermoid tumor.

Plain x-rays of the spine reveal an abnormality in 50-70% of children with intraspinal tumors (Table 8-5). Electromyography is occasionally

Table 8-3 Intraspinal Tumors Arising in Children*

Tumor type	Incidence (%)
Intradural tumors	
Intramedullary	
Gliomas (astrocytoma, ependymoma, glioblastoma, unclassified)	24.3
Extramedullary	
Meningioma	3.2
Neurinoma†	8.3
Lipomas	3.6
Epidermoid/dermoid†	8.9
Teratoma	2.5
Blood vessel tumors	3.1
Ganglioneuromas	1.3
Subarachnoid	
Medulloblastoma	1.9
Extradural tumors	
Sarcoma†	14.9
Lymphoma	1.8
Carcinoma	0.4
Neuroblastoma	13.1
Miscellaneous	12.7

*Adapted from Boggan JE, et al: Intraspinal tumors in children. Western J Med 133:108-114, 1980.
†May be intradural and extradural.

Table 8-4 Symptoms and Signs of Intraspinal Cord Tumor in Children

Clinical signs	Incidence (%)
Most prominent symptoms	
Gait disturbance	66
Pain (back and/or radicular)	51
Sphincter disturbance	31
Most frequent physical findings	
Altered deep tendon reflexes	57
Motor weakness	56
Sensory dysfunction	41

helpful in making the diagnosis, and cystometrograms should be obtained if sphincter dysfunction is suspected. Myelography is the definitive diagnostic test. Most recently, myelography, performed using water-soluble contrast agents, in combination with CT scanning has proved to be the most sensitive technique for determining the position and characteristics of intraspinal lesions and the extent to which the lesion involves the bony spine. Lumbar puncture and CSF analysis for glucose, protein cell count, and cytology should be delayed until it is determined that myelography is necessary to confirm the diagnosis.

INTRAMEDULLARY TUMORS

ASTROCYTOMA

This is a benign, slow-growing neoplasm that usually arises in the cervical and upper-thoracic spinal cord. It grows as a solid or cystic neoplasm and may involve a few spinal segments or the entire spinal cord. The tumor has a predilection for the cervical region. Males and females are equally affected. There is a slightly elevated incidence of astrocytoma in patients with classic neurofibromatosis.

Treatment should consist of decompressive laminectomy and, for low-grade tumors, gross total removal. It is classically taught that the margins of the tumor are indistinct. However, recent evidence suggests that total resection, even of extensive tumors, is feasible using microsurgical techniques. Subtotally resected tumors or those showing anaplastic histologic features should be irradiated postoperatively. In subtotally resected tumors treated with postoperative radiation therapy, the recurrence-free survival rate at 2-5 years is 61%. The long-term prognosis for totally resected tumors is uncertain at present.

EPENDYMOMA

Ependymomas tend to arise in the lumbosacral region at the conus medullaris, and may grow to involve the cauda equina. Less frequently, they occur in the cervical region. Those arising in the lumbosacral region tend to undergo mucoid degeneration which gives them their characteristic myxopapillary appearance. A significant incidence of spontaneous hemorrhage has been associated with these tumors. They tend to be well encapsulated, and complete surgical removal is usually possible using microsurgical techniques. Postoperative radiation therapy is indicated only in subtotally resected tumors. The rate of recurrence-free survival at 5 years in irradiated patients is 85%.

HEMANGIOBLASTOMA

Intraspinal hemangioblastomas are extremely rare. Over 60% arise within the cord; the other 40% are extramedullary or extradermal. Approximately one-third of patients have von Hippel-Lindau disease. Treatment consists

Table 8-5   Abnormalities Associated with Spinal Cord Tumors
Visible on Plain x-rays

Scoliosis	Soft tissue mass
Pedicle erosion	Ventral scalloping
Widening of interpedicular distance	Enlarged nerve-root foramina

of total resection. Radiation therapy for subtotally resected tumors has not produced prolonged recurrence-free survival.

EPIDERMOID/DERMOID CYSTS

Both of these lesions result from inclusion of epithelial elements at the time of closure of the neural tube (at the third to fifth week of fetal life). Epidermoid cysts are lined only by stratified squamous epithelium, whereas dermoid cysts include skin appendages, such as hair follicles, sebaceous glands, or sweat glands. Lower spinal cysts have been reported secondary to iatrogenic penetration of skin fragments in that region, usually due to tests for meningitis requiring repeated spinal puncture.

Dermoid cysts are slightly more common than epidermoid cysts in the spinal cord. Dermoids are most commonly found in the lumbosacral region. Their location may be intramedullary or extramedullary. Symptoms usually begin in the first two decades of life. There is frequently co-existing spina bifida occulta and, on occasion, associated syringomyelia has been noted. These cysts are frequently associated with a dermal sinus overlying the cyst that may act as a source of recurrent meningitis. They are usually well localized, and calcification may be noted. Multiple cysts are occasionally found.

Epidermoid cysts are also associated with spina bifida occulta and dermal sinuses. The cystic contents consist of desquamated keratin that, if it spills into the CSF pathways, may cause a chemical meningitis. Treatment of both entities consists of total resection; however, this approach is often not technically feasible following recurrent episodes of meningitis due to dense arachnoiditis. Subtotally resected lesions recur after a variable period of latency.

NEUROENTERIC CYSTS

These tumors are a result of faulty separation of primitive entoderm from the notochordal plate. This may result in a neuroenteric fistula or sinus tract that enters the spinal canal through an anterior bony defect and ends as an intraspinal cyst, although more often there is only an intraspinal cyst. Neuroenteric cysts most commonly occur at the level of the primitive lung bud (C5-T2) but they have been reported to occur throughout the spinal axis. They are most frequently intramedullary, but they may present as an extramedullary or extradural mass.

The cysts are variable in size. They are lined by a single layer of columnar or cuboidal epithelium resembling primitive lung-bud tissue or pseudostratified, mucus-secreting epithelium of intestinal origin. They may contain cloudy or clear fluid. Patients present with symptoms and signs of spinal cord compression or recurrent bouts of sterile meningitis. Plain x-rays of the spine and CT scans may reveal a circular defect in the anterior portion of the vertebral body. Treatment consists of complete removal of the cyst and closure of the anterior dural defect, if present.

LIPOMA

Lipomas are rare tumors. The majority are situated in the thoracic region. At least one-third of patients have other accompanying congenital anomalies, particularly spina bifida occulta. Lipomas are usually intradural extramedullary masses. However, intramedullary tumors have been reported. Histologically, they consist of benign adipose tissue with occasional striated or unstriated muscle fibers, neuroglia, and ganglion cells. They frequently calcify or form bone. Treatment consists of laminectomy and resection of as much of the lipoma as is technically safe and feasible. However, lumbar lesions are usually deeply embedded in the conus medullaris, making total removal impossible. The dura is usually repaired using a dural graft to allow for a generous decompression of the spinal elements.

NEURINOMA

When encountered in the child, neurinomas are usually associated with neurofibromatosis. These tumors may be single or multiple, and they usually arise from the posterior sensory rootlets. They may extend through the intravertebral foramina as dumbbell tumors. Histologically, they resemble acoustic neuromas. They do not undergo malignant degeneration.

Treatment consists of total removal, except in patients with neurofibromatosis, who frequently have multiple lesions. In these patients, surgery should be performed only on those lesions that are producing intractable pain or spinal cord compression. What benefit radiation therapy may have against subtotally resected tumors is uncertain.

MENINGIOMA

These tumors, which are frequent in adulthood, rarely occur in children. Female children are more often affected than males. The majority of meningiomas arise in the thoracic region. Treatment consists of total surgical removal.

SECONDARY TUMORS

METASTATIC BRAIN TUMORS

Cerebral metastases occur in approximately 6% of children with systemic malignancies. The most common tumors to metastasize to the brain are neuroblastoma, embryonal carcinoma, sarcoma, and Wilm's tumor. They most often involve the central hemispheres. Involvement of the pulmonary system usually precedes metastasis to the CNS, suggesting that metastasis occurs primarily through the vascular system. Surgery is indicated when the diagnosis is in question or if the lesion is solitary and accessible in an otherwise healthy patient. Whole-brain irradiation should follow surgery. With radiosensitive tumors or multiple lesions of known etiology, irradiation should be the primary therapy. The usual radiation dosage is 3000-4000 rads administered over the course of 3-4 weeks.

METASTATIC SPINAL CORD TUMORS

Spinal neuroblastoma is the most common cause of nontraumatic paraplegia in childhood. The tumors may be either solitary or multiple, and they involve the spine by extension through the intravertebral foramina. Their primary site is in the suprarenal area or along the sympathetic chain. They cause extradural spinal compression. Plain x-rays and CT scans of the spine usually demonstrate bone erosion associated with a paraspinal mass. Myelography is essential to delineate the extent of spinal cord involvement. Treatment consists of radical excision of the tumor, when feasible, followed by radiation therapy. Corticosteroids should be administered if the physical examination reveals spinal cord compression. Steroids are tapered rapidly during the course of radiation therapy. The prognosis is excellent in children under 2 years of age.

Lymphoma/sarcoma These tumors are rapidly growing, invasive lesions that may involve the spine by direct extension or by blood-borne metastases. In cases of lymphoma, involvement of the spinal cord may develop from the extension of tumor along nerve roots through the intravertebral foramina. In this instance, plain x-rays will show no spinal abnormality. CT scanning is more sensitive in diagnosing involvement of the bony spine and small paraspinal masses or invasion of the paraspinal muscle. As these tumors are very radiosensitive, radiation therapy is usually the primary mode of therapy. However, laminectomy is indicated if the diagnosis is uncertain or if rapid spinal cord compression is observed.

CNS leukemia In cases of acute lymphocytic leukemia, there is frequently subarachnoid seeding to the spine. Children usually present with radicular pain or signs and symptoms of multiple lesions located at various sites throughout the CNS (spine and brain). Myelography is often unrevealing. CSF analysis for glucose, protein, cell count, and cytology are usually diagnostic. Although the cytology determinations may be negative, there is often an increase in CSF protein content and/or decrease in CSF glucose levels. Repeated lumbar punctures for CSF cytology may be necessary to confirm the diagnosis. Treatment consists of craniospinal irradiation and/or intrathecal chemotherapy (methotrexate, cytosine arabinoside, thio-TEPA). Intrathecal chemotherapy is administered most effectively by placement of drug into the lateral ventricle using an Ommaya reservoir.

REFERENCES

Boggan JE, et al: Intraspinal tumors in children. Western J Med 133:108-114, 1980.

Matson DD: *Neurosurgery of Infancy and Childhood.* Charles C. Thomas, Springfield, 1969, pp 403-693.

Menkes JH: *Textbook of Child Neurology,* 2nd Ed. Lea & Febiger, Philadelphia, 1980.

Milhorat TH: *Pediatric Neurosurgery.* Davis, Philadelphia, 1978, pp 211-310.

Russell DS, Rubinstein LJ: *Pathology of Tumors of the Nervous System,* 4th Ed. Williams & Wilkins, Baltimore, 1977.

Wilson CB: Diagnosis and surgical treatment of childhood brain tumors. Cancer 35: 950-956, 1975.

9

Neurocutaneous Disorders

Bruce O. Berg, MD

The neurocutaneous syndromes, or phakomatoses (Gr. *phakos* = lens-shaped, mole, mother-spot, freckle) are characterized by their dysplastic nature and proclivity to tumor formation of the central and peripheral nervous systems, skin, and viscera. Except for Sturge-Weber syndrome, the phakomatoses are inherited, although sporadic cases do occur. There are reports of 'overlap' or 'crossover' of clinical manifestations of these syndromes but this can be explained on the basis of chance. Each syndrome should be considered as a distinct entity (see Table 9-1).

TUBEROUS SCLEROSIS

SEIZURES

Convulsive phenomena are common and may appear shortly after birth or anytime thereafter. In one large series of patients with tuberous sclerosis, convulsive phenomena occurred in 88%. Infantile spasms are particularly common in the infant or very young child and later assume the quality of other seizure types.

Though most patients with tuberous sclerosis who are mentally deficient have seizures, there appears to be no correlation between severity of convulsive phenomena and the degree of mental subnormality. However, mental retardation occurs more frequently in patients with seizures occurring before the age of 2 years. There is no one seizure type, other than infantile spasms in the very young patient, thought to be typical or particularly common in tuberous sclerosis. Although often recalcitrant to treatment, responsiveness to anticonvulsant medication cannot be predicted. There is no characteristic or typical EEG pattern other than hypsarrhythmia found in patients with infantile spasms.

MENTAL RETARDATION

Though mental retardation was earlier thought to be an essential component of this disease, about one third of affected patients have normal intelligence; however, some patients may appear quite normal early in life and only later in the first decade manifest signs of mental subnormality and/or convulsive disorder.

SKIN LESIONS

Skin abnormalities are common and occur in about 90% of patients. The most common lesion is adenoma sebaceum, which is usually seen between the ages of 2 and 5 years, appearing initially as a faint erythematous papular rash over the cheeks, nasolabial folds, and/or chin. Other parts of the face can also be affected. The lesions are angiofibromatous in nature rather than being truly adenomatous, and they frequently enlarge with time so that some may become 5-10 mm, or larger, in diameter; uncommonly, some patients have no adenoma sebaceum.

Another common skin lesion is the hypopigmented leaf-shaped macule which occurs in about 85% of patients and is seen more commonly on the trunk than limbs. These hypopigmented spots are often the first cutaneous clue of the disease; they are particularly enhanced under a Wood's light. The lesions have a normal number of melanocytes, but decreased tyrosinase activity and a reduction in melanosomes.

Other skin lesions include the shagreen patch, an isolated 'leathery' plaque usually found over the lumbosacral or gluteal region, cafe-au-lait spots, fibromas, and angiomas. Subungual or periungual fibromas (Koenen tumors) are found in about 20% of patients, usually first noted during adolescence, involving toes more often than fingers.

TUMORS

Cerebral lesions, or tubers, may be found within the cortical gyri, but are more often found in the region of the lamina terminalis or embedded within the basal ganglia or thalamus, often projecting into the ventricle. These subependymal hamartomas may slowly increase in size and some may undergo malignant transformation, in rare instances to glioblastoma multiforme. In one reported series, intracranial tumors occurred in 15% of patients. Unilateral megalencephaly (enlargement of one hemisphere) with microscopic features of tuberous sclerosis has been reported.

The microscopic features of the tuber are notable for decreased numbers of neurons and an increase in astrocytic nuclei with groups of large, bizarre-shaped cells, containing two or three nuclei with prominent nucleoli. Some of the cells contain cytoplasmic vacuoles. These giant, or 'monster' cells are more frequent near the center of the tuber. There is commonly a proliferation of fibrillary astrocytes, and abnormalities of myelination and cortical stratification.

Tumors may also occur in other organs including the kidney and heart; hamartomas are less often found in other organs. Renal tumors have been reported in 60-80% of patients, are relatively indolent, and may be unrecognized unless a search is made for them. These tumors are often histologically complex, containing elements of smooth muscle, fat, and blood vessels. Some may undergo degeneration.

Cardiac rhabdomyomas occur in one-third to one-half of patients, and are single, multiple, or the myocardium may be diffusely involved. This tumor has been found in patients as young as 4 days old. Echocardiography has greatly increased the ability to detect the tumor and has improved understanding of their natural history. Clinical presentation depends upon the number, size, and location of the tumor(s). They are commonly asymptomatic, but may be associated with cardiac dysrhythmias.

Table 9-1 Neurocutaneous Syndromes

Syndrome	Clinical features	Inheritance
Albright's syndrome (fibrous dysplasia)	Cutaneous pigmentation, polyostotic fibrous dysplasia, precocious puberty in females. Mental subnormality & convulsions sometimes present.	Not inherited female predominance
Bloch-Sulzberger syndrome (incontinentia pigmenti)	Vesicular or bullous pigmented skin lesions; grey-tan colored whorls or waves of skin pigmentation. CNS anomalies with possible mental deficiency, fits, & ocular lesions. Increased number of chromosomal breaks.	x-linked dominant
Bonnet-Dechaume-Blanc syndrome (Wyburn-Mason syndrome)	Retinal arteriovenous malformations associated with other cerebrovascular anomalies; facial angioma may be present.	Not inherited
Bregeat syndrome	Angiomas of the oculo-orbital vessels, ipsilateral cerebral angioma, contralateral facial angioma.	Not inherited
Cobb's syndrome (cutaneomeningeal angiomatosis)	Cutaneous angioma associated with spinal angioma of corresponding spinal level.	Not inherited
De Sanctis-Cacchione syndrome	Xeroderma pigmentosum, ataxia, dysarthria, mental deficiency. Hypoplastic genitalia are commonly seen.	? Autosomal recessive
Divry-van Bogaert syndrome	Cutis marmoratus, leptomeningeal angiomatosis, & leukodystrophy with spasticity, dementia, & fits.	x-linked recessive
Fabry's syndrome (angiokeratoma corporis diffusum)	Red-black papular eruption over trunk, limbs, & genitalia; sensory neuropathy with burning or shooting pains; cerebrovascular episodes & progressive renal & cardiovascular disease. Deficiency of α-galactosidase A.	x-linked

Syndrome	Description	Inheritance
Gruber's syndrome (splanchno-cystic dysencephaly)	Craniofacial abnormalities (microcephaly, encephalocele, meningocele, facial clefts), ocular anomalies; associated cystic changes of kidney, liver and/or pancreas; skeletal abnormalities, polydactyly and hypoplastic genitalia are commonly seen.	Autosomal recessive
Hemorrhagic telangiectases (Osler-Weber-Rendu syndrome)	Telangiectasia of skin & mucous membranes commonly associated with recurrent epistaxis. Vascular anomalies are found in lung, liver, & less commonly in brain & spinal cord.	Autosomal dominant
Klippel-Trenaunay-Weber syndrome	Limb hypertrophy with cutaneous & subcutaneous hemangiomas, varicosities, phlebectasia & occasionally arteriovenous fistula. Usually unilateral but any or all limbs can be affected. Other abnormalities include lymphangiomas, macrodactyly, syndactyly, or polydactyly. Most patients have normal mentality. Relationship to Sturge-Weber syndrome is unclear.	Not inherited
Krabbe-Bartels syndrome (multiple circumscribed lipomatosis)	Multiple lipomas, pigmented nevi & fibromas of proximal limbs & upper trunk (peripheral). Dysraphic abnormalities, (cerebral & spinal) with mental deficiency.	Not inherited
Linear nevus syndrome	Linear facial epidermal nevus, convulsions, & mental retardation. Hydrocephalus has been described.	Not inherited
Maffucci's syndrome	Asymmetrical dyschondroplasia, limb malformations, cutaneous nevi, angiomas of skin, viscera, & CNS. Malignant tumors can develop.	Not inherited
Neurocutaneous melanosis	Large, sometimes multiple, cutaneous pigmented nevi with melanotic cells in meninges; no evidence of malignant melanoma.	Not inherited
Xeroderma pigmentosum	Cutaneous telangiectases, atrophy, ulcerations, & extreme photosensitivity; mental deficiency, ataxia, dysarthria, & convulsions; associated with endocrine abnormalities.	Autosomal recessive

Reproduced with permission from Berg B: Neurocutaneous syndromes. *In* Swaiman KF, Wright FS (Eds.) *The Practice of Pediatric Neurology.* Mosby, St. Louis, 1982.

Gingival fibromas or papillomas are found in about 10% of patients; and dental abnormalities, characterized by pitting, indentations, or craters in the enamel, have been reported from scanning electron microscope observations.

OCULAR LESIONS

Abnormalities of the eye may occur and assume several forms, including a flattened yellow-green patch, found either centrally or peripherally in the fundus, or a nodular tumor (hamartoma) mass found in the region of the nerve head. The larger mulberry shaped tumor may be cystic.

PULMONARY ABNORMALITIES

Occasional involvement of the lung is seen, more commonly in females of normal intelligence; the average age of onset of respiratory symptoms is about 34 years. Exertional dyspnea is the most common symptom but cough and hemoptysis may occur. Cor pulmonale and spontaneous pneumothorax may be the cause of death. Radiographic findings include a fine reticular infiltration, occasionally seen in patients as young as 5 years.

ASSOCIATED CLINICAL ABNORMALITIES

Nonspecific endocrine abnormalities have been reported, including goiter, hypothyroidism, Cushing's syndrome, abnormalities of glucose tolerance tests and pituitary-adrenal function. There are also reports of hypoglycemia with associated pancreatic islet cell tumors and patients with acromegalic gigantism. Endocrine abnormalities appear to be more common than earlier reported.

RADIOGRAPHIC FINDINGS

Skull radiographs demonstrate intracranial calcification in about 60% of patients; other skull changes include areas of increased or decreased bone density. Computerized brain tomography has increased diagnostic accuracy to about 85%, demonstrating hamartomas, some of which are calcified, ventriculomegaly, and subependymal tumors. Mineralization of intracerebral hamartomas has been demonstrated in patients as young as 3 months old; this usually becomes more prominent with time. Areas of diffuse demyelination have been also described, but mineralized subependymal nodules are the most reliable of all CT findings. Periventricular calcification is less specific and cannot be distinguished from other conditions including toxoplasmosis, cytomegalic inclusion disease, and Fahr's syndrome.

Additional abnormal radiographic findings, typical of tuberous sclerosis, include cystic changes of the phalanges and/or metacarpals, usually found in older patients, and sclerotic areas of long bones.

TREATMENT

The incidence of mental retardation in the off-spring of familial cases appears to be no different from that of sporadic cases. Rarely, parents of two affected siblings have no obvious evidence of tuberous sclerosis on physical examination. In this circumstance, a CT brain scan, renal sonography, or echocardiography may be useful to demonstrate the typical lesions associated with the disease.

Management of patients with tuberous sclerosis is often difficult, not only for the patient and family but also for the physician. Convulsions are treated with anticonvulsant medications (see Chapter 10) in accordance with accepted therapeutic standards. Some convulsive disorders are recalcitrant to treatment however. The patient and entire family should have the benefit of genetic counseling but only after a diagnosis has been properly established.

VON RECKLINGHAUSEN'S DISEASE (Neurofibromatosis)

von Recklinghausen's disease is a pleomorphic condition characterized by a variety of skin changes, single or multiple tumors of the peripheral and/or central nervous systems, and abnormalities of bone as well as endocrine and vascular systems. It is inherited as an autosomal dominant trait with a penetrance approaching 100% and is notable for its marked variability of clinical expression. The frequency of disease is 1 in 2000-3000 births and although both sexes are affected, a slight male preponderance has been reported.

SKIN

Abnormalities of skin are usually present before neurofibromas are recognized, and include cafe-au-lait spots, pendulous fibroma molluscum, hypopigmented spots, or diffuse areas of hyperpigmentation. Some of these hyperpigmented spots are present at birth, but they commonly appear later in the first decade; the number and degree of pigmentation continues to increase during the second decade.

Cafe-au-lait spots, brown pigmented macules, are the most common and characteristic skin lesion of neurofibromatosis. They are oval or irregularly shaped and vary in size from millimeters to centimeters. Persons with six or more cafe-au-lait spots greater than 1.5 cm in the greatest diameter have a presumptive diagnosis of von Recklinghausen's disease. Axillary freckling is another important clinical sign. About 10% of the general population has one or more cafe-au-lait spots.

TUMORS

Neurofibromas may affect any nerve and vary markedly in size. Generally, if peripheral nerves are affected, there is less likelihood of central involvement. Peripheral neurofibromas are usually subcutaneous, readily palpable, and are more commonly found on the trunk than limbs. The lesions are probably more easily observed in tangential view in subdued light, or felt by gentle fingertip palpation of the skin. Plexiform neuromas, a characteristic lesion of neurofibromatosis, affect the limbs more often than trunk and are associated with hypertrophy of involved extremities. Large areas of limbs can be affected by the tortuous nerve trunks which are entwined in a fibrous matrix. Occasionally, neurofibromas affect the autonomic nervous system.

Less commonly involved areas include the tongue, adrenal medulla, and ganglioneuromas may be found particularly in the posterior mediastinum. About 10% of patients have neurofibromas of the gastrointestinal tract. Although it is commonly believed that 13% of patients have neurofibromas which undergo sarcomatous changes, the incidence of malignant change is more realistically 3-5%.

Any cranial nerve can be involved, but the optic nerve is most commonly affected, occurring in 20-30% of patients. The childhood **optic glioma** is usually an indolent tumor; it may involve the optic chiasm and/or hypothalamus and has been reported associated with the diencephalic syndrome of infancy. In this suprasellar site of tumor, one usually cannot distinguish histologically the specific site of tumor origin. Since the optic nerve is histologically different from other cranial nerves, some have included these tumors within the group of intracranial neoplasms.

Acoustic neuromas, particularly bilateral acoustic neuromas, are also associated with von Recklinghausen's disease, but occur less frequently than optic gliomas. They are sometimes associated with multiple meningiomas. There is an increased incidence of intracranial tumors including meningiomas, piloid astrocytomas, diffuse gliomas, glioblastoma multiforme, hamartomas, angiomas, and glial heteropias.

Intraspinal tumors are also more common in these patients compared with the general population, and occur most often in the thoracic region. They may be solitary or multiple, and are found in the intradural and/or extradural spaces. Associated vertebral bony defects and spinal cord anomalies are also found, including syringomyelia. These tumors usually occur in older adolescents or in young adults and are relatively indolent. Signs and symptoms of spinal cord dysfunction secondary to tumor may be easily overlooked.

ADDITIONAL CLINICAL FINDINGS

There is an increased incidence of pheochromocytomas, ranging from 2-5% of patients. Hypertension may also be secondary to dysplastic changes of the renal arteries; other vessels may be similarly affected. Macrocephaly and disorders of growth or sexual development are reported as well as anorexia nervosa. About 11% of patients have specific learning disabilities and 10-24% are mentally subnormal. Convulsions occur in 8-13% of patients.

RADIOGRAPHIC FINDINGS

A variety of abnormal bony radiographic findings occur in this disease. The changes are more commonly dysplastic rather than sequelae of erosion or pressure. The middle cranial fossae may be markedly enlarged or 'ballooned,' the sella turcica may be enlarged, or J-shaped. Missing portions or 'punched-out' lesions may be seen in the sphenoidal wings or frontal bones and are often found near the lambdoid sutures. The optic canals may be enlarged in the presence of optic gliomas. Radiographic abnormalities of the vertebral column include kyphosis, anterior meningocele, scalloping of vertebral bodies, and enlargement of the intervertebral foramina. Scoliosis is found in about 40% of patients.

Rarefaction of long bones can be seen in areas of subperiosteal neurofibromas and occasionally an unusually gracile bowing of the tibia and fibula is seen from early life. Spontaneous fractures and/or pseudarthroses may occur, usually in the middle or lower third of the tibia or fibula. Bones of limbs affected by plexiform neuromas may be enlarged.

TREATMENT

Because of the variety of lesions found in von Recklinghausen's disease, treatment must be individualized. Subcutaneous neurofibromas are best left untouched, unless their removal is indicated because of frequent irritation, abrasion, or for cosmetic reasons. Intracranial and intraspinal lesions are removed in accordance with appropriate neurologic judgement. The childhood optic glioma is usually an indolent tumor and some authorities have recommended long-term observation rather than active therapeutic measures; however, radiation therapy to the tumor site is generally recommended. A variety of orthopedic and plastic surgical procedures may be of benefit for other dysplastic processes.

It is essential that the patient have one primary physician to avoid fragmentation of medical and surgical care. Clinical information regarding the disease should be conveyed to the patient with accuracy and tact. Most patients with neurofibromatosis live relatively normal lives and are less likely to develop severe manifestations than earlier believed. Appropriate genetic counseling must be given.

STURGE - WEBER SYNDROME

The essential components of this syndrome include facial and leptomeningeal angiomas. It occurs sporadically, although one patient has been reported with translocation of the short arm of one D chromosome.

SKIN

The facial angioma is present at birth, usually unilateral and affects at least the supraorbital region. Cushing believed the angioma was confined to one or more divisions of the trigeminal nerve. This view is not completely accurate, however, for the facial angioma may not reach or may extend beyond the facial midline, and it may involve facial areas unrelated to divisions of the trigeminal nerve. The facial angioma is probably related to the configuration of developing facial processes and fissures. Occasionally, cavernous hemangiomas affect the nasopharyngeal mucous membranes.

OCULAR MANIFESTATIONS

Abnormalities of the eyes are common and include choroidal angiomas, congenital glaucoma, and buphthalmos; strabismus, optic atrophy, and iridic heterochromia where increased pigment is seen ipsilateral to the facial angioma. About one-third of patients have homonymous hemianopsia.

CONVULSIVE PHENOMENA

Most patients with Sturge-Weber syndrome have onset of convulsions before the age of 1 year. The child develops normally until the beginning of the seizures, but from that time there is commonly a leveling off, or even regression of development. The fits are usually simple partial (focal) in nature, but may become generalized (tonic/clonic). There is often a transient postictal weakness of the limbs involved in the focal fit (Todd's paralysis), but with increasing frequency and severity of seizures, the weakness usually becomes progressively severe or permanent, resulting in hemiparesis. About one-third of patients will be hemiparetic with concomitant hemiatrophy. One-half or more are mentally retarded and many have behavioral problems.

RADIOGRAPHIC FINDINGS

Of all neuroradiologic studies, CT brain scans have been most valuable to demonstrate structural intracranial changes in this syndrome. Areas of mineralization are more readily seen on CT scans than plain skull radiographs and have been observed as early as the neonatal period. Cerebral calcification has not been demonstrated on plain skull radiographs until after the first year of life. Cerebral hemiatrophy is a common finding.

Angiographic abnormalities include thrombotic lesions, decreased or absent cortical or superficial veins, enlargement of cerebral veins, prominent deep medullary veins, lack of filling the superior sagittal sinus and/or occlusion of the superior sagittal sinus.

NEUROPATHOLOGIC FINDINGS

Characteristic findings include unilateral thickening and increased vascularity of the leptomeninges, primarily overlying the occipital and/or parietal lobes. The frontal lobe is less commonly involved. Vessels within the subarachnoid space are remarkably convoluted or tortuous, lending a purplish-blue color to the area of the angioma. Abnormal vessels only rarely enter the cerebral substance. The hemisphere underlying the angioma is commonly atrophic; the molecular layer and some pyramidal cells are replaced by iron-calcium deposits, and laminar necrosis particularly notable in the calcarine region is seen. Ultrastructural examination of the calcific deposits are described as extracellular and extravascular filamentous and needle-like calcium apatite crystals. The reason for excessive mineralization is not known.

TREATMENT

The management of patients with Sturge-Weber syndrome may be difficult. Seizures are commonly intractable, despite careful therapeutic trials with a variety of anticonvulsant medications. From the time of onset of convulsive activity, it is common for the patient to have delayed aquisition of developmental milestones.

Hemispherectomy Once it becomes apparent that seizure control is a severe problem, hemispherectomy should be considered. A small number of children with Sturge-Weber syndrome has been reported in whom removal of the affected hemisphere resulted in marked improvement of seizure control, as well as the patient's general neurologic status. Caution must be exercised in recommending hemispherectomy early in the course of the disease until there is greater documentation of clinical experience.

HIPPEL - LINDAU DISEASE

This disease, characterized by the presence of retinal and/or cerebellar hemangioblastomas, is transmitted as an autosomal dominant trait with incomplete penetrance. Patients may have cystic tumors of the pancreas, kidneys, and epididymis, and there is an increased incidence of associated spinal cord angiomas and syringomyelia. Skin lesions are relatively uncommon.

TUMORS

Retinal hemangioblastomas occur at any time as groups of enlarging capillaries with grey exudate surrounding the vessels. The vessels are typically tortuous with an afferent arteriole and efferent venule leading to a raised tissue mass. The lesions are found in any part of the retina but are more commonly seen in the periphery; some lesions are small and easily overlooked.

Retinal lesions have been divided into 3 groups: (1) Those which are pink-red in color found in the mid-periphery of the retina with visible dilated feeder vessels and variable amount of exudate. (2) Pale grey lesions without dilated feeder vessels but with associated retinal vessels. (3) Lesions similar to those of group (2) but resembling diabetic microaneurysms without associated retinal vessels.

Fluorescein angiography is useful in delineating the lesions. There is a direct relationship between increasing age of the patient, the size and appearance of the retinal hemangioblastoma, and other visceral involvement. Patients with peripheral retinal lesions usually have no ocular complaints, but there is progressive visual loss if the macula is affected. Some patients have retinal detachment.

Cerebellar hemangioblastomas account for about 2% of brain tumors and 7-10% of all posterior fossa tumors. About 40% of hemangioblastomas are solid and 60% are cystic, often with a small vascular nodule as part of the tumor. The cerebellar tumor is usually paramedial, at or near the external cerebellar surface, and commonly associated with prominent cortical vessels. The tumor has also been found in the medulla oblongata, spinal cord, and rarely in the cerebral hemisphere or involving the pituitary gland. **Spinal hemangiomas** are usually in the cervical or thoracic regions. An increased incidence of syringomyelia has been reported.

Patients with **posterior fossa hemangioblastomas** may have signs and symptoms of increased intracranial pressure and/or cerebellar dysfunction. Polycythemia is present in 10-20% of patients; after tumor removal, the hematocrit falls but may increase with tumor recurrence. The CSF protein is usually elevated.

Other tumors that may occur in this disease include benign or malignant pancreatic and/or renal neoplasms, epididymal cysts or adenomas, and adrenocortical tumors. Angiomas and, rarely, hemangioblastomas may also be found in the pancreas. There is an increased incidence of pheochromocytomas and some patients have signs and symptoms of this tumor years before there is clinical evidence of retinal or cerebellar hemangioblastoma.

TREATMENT

Patients must be carefully evaluated and followed on a long-term basis. The possibility of tumor occurrence in other organs must always be kept in mind. Retinal hemangioblastomas are treated with a variety of therapeutic measures including photocoagulation, cryotherapy, or by laser beam.

Cerebellar tumors are treated surgically by incision of the cyst and removal of as much tumor tissue as possible. Removal of the tumor nodule is curative in some cases.

ATAXIA - TELANGIECTASIA (Louis-Bar's Syndrome)

Ataxia-telangiectasia (A-T) is a disease inherited as an autosomal recessive trait which affects multiple organs. It is characterized by ataxia, oculocutaneous telangiectasias, recurrent sinopulmonary infections, and immunoincompetency associated with an underdeveloped or absent thymus gland and lymphoreticular neoplasia. The pathophysiology remains obscure.

ATAXIA

Affected patients are usually normal until the onset of ataxia which is apparent during the first several years of life. At this time there are commonly no other physical abnormalities present. Progressive truncal instability and then limb ataxia become apparent. Occasionally, choreoathetotic movements are seen, even at an early age; rarely progressive dystonia can mask the ataxia. The development of signs is insidious and patients usually appear remarkably pleasant or sometimes apathetic. They are not particularly verbal and there is often excessive drooling; the child may be dysarthric.

ASSOCIATED NEUROLOGIC ABNORMALITIES

Many patients have abnormal ocular motility characterized by slow voluntary movements that may have a vertical component erratically interspersed. Impaired upward gaze, eye blinking, and concomitant 'jerky' head movements may be seen. This combination of head movement, eye blinking, and abnormal ocular motility is similar to the findings seen in oculomotor apraxia (see Chapter 13).

Young patients are commonly hypotonic and may have decreased muscle bulk. They are weak and the stretch reflexes are decreased to absent. Signs of a mild polyneuropathy may be present. There are usually no abnormalities of sensation. Although appearing a bit mentally dull early in the disease, patient performance on mental testing at that time is usually within normal limits; however, as the disease progresses there is a decline in mental function.

TELANGIECTASES

These dilated tortuous capillaries and very small arteries are usually apparent from 2-6 years of age and initially may not be particularly striking to careful observers. The bulbar conjunctivae are often first affected, but telangiectases can be found on the eyelids, nasal bridge, cheeks, and ears. They are also found in the antecubital and popliteal spaces. Cafe-au-lait spots, vitiligo, and 'sclerodermoid' changes are seen as well as progeric changes in skin and hair.

IMMUNOINCOMPETENCY

Chronic skin infection and blepharitis are common. Recurrent sino-pulmonary infections are a conspicuous component of this disease, affecting 80-90% of patients, resulting in chronic bronchitis and/or bronchiectasis. The infectious agents are bacterial.

Abnormalities of cell mediated or humoral immune systems are common. Examples of abnormalities of the cell mediated immune system include delayed skin graft rejection, poor response to skin test antigens, and lymphopenia. Impairment of the humoral immune system is characterized by decreased to absent serum levels of IgA, reduced levels of IgE, and impaired antibody response to antigen stimulation. Hypogonadism is seen in some patients, both male and female, and growth retardation is notable despite normal serum levels of growth hormone.

Some patients have an unusual hypersensitivity to immunosuppressive agents and radiation therapy, examples of which include ulcerative dermatitis, severe esophagitis, and deep-tissue necrosis. Fibroblastic strains from patients with A-T have been subjected to acute γ and x-radiation exposure, resulting in impairment of their ability to form colonies compared with normal controls.

Although there has been no indication of chromosomal imbalance in A-T, there is an increased incidence of spontaneous and x-ray induced chromosomal aberrations in mitogen stimulated lymphocytes and dermal fibroblasts. The frequency of induction of resistant mutants to antimetabolites following x-irradiation exposure is lower in A-T cells than normal cells. Ionizing radiation produces an increased chromosomal aberration compared to normal cells.

These studies are consistent with an anomaly or defective repair in DNA as a causal factor of abnormal radioresponsiveness of A-T cells. The predisposition to lymphoproliferative tumors appears related to an immunodeficient state, but defective DNA repair may also play a causal role.

DIAGNOSTIC TESTS

Abnormal elevation of serum alphafetoprotein appears to be a consistent finding in patients and is a most useful laboratory diagnostic test. Other useful diagnostic tests include demonstration of abnormal serum immunoglobins and impairment of delayed hypersensitivity responses.

178 NEUROCUTANEOUS DISORDERS

NEUROPATHOLOGY

Cerebellar atrophy is notable with loss of Purkinje cells and, to a lesser degree, granular cells. Neuronal loss has been described in the dentate and olivary nuclei, substantia nigra, and nuclear changes have been found in the hypothalamus and oculomotor complex. There may be a loss of some myelinated fibers in the posterior columns, spinocerebellar tracts and peripheral nerves. Decreased numbers of anterior horn cells may be found in older patients.

TREATMENT

A wide variety of abnormalities have been uncovered but the pathogenesis of A-T remains obscure. Patients must receive vigorous supportive therapy with particular attention directed to recurring infection and pulmonary function. Attempts to improve the immunological status, including plasma transfusion, administration of thymosin, and/or fetal thymus transplants have, thus far, not substantively altered the course of the neurologic signs and symptoms of this disease.

Physical therapy to avoid joint contractures is beneficial. Special educational placement should be arranged, if possible, to accommodate to the patient's particular needs.

In this disease, as in all chronic multiply handicapping diseases, parental and family counseling is important and beneficial. Appropriate genetic counseling is essential.

REFERENCES

Berg B: Neurocutaneous syndromes. In Swaiman DF, Wright FS (Eds.): The Practice of Pediatric Neurology. Mosby, St. Louis, 1982.

Berg B: Current aspects of neurocutaneous syndromes. In Moss AJ (Ed.): Pediatric Update 1982. Elsevier/North-Holland, New York.

Vinken PJ, Bruyn GW (Eds.): The phakomatoses. In Handbook of Clinical Neurology vol 14. North-Holland, Amsterdam, 1972.

10

Convulsive Disorders

Bruce O. Berg, MD

GENERAL CONSIDERATIONS

Epilepsy is a recurring alteration of brain function that begins and ends spontaneously and has a tendency to recur. It is not a specific disease but rather a symptom complex secondary to abnormal brain function. Prospective studies suggest that recurring nonfebrile convulsions affect 1-2% of our child population. Febrile seizures are slightly more frequent and usually affect infants and children 3 months to 5 years of age; these seizures are associated with fever without evidence of intracranial infection or defined cause.

Since convulsions are symptomatic of brain dysfunction, patients must be carefully evaluated to rule out the presence of infection, intracranial tumor, or structural malformation, as well as biochemical abnormalities or other potential causes of convulsive disorders. Despite careful clinical evaluation, the etiology of convulsive activity remains unknown in over one-half of patients, both child and adult.

When considering epilepsy as a possible cause of recurring alteration of consciousness, particular attention must be paid to the details of an accurate prenatal, perinatal, and developmental history as well as careful family history (see Chapter 1). It must be carefully established how the event begins, what actually happens during that event, and what is its duration and frequency. This information is obtained from the parents, other reliable observers of the event, and the child, if old enough to communicate. Complete general and neurodevelopmental examinations are required.

LABORATORY INVESTIGATION

Laboratory studies should include a complete blood count, urinalysis, and determination of serum electrolytes, calcium, magnesium, phosphorus, protein, and fasting blood sugar. Hypoglycemia, as a cause of convulsions, is more commonly seen in infants and young children with specific abnormalities of carbohydrate metabolism, but its presence must be ruled out in each patient regardless of age. Examination of the cerebrospinal fluid (CSF) should be performed if there is any question of CNS infection or brain degenerative disease. If there is clinical evidence of increased intracranial pressure, and particularly in cases of suspected intracranial mass lesions, a lumbar puncture (LP) should be performed only if neurosurgical facilities are readily available. In these circumstances of potential brain herniation, both physician and neurosurgeon should decide when and if an LP should be carried out. A computerized tomographic (CT) brain scan may be of great usefulness in this regard.

ELECTROENCEPHALOGRAPHY

An electroencephalogram (EEG) should be recorded in each patient during periods of alert wakefulness and sleep as well as during hyperventilation and photic stimulation. The presence of abnormal electrographic activity does not necessarily establish a diagnosis of epilepsy, for similar findings may be recorded in patients who have never had a seizure. The EEG, however, helps to corroborate a clinical diagnosis of convulsive disorder, while at the same time, assists in classifying the seizure type. When requesting an EEG it is important to let the electroencephalographer know what is the specific clinical problem and whether or not the patient is on medication.

The EEG is recorded during a finite period in the flow of time, but if patients have a convulsive disorder, abnormalities are usually apparent during the interictal period. Occasionally, a prolonged EEG is required with recording periods of 12-24 hours, to document abnormal electrical activity otherwise not recorded on a routine tracing. Administration of anticonvulsant medications may influence the EEG either by reducing, or in some cases enhancing, epileptiform activity; however, it is generally unnecessary and inadvisable to alter or discontinue any drug administration before obtaining an EEG.

Once the EEG has been obtained and the clinician is satisfied with the diagnosis and treatment plan, it is generally not necessary to follow patients with routine or serial tracings. Repeat EEGs are indicated if convulsions become uncontrolled or the quality of the fit has changed.

CLASSIFICATION

Convulsive disorders are generally classified in accordance with the International Classification of Convulsions (Table 10-1).

PARTIAL SEIZURES

Partial seizures are those in which the first clinical changes suggest activity of an anatomical and/or functional system of neurons located in a portion of one hemisphere. **Partial seizures with elementary symptoms** are a reflection of cerebral lesions that may be congenital malformations, tumor, or secondary to trauma, infection or ischemia. The fit begins locally, contralateral to the lesion, and symptoms may be motor, sensory, autonomic, or combinations thereof. Focal motor seizures commonly affect the fingers, hand, and face, probably because of the great cortical representation of these body parts. Adversive fits, more appropriately called contraversive, are also common focal motor seizures and are characterized by turning the eyes and head contralaterally to an irritative cerebral focus. **Partial seizures with simple sensory symptoms** are less common and require cautious interpretation, particularly in the older patient.

COMPLEX PARTIAL SEIZURES

Complex partial seizures are notable for recurring, episodic alterations of behavior, associated with motor and/or psychosensory symptoms. During the spell, patients have an altered responsiveness to their environment and are amnesic for the event. If an observer were to first witness the seizure after its onset, the patient's behavior or automatisms may seem quite purposeful; however, when observing the entire seizure, thrust upon the patient and interrupting his normal behavior in the flow of time, there is usually no question of its epileptic genesis. If attempts are made to restrain some patients during a complex partial seizure, they become obstreperous and flail their arms about. Such resistance is nondirected and should not be interrupted otherwise. The so-called episodic rage reactions directed at someone or something are virtually never a manifestation of epilepsy and these patients must be carefully evaluated with particular regard to personality and behavioral pathology. Complex partial seizures are typically associated with lesions of the temporal lobe. In some cases, EEG abnormalities are identified only after sleep deprivation, or by using nasopharyngeal or sphenoidal electrodes.

GENERALIZED SEIZURES

Generalized seizures are those in which the clinical features do not manifest any sign or symptom referable to an anatomical and/or functional system localized in one hemisphere. There is usually an initial impairment of consciousness and motor activity is generalized or at least bilateral, more or less symmetrical, and may be accompanied by an autonomic discharge. The EEG patterns from the start are bilateral, synchronous, and symmetrical over the two hemispheres.

Absence spells are usually first apparent between the ages of 5 and 9 years and are more frequent in females than males. They are relatively uncommon, comprising about 3% of all idiopathic convulsive disorders, and are characterized by a momentary cessation of activity. Some patients have minor eyelid fluttering or slight movement such as a facial twitch or licking the lips. They do not fall during the attack. The duration of the spell is 5-10 seconds and the patient then carries on with the activity in which he had been earlier engaged. The spells often occur during periods of inattention and may be so frequent that school performance is impaired for long periods of time without the cause being identified. Once the diagnosis has been established and the child appropriately treated, there is usually cessation of convulsive activity and a dramatic improvement in school performance. The term **pyknolepsy,** introduced in the distant past, was used to identify patients who had very frequent absence spells, sometimes many hundreds daily, and who were usually seizure-free by the time of puberty.

The frequency of absence spells is commonly greater than observed because their duration is brief and the spells are usually initially overlooked. The EEG shows paroxysmal activity of well-organized 2.5-3 Hz spike and wave activity, found in over 75% of interictal tracings, particularly during hyperventilation.

Myoclonic seizures are quick paroxysmal contractions of part of a muscle, a muscle, or groups of muscles. These convulsive manifestations

Table 10-1   International Classification of Convulsions*

Partial seizures (seizures beginning locally)

(a)   Partial seizures with simple symptoms (generally without impairment of consciousness).
   1.   With motor symptoms
   2.   With special sensory or somatosensory symptoms
   3.   With autonomic symptoms
   4.   Compound forms

(b)   Partial seizures with complex symptoms (generally with impairment of consciousness).
   1.   With impairment of consciousness only
   2.   With cognitive symptoms
   3.   With affective symptoms
   4.   With psychosensory symptoms
   5.   With psychomotor symptoms
   6.   Compound forms

Generalized seizures (bilaterally symmetrical and without local onset)
   1.   Absence (petit mal)
   2.   Myoclonic seizures
   3.   Infantile spasms
   4.   Clonic seizures
   5.   Tonic seizures
   6.   Tonic/clonic seizures (grand mal)
   7.   Atonic seizures
   8.   Akinetic seizures

Unilateral seizure (or predominantly unilateral)

Unclassified epileptic seizures

---

   * Gastaut H: Clinical and electroencephalographical classification of seizures. Epilepsia 11:102-119, 1970

may effect a slight movement of one digit, an entire limb, or head and neck flexion or extension. They may occur as one single myoclonic jerk or intermittently in the same or different place.

   Infantile spasms, known by a variety of names including West syndrome, massive myoclonus, jack-knife or salaam seizures, has an onset in 75% of cases before the age of 1 year. It is twice as common in boys than girls. This seizure disorder may first make its presence known by a momentary head nod or a brief flexion of legs upon the tummy and is commonly mistaken for colic. With passage of time the disorder will unequivocally declare itself by massive myoclonus with head flexion and legs abruptly drawn upon the abdomen. These massive muscular contractions occur singly or in a series, with one massive jerk after another, often punctuated by an unusual giggle or piercing cry that often makes parents think incorrectly that the child is in pain. Less commonly there is a massive extensor spasm. A third type is a 'lightning spasm' (blitzkrampf), notable for its extreme brevity. These seizures are particularly common upon waking from sleep or shortly thereafter.

The typical EEG found in about two-thirds of patients is characterized by a diffusely disorganized background and comprised of high amplitude delta (less than 4 Hz) activity with multifocal spikes and sharp waves. Because of the high voltage slow waves, this type of EEG has been called 'hypsarrhythmia' (Gr. *hypsa* = mountain, elevation). Hypsarrhythmia refers to the EEG and not the convulsive disorder.

Infantile spasms have been considered **cryptogenic** when the infant has been normal before the onset of seizures and **symptomatic** in cases of brain anomaly, congenital infection, prematurity and/or birth injury or, occasionally, following immunization. This seizure type may also be present in patients with tuberous sclerosis, female patients with agenesis of the corpus callosum (Aicardie's syndrome) and some metabolic disorders (phenylketonuria and maple syrup urine disease). Infantile spasms are difficult to control, but even in those patients with some modest seizure control and improvement in the EEG, over two-thirds of patients are significantly delayed in development.

Clonic and tonic/clonic convulsions are the usual seizure types associated with 'grand mal epilepsy.' These spells can occur without warning, or the patient may exhibit behavioral changes such as irritability, irascibility, or lethargy (the prodrome) hours before the fit. Commonly, because of this repetitive behavioral change before the apparent seizure, mothers know when the child is about to have a convulsion. Some patients perceive an unusual sensory experience (the aura) such as an unpleasant smell, abdominal cramping, a feeling of fear, or an ill-defined unpleasant feeling just before losing consciousness. Small children may sometimes come to their mother or father 'before' the fit and only later, when better able to communicate, are able to describe the aura. The onset of this sensory perception is actually the beginning of the convulsion.

The patient's eyes are open, usually directed upward or to the side and there are associated massive muscular contractions. The tonic phase usually persists 5-15 seconds and is followed by a clonic phase of generalized trembling or violent muscular jerks. Incontinence of bowel and/or bladder may occur and an occasional patient will bite the tongue. Unless it is well established that the patient bites the tongue as part of the seizure, it is inadvisable to jam an object between the patient's teeth; usually more damage is done to the soft tissues of the mouth in this way than by leaving the patient alone. The entire episode usually lasts 1 or 2 minutes and the patient then remains in a postictal state of headache, confusion, unresponsiveness, or all of the above. The interictal EEG commonly shows bilateral synchronous spike discharges and/or bursts of slow wave and spike or polyspike activity. It should be noted that the EEG may be normal.

Tonic fits are notable for forceful contraction of limb and axial musculature. The posture assumed during the spell varies among patients and in each patient may be the same or different during individual attacks. They are commonly refractory to all therapeutic measures.

Atonic seizures are usually of very brief duration and characterized by a sudden loss of a muscle tone, resulting in the patient abruptly plummeting to the ground. Occasionally they are associated with myoclonic jerks. The extent of impairment of consciousness is undetermined because the episode is so brief; however, some patients claim to be able to describe the incident. **Akinetic seizures** are described as those with loss of movement but without atonia.

UNILATERAL SEIZURES

Unilateral or predominantly unilateral seizures are those in which clinical and electrographic aspects are similar to those of the groups noted above, with the exception that clinical signs are restricted principally, if not exclusively to one side of the body. The EEG discharges are noted over the contralateral hemisphere. These seizures presumably depend upon generalized or at least diffuse neuronal discharge restricted to a single hemisphere and its neuronal connections.

UNCLASSIFIED SEIZURES

This category includes all convulsive phenomena that cannot be classified because of inadequate or incomplete data.

LENNOX - GASTAUT SYNDROME

Lennox initially described the clinical characteristics of atypical absence, atonic, and myoclonic fits and noted their association with slow waves and spike/polyspike activity in the EEG. This association of convulsive activity was called the 'petit mal triad.' Gastaut later described the syndrome as an epileptic encephalopathy of childhood, emphasizing the frequency of tonic and atypical absence seizures. The syndrome has become known as the Lennox-Gastaut syndrome and is characterized by atypical absence spells, myoclonic, atonic, and tonic fits in varying combinations. Most patients, after having developed normally, have a sudden onset of seizure activity that remains recalcitrant to treatment. There is usually a gradual deterioration of intellect. The EEG is characterized by interictal slow waves with spike/polyspike activity.

DIFFERENTIAL DIAGNOSIS

Breath-holding spells are common in childhood, usually starting between the ages of 6 and 18 months, varying in frequency during the next several years, and then disappearing by the age of 5 or 6 years. There are two types, described as either cyanotic (blue) òr pallid (white). The cyanotic type usually follows a period of lusty crying that has been provoked by anger or frustration. Breath is usually held in expiration and the child becomes cyanotic and then limp, often having a few associated muscle jerks. The pallid type of spell is vasovagal in nature. Following a minor or sudden fright, the child may or may not cry, appear surprised or fearful, fall to the ground limp and assume a transient posture of opisthotonus which is often preceded by a few muscle jerks.

Breath-holding spells are usually of short duration but if prolonged may result in generalized tonic, clonic, or tonic/clonic convulsions. The EEG is normal. It is essential to discuss the nature of the problem with the parents emphasizing that the episodes are self-limiting and of no danger to the child. The administration of anticonvulsant medications is of no significant benefit.

Syncope (fainting) is uncommon in childhood but increases in frequency during adolescence, particularly in females. It is secondary to decreased brain perfusion and hypoxia, usually following fatigue or acute emotional distress. The possibility of cardiopulmonary abnormalities must be ruled out. Patients generally experience a feeling of restlessness, sweating and/or impaired vision before the faint which, in the majority of cases, lasts for only a few minutes. There may be associated clonic muscle jerks.

Sleep disorders may also be confused with convulsive phenomena. Myoclonus during sleep is commonly seen in normal persons of all ages. These quick muscle jerks are often seen, particularly in the limb muscles, during periods of drowsiness or just after falling asleep. They are benign. Myoclonic jerks that appear shortly after walking, however, are a different matter and are probably a manifestation of an underlying convulsive disorder. **Night terrors** (pavor nocturnus), a nonREM dyssomnia, is another type of sleep-related event often thought to be a seizure activity. It occurs during stages III-IV of sleep, usually within the first or second sleep cycles and is characterized by an appearance of being awake, fear, terror, and confusion. Patients do not recall the event the next morning. Sleep-walking or enuresis may be associated phenomena. These nonREM dyssomnias are self-limiting. They usually occur only occasionally, and once identified as night terrors will greatly lessen parental anxiety and worry. If the episodes occur frequently, diazepam given at bedtime in low doses, will usually effect their disappearance.

Benign paroxysmal vertigo is a disorder usually with onset from 1-4 years, characterized by paroxysmal attacks of vertigo associated with sweat, pallor, and nystagmus; some children will fall during an attack which lasts only several minutes. There is no loss of consciousness. Important features which distinguish benign paroxysmal vertigo from complex partial seizures include a normal EEG and the demonstration of abnormal labyrinthine function.

Familial paroxysmal choreoathetosis is a rare condition notable for abrupt episodes of chorea, athetosis, and/or dystonic posturing that are usually precipitated by movement after a period of immobility. The duration of episode is usually a matter of minutes and there is no alteration of consciousness. The etiology of this disorder is unclear. Most patients respond to administration of phenytoin or clonazepam. (See Chapter 18.)

Pseudoseizures are more common than generally presumed in both epileptic and nonepileptic patients. There are no totally reliable diagnostic criteria, but most patients have some emotional disturbance. The episodes may be frequent, are usually indoors or at home when other persons are present, and only rarely occur during evening hours. Patients often talk or scream during the attack, the duration of which is usually minutes or longer. Incontinence or lip biting during the episode does not separate a pseudoseizure from true convulsive activity.

TREATMENT

The purpose of attempting prevention of convulsions is to maintain the patient's life activity as normal as possible and to avoid potential brain injury. Those patients in whom a specific cause of convulsions has been established, should receive appropriate treatment. However, despite careful, complete clinical evaluation, no etiology for recurring nonfebrile seizures can be established in over one-half of patients.

The clinician must be confident that the patient has an idiopathic convulsive disorder, or epilepsy, before attaching that diagnostic label, for the diagnosis implies a major commitment to at least 4 years of daily administration of medication and potential limitations of personal activities, employment, and driving privileges. The decision to treat the patient with a single fit depends upon the seizure type, circumstances regarding that convulsion and the concurrence of opinions of physician, parent and child.

After the seizure type has been determined, the most appropriate anticonvulsant drug is selected; that drug is administered·in gradually increasing dosages until the serum therapeutic level is reached (see Tables 10-2, 10-3, 10-4). If the seizures are controlled, that dosage of medication is continued; however, should the seizures recur, the drug dosage is increased until side-effects of that drug are apparent. If seizures remain uncontrolled, a second appropriate drug should be introduced, again in gradually increasing dosages until serum therapeutic levels of that drug are attained. Alterations of drug dosage should be made at intervals no less than about 7 days. *Use as few drugs as possible to control convulsive disorders.*

In occasional patients there is a fine line between seizure control and side-effects of the medication. Some patients would prefer to be free of all convulsive activity at the expense of experiencing unpleasant side-effects of higher drug dosage. Other patients would rather run the risk of having an occasional seizure and avoid the side-effects of medication at dosages that would otherwise control those seizures. *Generally, attempt to keep the patient free from all convulsive activity.*

Partial seizures, both simple and complex, as well as **generalized (tonic/clonic) seizures** are usually well controlled by phenobarbital, phenytoin, carbamazepine, or combinations thereof. Primidone is another drug that may be used for these seizure types although some patients complain of lethargy and/or unsteadiness while taking the drug.

Generalized seizures include a variety of seizure types some of which are readily controlled by medication while others are recalcitrant to treatment. **Absence spells** are usually well controlled by ethosuximide. If that drug does not control the spells, other drugs that have been effectively used include valproic acid or clonazepam.

The multiple seizure types as seen in Lennox-Gastaut syndrome are often difficult to control and a variety of anticonvulsant medications have been used including clonazepam, ethosuximide, phenytoin, and valproic acid. In some patients with seizures recalcitrant to treatment, a ketogenic

Table 10-2   Anticonvulsant Drugs used for Partial and Generalized (Tonic/Clonic) Seizures

	Total dosage/day	No. of doses/day	Half-life	Therapeutic blood level
Carbamazepine (Tegretol)	To 25 mg/kg	3-4	15 hours	4-12 μg/ml
Phenobarbital	4-6 mg/kg	1	4 days	20-40 μg/ml
Phenytoin (Dilantin)	4-8 mg/kg	1 (capsule) 2-3 (infatabs, suspension)	22 hours	10-20 μg/ml
Primidone (Mysoline)	10-25 mg/kg	3	10 hours	5-12 μg/ml
Valproic acid (Depakene)	15-60 mg/kg	3	8 hours	50-120 μg/ml

diet may be of benefit particularly when both patient and parent are well-motivated. The diet provides most calories as fat with little carbohydrate. The use of medium-chain triglyceride (MCT) oil in food preparations has made the diet more palatable, but it is still difficult to maintain a child on the diet for any length of time because he yearns, if not pilfers, other foods of his preference.

Infantile spasms are difficult to control with any therapeutic regimen, even though there may be improvement in the EEG. Over two-thirds of patients are significantly delayed in development. Either ACTH (IM) or prednisone (orally) is given daily for 4-6 weeks and then gradually discontinued over a period of several weeks. ACTH seems to be the preferred drug in many centers for reasons which are unclear at this time. Be mindful of possible signs and symptoms of a pseudotumor cerebri appearing during the reduction of steroid dosage. Anticonvulsants that may effect convulsive control on a long-term basis include valproic acid, clonazepam, and nitrazepam, when available. As patients become older the quality of the convulsion changes from that of massive myoclonus to other forms of generalized epilepsy including tonic/clonic, myoclonic, and/or akinetic seizures.

Drug interactions   When multiple anticonvulsant drugs are given, be mindful of potential drug interactions. For example, when using combinations of phenobarbital and phenytoin in usual dosages, the serum level of phenobarbital may be in the therapeutic range but the level of phenytoin may be less than otherwise expected. Similarly, valproic acid administered with phenobarbital and/or phenytoin, again in usually administered dosages, may result in therapeutic serum levels of valproic acid, but serum levels of phenobarbital may be higher, and phenytoin lower than expected. If the patient complains of lethargy it may be incorrectly presumed the lethargy is secondary to a high serum level of valproic acid when it is actually related to a high serum level of phenobarbital. *Be alert for all potential drug interactions.*

Table 10-3 Anticonvulsant Drugs used for Generalized (Absence) Seizures

	Total dosage/day	No. of doses/day	Half-life	Therapeutic blood level
Clonazepam (Clonopin)	0.01-0.2 mg/kg	2-3	18-50 hours	20-80 μg/ml
Ethosuximide (Zarontin)	20 mg/kg	2	55 hours	40-120 μg/ml
Trimethadione (Tridione)	20-40 mg/kg	3-4	16 hours	Not established
Valproic acid (Depakene)	15-60 mg/kg	3	8 hours	50-120 μg/ml

STATUS EPILEPTICUS

This is one of the few medical emergencies and is characterized by prolonged continuous partial or generalized seizures. The patient is unconscious. It may be the first clinical experience of a convulsive disorder or may occur in patients already identified as having epilepsy. Immediate attention must be directed to those circumstances that may result in permanent brain injury if not recognized and appropriately treated, including anoxia, hypoglycemia, hypocalcemia, CNS infection, and head injury.

Emergency treatment

(a) A patent airway must be assured. The patient should be placed in a position of comfort to avoid self injury and aspiration of secretions.

(b) An intravenous line should be established to remove blood for determination of glucose, calcium, magnesium, electrolytes, levels of anticonvulsant medications, screen for toxic substances, and blood cultures. After this blood sample has been obtained, a solution of 50% glucose should be given (1 mg/kg).

(c) The blood pressure, pulse, and respiration should be monitored and a careful record of all medications administered must be maintained.

1. *Diazepam* is rapidly effective with relatively few side-effects if given as the initial drug. Infants should receive 0.3 mg/kg up to 5 mg; children should receive 1 mg/year of age up to 10 mg. This undiluted drug should be given showly, IV, at 1 mg/minute. Particular attention should be paid to the possibility of respiratory depression; other complications include hypotension and bradycardia.

2. If the one-dose administration of diazepam does not control the prolonged convulsion, other longer-acting anticonvulsant drugs should be used; either phenytoin or phenobarbital.

   Phenytoin should be administered slowly, IV, at a dosage of 25-30 mg/kg at 1 mg/kg/minute. The drug cannot be given with dextrose solutions and should not be given IM because of slow absorption. There is generally no respiratory depression or sedation, and therapeutic drug levels are achieved in the brain within 30-60 minutes.

Phenobarbital is another useful drug and is slowly administered IV at 10 mg/kg. If the convulsive activity is not controlled within 20-30 minutes, the same dosage can be repeated. Be aware of possible respiratory depression and hypotension with increasing dosage.

Should continuous convulsive activity remain uncontrolled, general anesthesia may be required. *Meticulous attention must be given to the monitoring of patient's vital signs as well as accurately recording all medications administered.*

DURATION OF TREATMENT

Once the diagnosis has been made and it has been determined to start anticonvulsant medication, it is essential to clarify with parents and child that medication must be taken daily and as specifically recommended by the physician. It should be understood that drug dosage may require adjustment and that other anticonvulsant medications may be required in the future. The matter of compliance with drug schedules must be established at the very beginning of patient-physician relationship.

PSYCHOSOCIAL CONSIDERATIONS

Never underestimate the fears and supernatural beliefs patients and parents may have regarding epilepsy; if not recognized, these factors may unnecessarily complicate patient management. Information regarding the diagnosis and plans for management should be completely and tactfully discussed with the parents in an uncomplicated manner as well as with child patients at their level of understanding. Synonyms for recurring convulsions including seizure, fit, spell, and epilepsy should gradually be introduced during the discussion and fully explained. Both patient and parent should have their questions answered and the common fears of possible brain tumors, brain degenerative diseases, mental illness, or retardation should be allayed, if appropriate.

Each family has its own house rules and the patient should be treated as normally as possible within that frame of reference. Limitations of normal activity are few but include swimming unless accompanied by someone who is proficient in life-saving measures and understands that the patient has a convulsive disorder. It is generally advisable to avoid potential convulsive precipitants such as inordinate fatigue, stress, and certain drugs (alcohol and psychotropic drugs).

A medical social worker can be of great assistance in the assessment and management of patients. Additional useful resources include the Epilepsy Foundation of America and local chapters of the Epilepsy Society.

PROGNOSIS

The prognosis of childhood epilepsy is generally good, particularly for those whose neurodevelopmental examinations are normal and whose seizures are readily brought under control. It is generally accepted that after 4 years of seizure-free activity in patients who have no significant neurologic deficits, the anticonvulsant medication can be gradually withdrawn. The risks of recurrence vary, depending upon the type(s) of seizure and are most likely to occur during the first year after anticonvulsant drugs have been discontinued.

Table 10-4 Anticonvulsant Drugs

Drugs	Daily dosage	Preparations	Comment
Barbiturates			
Mephobarbital (Mebaral)	6-12 mg/kg	Tablets 32, 50, 100, 200 mg	Used for partial & generalized (tonic/clonic) seizures. Has less sedating & anticonvulsant properties than phenobarbital; but is effective in seizure control. Contraindications are same as for phenobarbital.
Metharbital (Gemonil)	5-15 mg/kg	Tablets 100 mg	Not a first-choice anticonvulsant drug, but has been used for partial & generalized (tonic/clonic) seizures. May be effective in controlling myoclonic jerks. Contraindications as for phenobarbital.
Phenobarbital	4-6 mg/kg	Tablets 15, 30, 60, 100 mg Elixir 20 mg/5 ml	Effective & relatively inexpensive drug particularly useful in partial seizures & generalized (tonic/clonic). 25-33% of children may have varying degrees of behavioral change (irritability, hyperactivity, disturbance of sleep patterns, & rarely, somnolence) or interference with higher cortical function (attentional deficit, impairment of short-term memory & comprehension). Nystagmus & ataxia may occur at excessive dosages. Scarlatiniform or morbilliform rashes occur in 1-2% of patients. Contraindicated in severe renal or hepatic disease & porphyria.
Primidone (Mysoline)	10-25 mg/kg	Tablets 50, 250 mg Suspension 50 mg/ml	Useful in control of partial seizures & generalized (tonic/clonic). Administer in gradually increasing doses to maintenance level. Side-effects: lethargy, ataxia, dizziness, & occasional headache.
Benzodiazepines			
Clonazepam (Clonopin)	0.01-0.2 mg/kg	Tablets 0.5, 1, 2 mg	For generalized seizures (absence, myoclonic, & infantile spasms).. Primary side-effects are CNS depression including drowsiness & ataxia. Others include skin rash, hair loss, nausea, anorexia, increased salivation, anemia, &/or leukemia, & behavioral change.
Diazepam (Valium)	0.25-0.4 mg/kg	Ampuls: 2 ml Vials: 10 ml Tablets 2, 5, 10 mg	Has little value as an oral anticonvulsant. Primarily used in status epilepticus. Side-effects include respiratory depression & occasionally hypotension. When used as adjunctive medication common side-effects include drowsiness, fatigue, & ataxia. Contraindicated in

Phenytoin (Dilantin)	4-8 mg/kg	Tablets: 50 mg Capsules: 30, 100 mg Suspension: 30, 125 mg/5 ml Vial: 100 mg/2.2 ml (solvent) 250 mg/5.2 ml (solvent)	A major anticonvulsant useful in controlling partial & generalized (tonic/clonic) seizures. Has occasionally been used for akinetic or myoclonic attacks. Capsules can be given in a single daily dose, but tablets (Infatab) & suspension should be given 2-3 doses/day. Side-effects include gingival hyperplasia, dermatitis, hirsutism, lymphadenopathy, megaloblastic anemia, & leukopenia. Pulmonary fibrosis, hepatitis, & polyneuropathy have been reported. Nystagmus, ataxia, & lethargy are seen in drug overdosage. Contraindicated in patients with known hypersensitivity to the hydantoins.
Ethotoin (Peganone)	0.5-1 gm/day	Tablets 250, 500 mg	Of little usefulness in convulsive disorders. Has been used in combination with other anticonvulsants for partial & generalized (tonic/clonic) fits. Side-effects include dermatitis, lethargy, or GI disturbances. Blood dyscrasias have been reported & when given with phenacemide, paranoid symptoms have been noted. Contraindicated in patients with hepatic or hematologic disorders.
Mephenytoin (Mesantoin)	100-400 mg/day	Tablets 100 mg	Used in partial or generalized (tonic/clonic) seizures not well controlled by other drugs. Adverse side-effects include blood dyscrasias, skin-mucous membrane lesions, & CNS effects. Complete blood count should be done before therapy, after 2 weeks of full maintenance dosage & every month for 1 year, then every 3 months. If neutrophil count drops between 2400-1600/mm^3, WBCs are obtained every 2 weeks. Patient or parents must be well informed about symptoms & signs of agranulocytosis. Patient must be closely followed.

Oxazolidinediones

Paramethadione (Paradione)	20-60 mg/kg	Capsules 150, 300 mg Solution: 300 mg/ml	Rarely used in the treatment of absence seizures (see trimethadione).
Trimethadione (Tridione)	20-30 mg/kg	Tablets: 150 mg Capsules: 300 mg Solution: 200 mg/5 ml	For control of absence seizures in patients who do not respond to ethosuximide. Adverse effects: lethargy, photophobia, anorexia, nausea, vomiting, & weight loss. Less common adverse effects: blood dyscrasias, nephrotic syndrome, hepatitis, lupus erythematosus, & myasthenia gravis syndrome. Patient should have CBCs & urinalyses at monthly intervals. Use of drug is contraindicated in patients with hepatic or renal disease, blood dyscrasias, or in pregnancy.

Table 10-4 (continued)   Anticonvulsant Drugs

Drugs	Daily dosage	Preparations	Comment
Succinimides			
Ethosuximide (Zarontin)	20 mg/kg	Capsules: 250 mg Syrup: 250 mg/5 ml	Drug of choice for control of absence spells. Because of GI complaints, begin in low doses, gradually increasing to maintenance dose. Side-effects: headache, restlessness, or drowsiness. Adverse reactions: leukopenia, agranulocytosis, aplastic anemia, & lupus erythematosus.
Methsuximide (Celontin)	10-20 mg/kg	Capsules: 150, 300 mg	For generalized epilepsies (absence spells, myoclonic, & akinetic) not well controlled by other drugs. Adverse reactions: headache, drowsiness, irritability, ataxia. Hematologic disorders include eosinophilia, leukopenia, monocytosis, pancytopenia.
Phensuximide (Milontin)	20-40 mg/kg	Capsules: 500 mg	For generalized epilepsies not well controlled by other drugs. Patient may complain of anorexia, vomiting, drowsiness, dizziness, or ataxia. Granulocytopenia, aplastic anemia, & skin rash have been reported.
Others			
Acetazolamide (Diamox)	15-20 mg	Tablets: 125, 250 mg Capsules: 500 mg	Used occasionally for generalized epilepsies (absence, akinetic, or myoclonic fits). Results have been mixed. Side-effects are few: paresthesias, anorexia, polyuria, & drowsiness.
ACTH	25-30 units/ 24 hours 4-6 weeks	Acthar gel (IM) 1-5 ml vials 40-80 USP units/ ml. Lyophilized powder 25-40 units/vial	For infantile spasms. Side-effects are those of hyperadrenocorticism. Contraindications: active tuberculosis, ocular herpes simplex, & psychoses.

Drug	Dosage	Formulations	Notes
Bromides	50-100 mg/kg	Triple bromide Tablets: 450, 900 mg Syrup: 1.2 gm/5 ml Elixir: 1.2 gm/5 ml	Considered when other drugs have failed to control partial or generalized (tonic/clonic) seizures. Toxic effects: drowsiness, psychosis, acneiform eruption, & nodular skin lesions. Adverse CNS symptoms & signs including ataxia & dysarthria have been described.
Phenacemide (Phenurone)	15-35 mg/kg	Tablets: 500 mg	*This drug is not used unless other anticonvulsant medications are proven ineffective.* Rarely used for partial or generalized (tonic/clonic) epilepsies. Personality changes, psychosis, & suicide attempts have been reported as well as toxic effects on liver, kidney, & hematopoietic system. CBC & urinalysis should be done before drug is started, and at monthly intervals thereafter. Contraindicated in pregnancy.
Prednisone	2 mg/kg	Tablets: 2.5, 5 mg	Preferred to ACTH by some for infantile spasms. Given for 4-6 weeks. Should be gradually discontinued over several weeks to avoid precipitation of symptoms & signs of pseudotumor cerebri.
Carbamazepine (Tegretol)	To 25 mg/kg	Tablets: 200 mg 100 mg (chewable)	Particularly useful for control of partial seizures with complex symptomatology, generalized tonic/clonic, and mixed seizure patterns. Common adverse effects: nausea, anorexia, drowsiness, visual disturbances, & ataxia. Leukopenia, aplastic anemia, & agranulocytosis have been reported. It is important to get a CBC & platelet & reticulocyte count before medication is started and periodically.
Valproic acid (Depakene) Divalproex sodium (Depakote)	15-60 mg/kg	Capsules: 250 mg Syrup: 250 mg/5 ml Tablets, enteric coated, 250 500 mg	Particularly useful in control of generalized epilepsies, especially absence seizures. Has also been used with fair to good results in partial seizures. Adverse effects generally mild (nausea, vomiting, lethargy) & usually occur shortly after drug has been started. Others are ataxia, headache, nystagmus, & diplopia. Minor elevations of transaminases & LDH are frequent & appear to be dose-related. Abnormal LFTs may indicate potentially serious hepatotoxicity. Hepatic failure resulting in fatality has occurred, but usually in the first 6 months of treatment. LFTs should be performed before therapy is begun, then at frequent intervals, especially during the first 6 months. Discontinue drug immediately in the presence of significant hepatic dysfunction, suspected or apparent.

FEBRILE CONVULSIONS

Febrile convulsions usually occur in children 3 months to 5 years old and are associated with fever but without evidence of intracranial infection or known cause. About one-third of patients who have had one febrile fit and who have not received prophylactic anticonvulsive treatment will have another febrile seizure. The recurrence of febrile fits does not necessarily increase the risk of epilepsy.

Risk factors have been identified which separate a group of children with febrile seizures at high risk for developing recurring nonfebrile seizures from a low-risk group. These factors include: (a) family history of nonfebrile seizures; (b) abnormal neurodevelopmental status prior to the febrile seizures; (c) atypical seizures or those followed by transient or permanent neurologic abnormalities.

Patients with two or more risk factors are at 'high risk' with a 13% chance of developing recurring nonfebrile seizures; whereas only 2 or 3% with one or none of the risk factors develop epilepsy.

Treatment of febrile seizures Several anticonvulsant drugs have been used for prophylactic administration including phenobarbital and valproic acid. Phenobarbital is generally the drug of choice, despite the fact that one-fourth to one-third of children who receive the drug have varying degrees of behavioral changes (irritability, hyperactivity, disturbance of sleep, or lethargy) or interference with higher cortical function (attentional deficit disorder, impairment of short-term memory and comprehension). Valproic acid, though effective, is less commonly administered. There have been few serious side-effects with this drug; however, some **toxic reactions** have occurred including gastrointestinal disturbances, toxic hepatitis, and pancreatitis. Liver function studies should be determined before the drug is started and at periodic intervals thereafter in those patients who recieve valproic acid on a prolonged basis.

If it is decided that prophylactic anticonvulsive treatment is required the standard duration of treatment is 2 years, or 1 year after the last seizure, whichever is longer. Medication is gradually discontinued over 1-2 months.

REFERENCES

Aminoff MF (Ed): *Electrodiagnosis in Clinical Neurology.* Churchill-Livingston, New York, 1980.

Browne TR, Feldman RG (Eds): *Epilepsy: Diagnosis and Management.* Little, Brown, Boston, 1983.

Laidlaw J, Richens A: *A Textbook of Epilepsy,* 2nd ed. Churchill-Livingston, Edinburgh, 1983.

Morselli PL, Pippenger CE, Penry JK (Eds): *Antiepileptic Drug Therapy in Pediatrics.* Raven Press, New York, 1983.

Thurston JH, et al: Prognosis in childhood epilepsy: additional follow-up of 148 children 15 to 23 years after withdrawal of anti-convulsant therapy. N Engl J Med 306:831-836.

11

Problems of the Newborn

Suzanne L. Davis, MB, ChB

ASPHYXIA AND HYPOXIC - ISCHEMIC ENCEPHALOPATHY

Asphyxia resulting in injury to the central nervous system is caused by both hypoxemia, a decrease in blood oxygen content, and ischemia, a decrease in cerebral blood perfusion. Complications of pregnancy, labor, delivery, and the neonatal course predispose an infant to hypoxic-ischemic encephalopathy (Table 11-1). The degree and distribution of brain injury depend on the duration and severity of hypoxia and ischemia as well as regional variations in metabolic activity and blood flow. Several patterns of central nervous system pathology have been described (Table 11-2). Periventricular leucomalacia, infarction of the deep cerebral white matter, occurs almost exclusively in preterm infants, in contrast to infarctions of the parasagittal cortex and that brain substance supplied by the middle cerebral artery, which are typically seen in the asphyxiated term newborn. However, in any single case, elements of more than one pathological pattern may be present. The malnourished infant who is small for gestational age is more susceptible to an hypoxic-ischemic insult, exacerbated by a tendency to develop hypoglycemia under stress. On the other hand, elevated blood glucose levels have increased permanent neurologic injury in animal models of asphyxia, because of enhanced lactic acid production and tissue acidosis.

CLINICAL CHARACTERISTICS

Prenatal asphyxia may be clinically silent although it usually causes changes in fetal heart rate and loss of the normal fetal respiratory pattern (Table 11-3). Although a nonspecific sign, the loss of beat-to-beat variation in heart rate is probably the most sensitive indicator of fetal distress. Meconium staining of the amniotic fluid is often associated with neonatal depression especially when it is heavy and occurs early. In the immediate newborn period, the Apgar score is a widely used indicator of neurologic status (Table 11-4). Apgar scores of 5 or less at 5 minutes are associated with increased neurologic morbidity.

The asphyxiated newborn shows signs of neurologic depression that may persist for hours or days (Table 11-5). The severity and duration of these signs are important predictors of subsequent mortality and morbidity. In a mild encephalopathy, signs of irritability may be followed by seizures within 12-24 hours. If symptoms resolve within several days there is gener-

Table 11-1   Causes of Fetal and Neonatal Asphyxia

Prenatal Maternal hypotension; maternal pulmonary insufficiency; maternal hypertension; maternal diabetes; placental infarction or separation; fetal hemolytic disease; postmaturity.

Intrapartum Maternal hypoventilation during anesthesia; maternal hypotension or compression of the inferior vena cava; umbilical cord prolapse; immaturity; placenta previa; cephalopelvic disproportion; malpresentation; shoulder dystocia.

Postpartum Respiratory depression from asphyxia, drugs, or airway obstruction; lung immaturity; respiratory distress syndrome; meconium aspiration; congenital abnormalities of the lungs, diaphragm, or airway; severe apnea; recurrent seizures.

Table 11-2   Pathology and Outcome in Hypoxic-Ischemic Encephalopathy

Type of hypoxic insult	Pathology	Outcome
Profound hypoxemia	Widespread neuronal necrosis of cortex, cerebellum, basal ganglia, and brain stem nuclei.	Mental retardation, facial diplegia, bulbar palsy, quadriparesis, and movement disorder.
Prolonged moderate hypoxemia with hypotension in term infant.	(1) Parasagittal cortical infarction. (2) Infarction-territory of middle cerebral artery.	Proximal hypotonia most severe in the shoulders. Hemiparesis.
Prolonged moderate hypoxemia with hypotension in preterm infant.	Periventricular white matter infarction (leucomalacia).	Spastic diplegia.

Table 11-3 Fetal Heart Rate Abnormalities

Type	Relation to contractions	Significance
Decelerations	(1) Early	Vagal response to head compression. Benign.
	(2) Variable	Intermittent umbilical cord compression. Usually benign.
	(3) Late, persisting for 30 seconds after contraction ends	Signifies asphyxia, often with metabolic acidosis.
Loss of beat-to-beat variation (normally 6-8 bpm).		Signifies fetal distress, drug depression.

Table 11-4 Apgar Score

Sign	Score		
	2	1	0
Color	Pink	Pale or blue extremities	Central pallor or cyanosis
Response to pain	Brisk response with crying	Sluggish or transient response	No response
Tone	Normal flexor tone	Decreased tone	Flaccid
Breathing	Established	Inadequate or periodic	Apnea
Heart rate	Normal	Bradycardia (less than 100 bpm)	Absent

Table 11-5 Clinical Signs of Asphyxia

Mild Hyperalertness and irritability; tachycardia and diaphoresis; jitteriness; seizures beginning at 12-24 hours.

Moderate Lethargy and decreased spontaneous movement; hypotonia; poor suck and swallow; absent acoustic blink and Moro reflexes; seizures.

Severe Coma; profound hypotonia; recurrent apnea; signs of brain stem dysfunction (unreactive pupils, loss of reflexive eye movements, facial palsy); seizures; signs of increased ICP beginning at 24-48 hours.

Table 11-6   Management of Hypoxic-Ischemic Encephalopathy

Prevention	Avoidance of premature delivery; fetal monitoring during labor; support of airway and ventilation in the depressed infant.
Supportive care	Monitor pO_2, pCO_2, glucose, electrolytes.
Early treatment of seizures	Consider prophylactic phenobarbital in the infant with a high risk for seizures.
Manage increased ICP	Fluid restriction; early detection of inappropriate ADH secretion; mannitol 0.25 mg/kg IV.

ally a good prognosis. The severely asphyxiated infant may deteriorate over 24-72 hours, manifest recurring seizures, progressing to signs of increased intracranial pressure and respiratory arrest. Evidence of myocardial, renal, and bowel ischemia is often prominent following severe asphyxia.

The extent of an acute hypoxic-ischemic injury in the newborn may be difficult to determine using current brain imaging techniques. In computerized tomographic brain scans, cerebral infarction is difficult to distinguish from normal white matter which, in the immature brain, has low x-ray attenuation. When hypodensity extends to involve the cortex there is a definite correlation with focal neurologic sequelae. Head ultrasonography may fail to show acute changes, but regions of decreased or even increased echogenicity have correlated with cerebral infarction demonstrated at autopsy.

Nonspecific EEG changes occur in hypoxic-ischemic encephalopathy. Severely abnormal background patterns (isoelectric, extreme low voltage or burst suppression), which are unresponsive to external stimuli, are associated with extensive and often irreversible encephalopathies. The outcome is especially poor when these EEG abnormalities persist beyond 1 week. Less severe changes, such as an immaturity of sleep-related EEG patterns, usually signify mild reversible encephalopathies or drug effect. The normal newborn EEG includes many sharp transients which resemble paroxysmal activity. When sharp waves or spikes are consistently focal they often signal underlying focal pathology. However, cortical infarction is usually associated with focal decrease in EEG amplitude.

Brain stem auditory evoked potentials (BAEPs) are often abnormal in severely asphyxiated newborns especially when there are clinical brain stem abnormalities. BAEP changes also occur in other metabolic encephalopathies such as hyperbilirubinemia and in some inherited metabolic defects.

MANAGEMENT AND OUTCOME

Prevention of hypoxic-ischemic encephalopathy in the newborn depends on early identification of the fetus and newborn at risk, and appropriate obstetrical and pediatric management (Table 11-6). Care of the asphyxiated newborn includes support of airway and ventilation, careful management of fluids, and the early treatment of electrolyte disturbances and hypoglycemia. Early recognition and treatment of seizures is important because they increase cerebral metabolic demands and may cause apnea and hypotension. Prophylactic use of phenobarbital for 1 week has been advocated for the asphyxiated infant.

Diffuse brain swelling and increasing intracranial pressure occur at 24-72 hours in the severely asphyxiated infant with widespread brain infarction. The role of steroids in reducing intracranial pressure in this situation has not been clarified and steroids are not recommended. Appropriate fluid restriction and use of hyperosmolar agents may be beneficial. The sequelae of neonatal hypoxic-ischemic encephalopathy are many (see Table 11-2).

INTRACRANIAL HEMORRHAGE

The major forms of primary intracranial hemorrhage in the newborn (epidural, subdural, subarachnoid, and intraparenchymal) may follow trauma to the head during delivery in which there is both compression and distortion of intracranial structures. Some degree of asphyxia usually accompanies significant head trauma. Secondary hemorrhage into infarcted brain usually occurs in the setting of a coagulation defect. Hemorrhagic infarction is usually located in the basal ganglia or the territory of the middle cerebral artery in the term infant, and in the periventricular white matter or cerebellum in the preterm infant.

Periventricular hemorrhage is a unique form of hemorrhage seen almost exclusively in the preterm infant. It arises from small vessels in the involuting germinal matrix. Secondary extension into the ventricular system is common. In most reports periventricular/intraventricular hemorrhage is detected in 40-50% of small premature infants studied by routine ultrasonography or CT scan.

CLINICAL CHARACTERISTICS

Early signs are frequently consistent with the accompanying hypoxic-ischemic encephalopathy (Table 11-7). Large hemorrhages which compress neighboring brain structures present with focal abnormalities such as hemiparesis (convexity subdural or cerebral hemorrhages) or brain stem dysfunction (posterior fossa subdural or cerebellar hemorrhages). Periventricular hemorrhage in the preterm infant may be initially silent.

A detectable fall in hematocrit often accompanies moderate intraventricular hemorrhage. An extensive intracranial hemorrhage with acute ventricular distention is often signaled by sudden neurologic deterioration with profound hypotonia, apnea, or seizures. Intracranial hemorrhage should be suspected in the presence of unexplained jaundice or signs of increasing intracranial pressure.

Extensive blood within the ventricular system or posterior fossa subarachnoid space prevents the normal flow of cerebrospinal fluid and causes acute hydrocephalus. However, hydrocephalus usually evolves more

Table 11-7   Clinical Presentation of Intracranial Hemorrhage in Newborn

Location	Etiology	Presenting signs
Epidural	Head trauma; skull fracture.	Silent; hemiparesis or focal seizures.
Subdural	Head trauma Asphyxia Convexity or interhemispheric—rupture of bridging veins. Posterior—rupture of veins draining into vein of Galen.	Silent; jaundice; hemiparesis or focal seizures (convexity) brain stem compression (posterior); increase in ICP—hydrocephalus; progressive head enlargement—chronic subdural effusion.

Subarachnoid
  Primary
  Secondary to subdural or intraventricular hemorrhage.
	Head trauma; asphyxia.	Silent; occasionally seizures.

Cerebellar	Preterm, associated with intraventricular hemorrhage. Associated with posterior subdural hemorrhage.	Brain stem compression; increase in ICP—hydrocephalus
Cerebral	Primary—cerebral contusion with head trauma, occasionally from vascular malformation or congenital aneurysm. Secondary—infarction with coagulation defect, rarely tumor.	Hemiparesis, diparesis, or focal seizures; increased ICP.
Periventricular	Preterm, from germinal matrix; asphyxia; respiratory distress; pneumothorax.	Silent; fall in hematocrit; acute increase in ICP with neurologic deterioration; gradual progressive increase in ICP—communicating hydrocephalus.

slowly and presents with increasing head circumference and fontanelle tension 1-3 weeks after birth. In this situation, communicating hydrocephalus results from the blockage of CSF absorption in the arachnoid villi by blood in the subarachnoid space. Periventricular/intraventricular hemorrhage has a varied outcome (see Table 11-8).

Acute intracranial hemorrhage is readily detected on CT scan as a region of increased attenuation. The persistence of signs of hemorrhage on CT scan depends on the size of the hemorrhage. CT scan may not reliably detect small intracranial hemorrhages more than 1 week after their occurrence. At ultrasonography, hemorrhage is visualized as a region of increased echogenicity which may persist for several weeks. However, hemorrhages located over the convexity or in the posterior fossa are not always readily detected by this method.

MANAGEMENT AND OUTCOME

Unless an intracranial hemorrhage is sufficiently large to endanger the infant's life by its mass effect and compression of neighboring structures, acute surgical drainage is usually not necessary. Acute hemorrhagic hydrocephalus in the preterm infant may require immediate ventricular drainage (Table 11-9). Permanent ventriculoperitoneal shunt placement is feasible even in the very small infant when the CSF protein content has fallen to 200 mg/dl or less, as the blood is absorbed. However, posthemorrhagic ventriculomegaly may be transient and resolve spontaneously. In these circumstances, efforts to decrease CSF production with diuretics or hyperosmolar agents or by repeated removal of CSF by lumbar puncture may stabilize ventricular size and render the placement of a permanent ventriculoperitoneal shunt unnecessary. When posthemorrhagic ventriculomegaly is accompanied by signs of increased intracranial pressure these temporizing measures are usually not successful in avoiding eventual shunt placement.

BIRTH TRAUMA

Extracranial traumatic hemorrhage occurs in one of three anatomic locations: within the subcutaneous tissues, the subgaleal, or the subperiosteal spaces (Table 11-10). In each case, a scalp mass is often accompanied by excessive molding and appears following a difficult or precipitous delivery, or after the use of forceps. Surgical drainage of an extracranial hematoma is contraindicated.

Skull fractures are usually parietal in location and may be accompanied by an epidural hematoma or cephalohematoma. Depressed skull fractures may be present as localized palpable bony defects following localized compression of the skull from maternal pelvis or forceps. Small uncomplicated depressed fractures may not require surgical intervention. Traumatic intracranial hemorrhages may also occur (Table 11-7).

Spinal cord injury is a rare cause of a flaccid quadriplegia without diaphragm involvement. Trauma is commonly localized to the low cervical

Table 11-8   Periventricular/Intraventricular Hemorrhage

	Locations	Outcome
Grade 1	Subependymal	Benign
Grade 2	Subependymal and intraventricular without ventrilar distention.	Benign or transient ventriculomegaly; occasional communicating hydrocephalus.
Grade 3	Subependymal and intraventricular with acute distention of ventricles.	Acute increase in ICP; progressive ventriculomegaly, communicating hydrocephalus.
Grade 4	Subependymal, intraventricular and parenchymal (hemorrhagic infarction).	As in grade 2 or 3, with persisting neurologic signs.

Table 11-9   Management of Posthemorrhagic Ventriculomegaly

Stable ventriculomegaly	Observe with 1-2 times weekly ultrasonography.
Progressive ventriculomegaly without signs of increased ICP.	Diamox 15-30 mg/kg/day; Furosemide 1-2 mg/kg/day; Glycerol; serial lumbar punctures.
Progressive ventriculomegaly with signs of increased ICP or neurologic deterioration.	Ventricular drain (CSF protein over 200 mg/dl) or ventriculoperitoneal shunt.

Table 11-10   Extracranial Traumatic Hemorrhage

	Location	Signs
Caput succedaneum	Edematous scalp	Soft, pitting mass.
Subgaleal hemorrhage	Beneath scalp aponeurosis	Firm, fluctuant mass; occasionally causes acute blood loss.
Cephalohematoma	Subperiosteal; commonly associated with skull fracture.	Firm, tense mass often not apparent at birth; usually parietal location.

Table 11-11 Signs of Brachial Plexus Injury

Proximal cervical roots (C5, C6, C7) (Erb's palsy)	Weakness of shoulder abduction and external rotation (C5); elbow flexion and supination (C5, C6); wrist and finger extension (C6, C7). The diaphragm may be involved (C4, C5). Biceps jerk is absent, triceps and brachioradialis jerks are often depressed. Sensory loss on the lateral aspect of the arm.
Total plexus injury (C5, C6, C7, C8, T1)	Weakness, in addition, of intrinsic hand muscles (C8, T1); flexors of the wrist and fingers (C7, C8, T1). Horner's syndrome is often present. Biceps, brachioradialis, and triceps tendon reflexes are absent. Extensive sensory loss in the limb.

and upper thoracic regions. It usually results from forceful delivery of the head during breech presentation when there is excessive longitudinal traction on the neck. Neuropathologic examinations have shown acute hemorrhage and disruption of the spinal cord with rupture of the spinal dura, the cause of the characteristic snapping sound which often accompanies this injury. Because of the nature of the injury, the neurologic deficit caused by cord transection is usually permanent.

The spinal roots which form the brachial plexus (C5, C6, C7, C8, and T1) are the most common sites of injury to the peripheral nervous system. Usually the nerve root sheath is torn by distracting forces. Actual root avulsion is less common. The clinical signs of brachial plexus injuries depend on which roots are involved (Table 11-11). Most infants with partial brachial plexus palsies have full recovery within 1 year. Infants with total plexus involvement have a less satisfactory outcome. The affected limb should be supported for at least 1 week before passive therapy and splints are used to prevent the development of contractures.

NEONATAL SEIZURES

Seizures occurring in the newborn are almost always symptomatic of a significant diffuse or focal encephalopathy. They rarely occur in an otherwise healthy infant as in idiopathic epilepsy of the older child (see Chapter 10). The more common causes of neonatal seizures include metabolic abnormalities, infections, toxic states, developmental defects, as well as drug withdrawal (Table 11-12).

Table 11-12   Causes of Seizures in the Newborn

Asphyxia	Prenatal; intrapartum; neonatal.
Intracranial hemorrhage	
Bacterial meningitis	Group B streptococcus; *Escherichia coli; Listeria monocytogenes.*
Nonbacterial meningoencephalitis	Cytomegalovirus; toxoplasmosis; rubella; herpes simplex; coxsackie B.
Metabolic disorders	Hypoglycemia; hypocalcemia; hypomagnesemia hyponatremia; hypernatermia; inherited metabolic defects; pyridoxine dependency.
Toxic conditions	Local anesthetic.
Drug withdrawal	Narcotic dependency; short-acting barbiturates.
Developmental defects	Schizencephaly; lissencephaly; pachygyria.

CLINICAL CHARACTERISTICS

Many of the clinical manifestations of seizures are unique to the newborn (Table 11-13). In the premature infant generalized tonic seizures are most often seen, while focal or multifocal clonic seizures are more common in the term infant. Subtle seizures are often difficult to distinguish from dystonic movements. They sometimes manifest no motor components at all and are recognized as seizures by their autonomic accompaniments.

Clinical seizures are usually, but not always, accompanied by electrographic seizure activity. Ictal EEG patterns include runs of periodic sharp, slow transients, or spikes, which may be diffuse or focal, or episodic rhythmical fast activity. Interictal EEG abnormalities involve the background activity (low voltage or burst suppression patterns) or epileptiform transients which are often focal or multifocal.

MANAGEMENT AND OUTCOME

Acute management of newborn seizures:

1. Maintain an adequate airway and ventilation.
2. Determine blood glucose, calcium, magnesium, and electrolytes.
3. Glucose 25% solution, 2-4 ml/kg IV, if indicated.
4. Calcium gluconate 5% solution, 4 ml/kg IV, if indicated.
5. Magnesium sulfate 50% solution 0.2 ml/kg IV, if indicated.
6. Phenobarbital 20-40 mg/kg IV; maintenance dose 2-5 mg/kg/day orally; therapeutic level 15-40 μg/ml.
7. Phenytoin 20 mg/kg IV; maintenance 6-10 mg/kg/day orally; therapeutic level 10-20 μg/ml.
8. Paraldehyde in oil rectally 0.03 ml/kg per dose, or 5% solution in 5% dextrose 150 mg/kg/hour IV (avoid plastics except polyethylene).
9. Pyridoxine 50 mg IV.

Table 11-13 Seizure Types in the Newborn

Generalized tonic seizures	Extension of arms and legs. Usual seizure type in the preterm infant.
Myoclonic seizures	Flexion jerks of the extremities.
Focal clonic seizures	Repeated flexion jerks of the extremities. Usual seizure type in term infants.
Multifocal clonic seizures	Usually clonic seizures recur at each site in sequence.
Subtle seizures	Eye deviation or jerking; eyelid fluttering; oral-buccal-lingual movements; dystonic swimming or peddling movements; apnea; autonomic changes, including increased blood pressure and tachycardia.

The outcome following newborn seizures is primarily determined by the etiology of the seizures. Transient reversible metabolic disturbances such as hypocalcemia have a benign prognosis and do not require treatment with anticonvulsants if they are uncomplicated. When seizures accompany hypoglycemic or hypoxic-ischemic encephalopathies, neurologic recovery depends on the degree and duration of the insult. If there is a recurrence of seizures beyond the neonatal period, it is usually within the first year of life.

APNEA

In the newborn, hypoventilation and apnea are major symptoms of both pulmonary and neurologic disorders. Apnea is often a symptom of a severe diffuse encephalopathy resulting from asphyxia, hypoglycemia, or depressant drugs. During apnea, the degree of hypoxemia depends on the duration of the episode, the infant's size and activity level. Hypoxemia is relatively greater during obstructive than central apnea.

Congenital central hypoventilation is a rare syndrome of respiratory failure due to hypoventilation or apnea during drowsiness and sleep. This failure to maintain adequate ventilation is most significant during non-rapid eye movement sleep. The syndrome is sometimes accompanied by defects in autonomic innervation of the bowel. Some infants with this syndrome may develop normally when treated with tracheostomy and assisted ventilation during sleep and daytime naps.

Preterm infants who have survived the acute complications of prematurity may suffer repeated respiratory pauses with significant hypoxemia. This apnea of prematurity usually has mixed central and obstructive components and is most common during drowsiness and active sleep. Theophylline usually reduces the apnea in premature infants.

REFERENCES

Dennis J: The implications of neonatal seizures. *In* Korobkin R, Guilleminault C (Eds): *Advances in Perinatal Neurology,* vol I. SP Medical and Scientific Books, New York, 1979, pp 205-224.

Dubowitz L, Dubowitz V: *The Neurological Assessment of the Preterm and Full Term Newborn Infant.* Clinics in Developmental Medicine, No 79. Spastics International Medical Publications, London, 1981.

Fitz CR: Computed tomography in the newborn. *In* Korobkin R, Guilleminault C (Eds). *Progress in Perinatal Neurology,* Vol I, Williams & Wilkins, Baltimore, 1981, pp 85-120.

Tarby TJ, Volpe JJ: Intraventricular hemorrhage in the preterm infant. Pediatr. Clin North America, vol 29, no 5. Saunders, Philadelphia, 1982, pp 1077-1104.

Tharp BR: Neonatal electroencephalography. *In* Korobkin R, Guilleminault C (Eds): *Progress in Perinatal Neurology,* vol I, Williams & Wilkins, Baltimore, 1981, pp 31-64.

Volpe JJ: *Neurology of the Newborn.* Saunders, Philadelphia, 1981.

12

The Dysmorphic Child

Bryan D. Hall, MD

Physicians trained in the discipline of clinical neurology usually approach patients with neurologic dysfunction and concomitant dysmorphic features as primarily having a neurologic disorder but dysmorphic features are thought to be secondary and of lesser importance. This approach to the clinical problem is generally imprudent for attention must be directed to both the neurologic disorder as well as the dysmorphic features. An organized diagnostic approach is essential to understand the nature of these problems.

CHARACTERISTICS OF A DYSMORPHIC PATIENT

It is generally accepted that a dysmorphic patient has one or more physical abnormalities in one or more external body areas. However, many physicians incorrectly consider a patient as dysmorphic only if craniofacial areas are abnormal; hence, the unfortunate terms 'FLK' or 'funny looking kid.'

Since most dysmorphic persons have multiple congenital anomalies that usually include the craniofacial area, physicians must develop an understanding of what defines a dysmorphic face. The person's face must differ significantly from his 'normal' siblings and parents to be considered potentially dysmorphic. Facial features are then compared with the accepted range of normal for racial and ethnic backgrounds. The characterization as dysmorphic is simple when malformations such as facial clefts or anophthalmia are noted, but it becomes more complicated when subtle differences such as a flat nasal bridge, epicanthic folds, or a simple philtrum are the only differentiating features.

Most dysmorphic features as isolated findings are not abnormal but when associated with other dysmorphic characteristics, the combined gestalt is different from that of other normal family members and features of the general population. Certainly, some individuals suspected of being dysmorphic may resemble a sibling or parent but this should alert the clinician to the possibility that those relatives with similar features may also be dysmorphic. In that circumstance, the questionably dysmorphic individuals must be critically compared to other family members, particularly if the suspected dysmorphic feature(s) exist in parent and child.

DYSMORPHIC TYPES

There are two basic types of dysmorphism: prenatal (congenital) and acquired (perinatal, postnatal). Prenatal dysmorphism suggests that fetal abnormalities developed during the gestation; while acquired dysmorphism

207

Table 12-1 Examples of Prenatal Dysmorphism under Primary
Secondary Categories

Primary defects (malformation, anomaly)	Secondary effects (deformation)	Secondary defects (disruption)
Polydactyly	Clubbed feet	Glossoptosis cleft palate
Congenital heart anomaly	Joint dislocation	Potter anomaly
Cleft lip/palate	Joint contracture	beak nose
Anophthalmia	Bowed limb	Amnion band limb
Omphalocele	Torticollis	amputation
Hypospadias	Cranial contour	Uterine compression
Phocomelia	abnormalities	limb deficiency
Absent radius	Plagiocephaly	Edema related nail
Spinal dysraphism	Cortical thumb	dysplasia
Anencephaly	Absent flexion creases	Edema related webbed
	Prune belly	neck

results from some perinatal or postnatal insult. This dichotomy is most important for it allows one to determine the onset of the dysmorphic features, a fact of great importance with ramifications for diagnosis, classification, treatment, and genetic counseling.

Prenatal dysmorphic features may consist of primary defects (malformations, anomalies), secondary effects (deformation), or secondary defects (disruption). A *primary defect* is the basic alteration of structural development of a body part during its critical period in organogenesis. Since the architecture of most body structures is defined by the tenth fetal week, a primary defect has usually occurred before this period. A *secondary effect* is the result of adverse effects of the primary defect, or an intrauterine environmental abnormality. In this circumstance, the basic structure of the body part is normal, but has become malpositioned or compromised as may be the case in club foot or hip dislocation.

Secondary defects occur when a 'normally formed' structure is so disrupted that it looks like a primary defect but existing evidence suggests that its derivation was the result of a separate malformation. An example of this is the Pierre Robin anomaly in which the primary defect (hypoplastic mandible) gives rise to a secondary defect (cleft palate) by lack of tongue support, which allows it to obstruct closure of the palatal shelves. Most secondary events classified under prenatal dysmorphism originate later than 10 fetal weeks although they may occur earlier. Table 12-1 lists some common examples of primary defects, secondary effects, and secondary defects.

Acquired dysmorphic features are those which become apparent only later in persons who earlier had a normal appearance but who sustained some perinatal or postnatal insult. *Perinatally acquired dysmorphism* occurs when an otherwise normal infant experiences some insult during labor, delivery, or the neonatal period, resulting in some neurologic impairment. This often results in microcephaly, spasticity, hirsutism, and an overall abnormal facial and body appearance.

Postnatally-acquired dysmorphism occurs more frequently in neuro-degenerative or other metabolic disorders, wherein normally appearing new-borns and infants have an acute or insidious onset of signs and symptoms of degenerative disease and, subsequently, an alteration of their appearance. These patients through mechanisms of neurologic damage and/or abnormal storage of neurochemical by-products, may be remarkably dysmorphic. Of great importance in this group of patients is the absence of any perinatal insult and the fact they were of normal physical appearance at birth. Only later will they become dysmorphic. The effects of acquired dysmorphism are considered secondary in nature.

DIAGNOSTIC CATEGORIZATION

It is important to understand and use a systematic approach to the recognition and diagnosis of dysmorphic persons who may also have neurologic disorders. Table 12-2 lists a simplified scheme for the diagnostic categorization of these patients. Appropriate categorization is essential in order to make a correct diagnosis, for it narrows the differential diagnoses considerably and focuses attention on the more important clinical and diagnostic laboratory features to be pursued. This table is based upon the assumption that patients with both dysmorphic and abnormal neurologic signs and/or symptoms, can be accurately diagnosed by pattern identification of the dysmorphic features, with some support from neurologic findings but only rarely by neurologic findings alone. This assumption is generally true since most abnormal neurologic features are secondary and, hence, less specific for diagnostic and etiologic considerations.

Dysmorphic features often include a significant number of primary defects which serve as solid clues to pattern or syndrome identification. Some neurologic features such as encephalocele, anencephaly, and spina bifida represent primary defects, and as such, carry equal importance when compared with nonneurologic prenatal dysmorphic characteristics. Emphasis on dysmorphic features is less useful when manifestations of dysmorphism have their origin secondary to perinatal or postnatal events. In these cases, the acquired dysmorphism usually relates to the basic neurologic abnormality and, consequently, identification of the pattern of neurologic features is more important.

METHOD OF DIAGNOSIS

The first step (Table 12-2) is the important process of determining whether the patient's abnormalities represent prenatal or acquired dysmorphism. It is essential to know whether or not the patient was anatomically normal at birth. A finding of any primary defect (step 2) immediately places the dysmorphic feature in the prenatal category. Secondary effects and secondary defects identifiable at birth also indicate a prenatal insult; certain secondary features like hypotonia or hypertonia are not easy to date. Usually, historical or clinical features such as body posture, muscle mass, dermal crease patterns, newborn head circumference, intrauterine fetal activity, etc., can be used to date this major secondary feature. If no prenatal dysmorphic features can be identified, the process is more likely acquired. Determining whether the insult occurred in the perinatal period or was postnatal is best established by carefully documenting the history of peri-

Table 12-2 Diagnostic Categorization of Dysmorphic Patients with Neurologic Abnormalities

	Prenatal dysmorphism					*Acquired dysmorphism*	
Step 1	*Prenatal dysmorphism*					*Acquired dysmorphism*	
Step 2	*Prenatal onset*					*Perinatal onset*	*Postnatal onset*
Step 3	*Primary defect(s)*		*Secondary effect*	*Secondary effect*	*Secondary defect*	*Secondary effect*	*Secondary effect*
Step 4	*Multiple*	*Single*	*Single or multiple*	*Single or multiple*	*Single or multiple*	*Single or multiple*	*Single or multiple*
Step 5	Associated with mental retardation, prenatal, postnatal growth deficiency.	Variable association with mental retardation, prenatal, postnatal growth deficiency.	Associated with problems in area of involvement or systems dependent on area of involvement.	Associated with primary defect. Attention directed to primary defect.	Associated with primary defect. Attention directed to primary defect.	Associated with perinatal insult.	Associated most frequently with neurodegenerative or other metabolic disorders.
	Example 1. Chromosomal disorders 2. Meckel-Gruber 3. Seckel dwarfism	*Example* 1. Single gene 2. Environmental 3. Developmental 4. Unknown	*Example* 1. Holoprosencephaly 2. Multifactorial (anencephaly, encephalocele) 3. Cleft lip	*Example* 1. Club foot (due to oligohydramnios) 2. Hip dislocation (breech delivery 2° to intrauterine hypotonia) 3. Expressionless face (congenital myotonic dystrophy)	*Example* 1. Syndactyly (2° to amniotic bands) 2. Limb deficiency (2° to intrauterine compression caused by cornuate uterus)	*Example* 1. Neonatal asphyxia 2. Neonatal hypoglycemia 3. Subarachnoid hemorrhage (all of above may later have microcephaly, spasticity & hypertrichosis)	*Example* 1. PKU 2. Hurler syndrome 3. Tay-Sachs 4. Neurofibromatosis 5. Tuberous sclerosis

natal trauma. Patients who have sustained some perinatal insult have a normal newborn phenotype. Those patients who have had some postnatal insult usually have an interval of normal activity and development, followed by progressive deterioration of their neurologic status and phenotype.

At this point (step 3) one must determine what features are primary or secondary. All primary features are defects of early prenatal onset. When properly identified, primary defects and their patterns are essential to establish a recognizable dysmorphic syndrome. Identification of primary defects dramatically reduces the complexity of malformation syndromes by minimizing the number of features to be emphasized.

For example, a child with (1) clubbed feet, (2) dilocated hips, (3) hypertonia, (4) intrauterine growth retardation, (5) microcephaly, (6) low-set ears, (7) cleft palate, (8) congenital heart defect, (9) syndactyly of 4th-5th fingers, and (10) scalp defect, has four primary defects (7-10). The remaining features (1-6) are secondary effects. The initial pursuit of the diagnosis in the above patient should be directed to the four primary defects, and the six secondary effects should not confuse the issue of diagnosis.

An important observation is that the less common the primary defect, the more valuable it is as a diagnostic clue. For example, rare primary defects such as a lateral facial cleft, scalp defect, multiple oral frenulae, lingual hamartomas, and absent tibias are much more valuable as individual features than the more common defects such as an omphalocele, unilateral cleft lip, micrognathia, congenital heart defect, or polydactyly.

The clinician must now determine (step 4) if the abnormalities are multiple or single under their primary or secondary categories. Multiple primary defects are generally considered to represent a *multiple congenital anomaly syndrome* such as trisomy 13, while a single primary defect is an *anomaly,* as in the case of unilateral absence of the thumb. A single primary defect with secondary effects or defects is an *anomaly sequence;* for example Pierre Robin syndrome. Whether there are single or multiple secondary effects or defects under prenatal dysmorphism is not particularly important because their identification only serves to point to the causative primary defect(s). However, the larger the number of secondary features, the more indirect clues one has to assist in making a final diagnostic decision.

All features of acquired dysmorphism are secondary, usually multiple, and often additive. A careful neurologic assessment is essential in patients with acquired dysmorphism, particularly in the early stage of phenotypic change when dysmorphic features are not present or distinct.

Finally (step 5) the clinician should reconsider each and all of the factors that suggest the patient's dysmorphic features are consistent with the functional diagnosis. Clinical examples are given (Table 12-2) for each category to illustrate some types of diagnoses one might consider.

Examples of dysmorphic states are listed under somewhat different but related categories (Table 12-3), when compared to those of Table 12-2. Neurologic syndromes are usually made up of entities with postnatally-acquired dysmorphic characteristics. Some obviously 'pure' neurologic syndromes such as I-cell disease and generalized gangliosidosis (Gm1) have prenatally-acquired dysmorphic features as well as postnatally-acquired dysmorphic features. Some relatively 'pure' neurologic syndromes such as neurofibromatosis or tuberous sclerosis occasionally have secondary pre-

Table 12-3   Examples of Pure Neurologic, Anomaly/Sequence, and Multiple Anomaly/Neurologic Syndromes

Neurologic syndromes	Anomaly/sequence neurologic states	Multiple anomaly/ neurologic syndromes
1. Neurofibromatosis (occasional prenatal dysmorphism).	1. Holoprosencephaly (+ midline cleft lip) with secondary hypotelorism, microcephaly.	1. Trisomy 13, 18 21.
2. Tuberous sclerosis (occasional prenatal dysmorphism).	2. Sturge-Weber syndrome (facial hemangiomatosis) with facial hypertrophy, glaucoma, seizures.	2. 4p-(Wolf-Hirschhorn).
3. Schwartz-Jampel syndrome.	3. Septo-optic dysplasia with growth failure, ± mental retardation.	3. Cornelia DeLange syndrome.
4. Tay-Sachs disease (Gm2 gangliosidosis).	4. Lumbar spina bifida with secondary dislocated hips, clubbed feet, and hydrocephalus.	4. Meckel-Gruber syndrome.
5. Hurler syndrome (MPSI).	5. Amniotic bands with secondary encephalocele, facial clefts.	5. Smith-Lemli-Optiz syndrome.
6. Myotonic dystrophy (congenital and adult onset).	6. Encephalocele (midline, occipital) with secondary frontal recession, microcephaly.	6. Oral-facial-digital syndromes (types I, II).
7. Huntington's chorea.	7. Encephalocele (midline, frontal) with secondary hypertelorism and nasal deformity.	7. Fetal alcohol syndrome.

natally-acquired dysmorphic characteristics. The anomaly-sequence neurologic status consists of a single primary defect with secondary effects and defects involving the nervous system. Holoprosencephaly, for example, is considered a single anomaly/sequence of undetermined etiology only if the midportion of the anterior brain, skull, and facies are involved. However, if additional body areas outside the craniofacial area display primary defects (anomalies), then the patient has a multiple anomaly/neurologic syndrome.

Accurate diagnosis is achieved only when each dysmorphic feature is critically considered regarding its primary or secondary nature, the time of onset, and how it relates to adjacent, proximal or distal features. Once this is done, an appropriate pattern can be established. Careful literature review at this point will usually assure the correct diagnosis, if one is at all possible.

REFERENCES

Dyken PR, Miller MD: *Facial Features of Neurologic Syndromes,* 1st ed. Mosby, St. Louis, 1980.

Gorlin RJ, Pindborg JJ, Cohen MM Jr: *Syndromes of the Head and Neck,* 2nd ed. McGraw-Hill, New York, 1976.

Potter EL, Craig JM: *Pathology of the Fetus and the Infant,* 3rd ed. Year Book, Chicago, 1975.

Smith DW: *Recognizable Patterns of Human Malformation,* 2nd ed. Saunders, Philadelphia, 1976.

Smith DW: *Recognizable Patterns of Human Deformation,* 1st ed. Saunders, Philadelphia, 1981.

Warkany J: *Congenital Malformations,* 1st ed. Year Book, Chicago, 1971.

13

Ophthalmic Problems
in Childhood

Creig S. Hoyt, MD

EVALUATION

Examination of the visual system of each patient must be carefully and systematically carried out for it may lead to the anatomic localization of a primary neurologic abnormality. Several attempts may be required, however, since infants and young children are often irritable and/or distractible.

A thorough sensory examination is warranted even in the very young child. Affections of the visual system may be manifest as loss of visual acuity, disorder of color vision, localized field defects, abnormal negative or positive visual phenomena, or as a higher integrative visual disturbance.

VISUAL ACUITY

The most common test of visual acuity is a standard set of letters of the alphabet of graded sizes, presented to the subject at a stated distance. Reading letters is a task of some complexity and may not be appropriate for children under the age of 5 years. Other means of determining visual acuity include the 'illiterate' E test, graded sized pictures of common objects, and electrophysiological techniques. Any degree of visual acuity loss implies a disturbance of the system's subserving central vision; namely, the papillomacular bundle and its connections.

COLOR VISION

Congenital disturbances of color vision, particularly red-green disorders, are common. Generally, all acquired disorders of the optic nerve selectively interfere with perception of red-green hues. Blue-yellow disorders occur in dominantly inherited optic atrophy and central retinal disorders result in blue-yellow dyschromatopsia.

VISUAL FIELDS

Consistent topographical arrangement of visual fibers projecting from the retina to the visual cortex enables one to make precise anatomical diagnoses by means of visual field testing (see Chapter 1). This may be done by confrontation techniques, with tangent screen, perimetry testing, or with newer automated field devices. (See Table 13-1.)

Table 13-1 Abnormalities of the Visual Fields

Central scotoma	Any central defect of the visual field encompassing primarily the fixation area is referred to as central or paracentral scotoma; the configuration is generally oval. These defects suggest disease processes affecting the macula or optic nerve. Rarely the disorder involves the chiasm or visual cortex.
Centrocecal scotoma	A defect involving both the fixation point and the blind spot; these are characteristic of diseases of the papillomacular bundle, especially metabolic disorders.
Arcuate scotoma	This field disorder reflects the anatomic configuration of the retinal nerve fiber layer. Although it is typical of the field disorder produced by glaucoma it is more commonly seen in children with congenital malformations of the optic nerve.
Ring scotoma	A field defect encircling the fixation point at some distance. This is pathognomonic for retinal diseases particularly degenerative disorders as in the case of retinitis pigmentosa.
Hemianopsia	This term implies a defect involving half of the visual field. It may be homonymous (field loss is identical in each eye), and is typical of a disease process posterior to the decussation of visual fibers in the chiasm. It may be bitemporal (temporal fields of both eyes are involved). This is the typical field disturbance found in chiasmal disorders, but may also be demonstrated in congenital optic nerve disorders (hypoplasia, dysplasia, etc.) Altitudinal hemianopsia represents involvement of the fibers of only the lower or upper half of the retina. This field defect is usually seen in diseases of the retina, optic nerve, occipital cortex, or rarely, the chiasm. True binasal hemianopsia probably does not occur but lesions primarily affecting the nasal fields may be seen in optic nerve malformations.
Quadrantopsia	Quadrant field defects are demonstrated in disorders posterior to the lateral geniculate body. Superior quadrantopsia is typical of temporal lobe pathology involving the optic radiations known as Meyer's loop; inferior quadrantopsia is less common and is usually a sign of parietal or occipital lobe disease.

POSITIVE PHENOMENA

Disorders of the visual system may be manifested by signs of excitatory activity; these are primarily photopsias or hallucinations.

Photopsias are flashes of light, usually secondary to retinal disease. The sensations may be flashes or 'banks' of light which are usually described as intensely white but they may contain color, commonly blue. Photopsias may also occur as a result of disease of the occipital cortex. This is usually an event confined to one hemi-field but may be so disturbing to the child that it is reported to involve one or the other eye. Migraine is the most common disorder associated with photopsias, although retinal detachment, arteriovenous malformations of the occipital cortex, and seizure activity must always be considered in the differential diagnosis.

Hallucinations are apparent perceptions of external objects when such objects are not present. It is generally believed that highly organized visual hallucinations, such as images of people or objects, usually indicate temporal lobe pathology; whereas, unformed hallucinations, such as zig-zag lines, signify occipital lobe disease.

NEGATIVE PHENOMENA

Obscurations are transient losses or blurring of vision that may occur in several settings. The visual loss associated with papilledema lasts only for seconds, that of migraine for minutes, and with cerebral ischemia, minutes to hours.

Amaurosis implies total or partial loss of vision. It is important to determine if this has been present since birth or has been recently acquired. Bilateral visual loss acquired in the perinatal period usually results in pendular nystagmus, except in cases of 'cortical blindness.'

Night blindness (nyctalopia) refers to a specific visual loss or deficiency that occurs in reduced illumination. It generally occurs with retinal disorders that primarily affect the rods, as seen in retinitis pigmentosa and vitamin A deficiency.

Day blindness (hemeralopia) refers to vision that is worse in good illumination; it is less common than night blindness. Day blindness reflects selective dysfunction of the retinal cones and is accompanied by photophobia, nystagmus, color vision loss, and reduced visual acuity.

DISORDERS OF HIGHER INTEGRATIVE FUNCTION

The act of 'seeing' is more complex than just the processing of visual signals by the occipital lobe. Disorders of the parietal lobe, temporal lobe, and corpus callosum may be manifested by specific integrative visual disturbances.

Alexia and dyslexia imply a specific inability to perceive the meaning of written words or symbols. Developmental dyslexia is of considerable importance to the pediatrician since children with learning disabilities are frequently brought to physicians for consultation. Although there is rarely any sign of primary ocular defect in these children, recent evidence suggests that at least some have minor dysplasias of the language-relevant areas of the brain.

Agnosia may be defined as the loss of ability to recognize the importance of sensory stimuli. Visual agnosia is the failure to recognize common object when the optic pathways are intact. Different types of visual agnosia may occur with lesions of various portions of the temporal or parietal lobe.

EVALUATION OF THE 'BLIND' CHILD

Although 'blindness' is not a common handicap in children, its early detection is of utmost importance so that rehabilitation and education may be initiated as early as possible. In the preverbal child, one often assesses the motor system and makes inappropriate conclusions about the sensory system. Clinicians should be cautious, therefore, in making the diagnosis of 'blindness.'

Normal visual acuity development It was once believed that children did not develop the potential to read 6/6 until 4 or 5 years of age. However, full-term infants have the capacity to fix and follow at birth and probably have a visual acuity of 6/36 or better.

Visual testing of the neonate Recent evidence suggests the ideal fixation target for testing neonatal visual function is the human face. Slight movement of the examiner's face in front of the infant will usually elicit following movements even when a flashlight, toy, or optokinetic test tape will not.

Multiply-handicapped children Normal visual development may be delayed in the child with other handicaps, especially of the central nervous system. Similarly, significant visual defects may cause delay in normal motor development.

Cortical blindness In this circumstance, it is implied that the visual system is entirely normal except for the occipital cortex. The diagnosis is made in a child with apparent blindness, normal pupillary responses, and no nystagmus. Most children with acquired cortical blindness have a good prognosis for significant visual recovery because of the incomplete destruction of the visual cortex and/or the ability of the extrageniculate striate system to subserve primary visual functions.

THE OCULAR MOTOR SYSTEM

The control of ocular movements involves the integration of input from several subsystems of the brain. Even when the eyes are looking straight ahead there is continual neuromuscular activity maintaining this eye position. A comprehensive model of the neuronal control of eye movements is yet unavailable but, at the same time, a great deal of information is known.

TYPES OF EYE MOVEMENTS

Saccadic These voluntary quick 'jerks' of the eyes are the primary movements involved in most visual activity including reading. They are initiated within the contralateral frontal region and descend to the brain stem via the frontomesencephalic neuronal pathway. Horizontal saccades are integrated in the pons and vertical saccades in the midbrain.

Pursuit movements are slow and elicited by a moving target. They play little function in ordinary ocular activity and are thought to be initiated from within the ipsilateral occipital lobe.

Vestibular ocular movements result from changes in the position of the head and neck. They are generated within the vestibular neuronal complex in the pons and play a constant role in coordinating eye movements with changes of head and neck posture.(See p. 14.)

Vergences are unique ocular movements that defy Hering's law (there is equal ennervation of yolk muscles of the two eyes). Convergence is undoubtedly mediated through a midbrain center. Whether there is an active divergence center or not (or whether divergence results from a relaxation of convergence) is yet to be determined.

Fusion is the shift of one eye (the deviating eye) in order to reestablish alignment of both eyes on a single target. A precise center for this type of eye movement is not known but is probably in the midbrain.

SYMPTOMS OF OCULAR MOTOR DISTURBANCES

Diplopia is the abnormal sensation of seeing one object as two and is usually secondary to ocular motor misalignment. In young children, suppression of vision (amblyopia) in the deviating eye may prevent the perception of diplopia despite a gross ocular motor disturbance.

Oscillopsia is the perception of movement of a stationary object. It results in some acquired forms of nystagmus particularly those of vestibular origin.

Head nodding and abnormal head positions Nodding of the head may occur as a compensatory adjustment in some forms of nystagmus. It is a central feature of spasmus nutans. Abnormal positions of the head may result from ocular motor misalignment or nystagmus. The head position may be an effort to compensate for a weakness of a vertically-acting extraocular muscle (primarily the obliques). In some forms of nystagmus, a head turn or more rarely, a tilt, may occur in order to place the eyes in the position of least nystagmoid movements (null point).

CRANIAL NERVE PALSIES

Third nerve The diagnosis of a third-nerve palsy is easy to establish and is characterized by ptosis, dilatation of the pupil, and downward and outward deviation of the eye. An isolated third-nerve palsy in children is rarely an ominous sign. It is usually of congenital or traumatic origin. Other less common causes include migraine, inflammation, and rarely a brain tumor.

Fourth nerve The diagnosis of a fourth-nerve palsy is not always simple. Paralysis of the superior oblique muscle produces upward deviation of the eye and limitation of depression in adduction. However, paralysis of intorsion is usually evident because it commonly results in compensatory head tilt toward the opposite shoulder. The etiology of most isolated childhood fourth-nerve palsies is usually congenital or secondary to trauma.

Sixth nerve   Because paralysis of the sixth nerve results in inward turning of the affected eye, this disorder can mimic a strabismus esotropia. It is essential that one evaluate the abducting power of the affected eye in order to make this distinction. In sharp contrast to palsies of the third and fourth nerves, sixth-nerve palsies are not always benign in children. They may occur with brain tumors, primarily intrinsic pontine lesions, or secondary to hydrocephalus. There are benign causes, however, including congenital, traumatic, and postinfectious etiologies. The last entity commonly occurs a few days after a mild respiratory or gastrointestinal disturbance and resolves without therapy within a period of 6-8 weeks.

SUPRANUCLEAR DISTURBANCES

Gaze palsies describe a defect in conjugate movements of both eyes; there may be a defect of horizontal or vertical gaze. Horizontal gaze palsies result in the inability to turn both eyes in one direction. Diplopia is not present. Lesions of either the frontal lobe or pontine gaze centers may produce this defect. The frontal lobe lesion produces a contralateral gaze palsy; whereas, a pontine lesion produces an ipsilateral disturbance. Frontal lobe gaze palsies are uncommon in children and are usually transient. Pontine gaze center palsies, however, may be a sign of an intrinsic mass lesion. Congenital gaze palsies are not uncommon and constitute part of the Mobius syndrome. Vertical gaze palsies are almost always a sign of midbrain pathology and are usually confined to upgaze only. The upward gaze center lies dorsal to the aqueduct; whereas the downward center is vertical. The most common causes of vertical gaze palsies in children are hydrocephalus, kernicterus, intrinsic and extrinsic lesions of the midbrain, and lipid storage diseases.

Internuclear ophthalmoplegia characteristically consists of ipsilateral paresis of the medial rectus muscle with normal convergence and variable nystagmus in abduction of the other eye. It is produced by a lesion in the medial longitudinal fasciculus carrying excitatory fibers from the pontine gaze center to the third-nerve nuclear complex in the midbrain. In children it is usually the result of a mass lesion or demyelinating disease, although it may rarely be on a congenital basis.

Gaze apraxia is a congenital disorder of voluntary horizontal gaze in which the child is unable to look quickly toward either side. It is distinguished by the presence of compensatory head thrusts that stimulate vestibular centers and allows the child to divert the eyes to the desired point of fixation. This is usually an isolated disorder although a similar ocular motor disorder is sometimes observed in patients with ataxia-telangiectasia (see Chapter 9).

Skew deviation refers to an acquired vertical divergence of the eyes which is secondary to supranuclear dysfunction. The degree of ocular separation may be constant or variable in different positions of gaze, and there may be an accompanying horizontal disconjugate separation. Skew deviation is generally considered a poor localizing sign of posterior fossa dysfunction. It is a common transient disorder in otherwise healthy neonates.

Dysmetria, ocular flutter, and opsoclonus These disorders are considered by most authorities to be a spectrum of abnormalities of a single eye movement system (cerebellar). **Dysmetria** is the over- or undershooting of a new target by the eyes while changing fixation. **Flutter** occurs spontaneously during fixation and consists of several rapid, small amplitude, horizontal pendular oscillations. Flutter commonly coexists with ocular dysmetria in cerebellar system lesions. **Opsoclonus** is characterized by irregular, chaotic, semiconjugate, rapid to-and-fro oscillations of the eyes in a horizontal or oblique direction. It is distinct from nystagmus in lacking the rhythmicity and regularity inherent to nystagmus. It is most frequently observed in encephalitis but may be present in child patients who have an occult neuroblastoma. (See Chapter 17.)

NYSTAGMUS

Nystagmus consists of rhythmic oscillations or tremor-like movements of the eyes. It is usually bilateral but may be unilateral. In rare instances it is voluntary.

Nystagmus due to poor vision Interference with visual function in the perinatal period may result in a typical form of nystagmus, which is largely pendular but may become 'jerky' in extremes of lateral gaze. Typically, the child's visual acuity is worse for distant vision compared with near. This is because nystagmus may be dampened with convergence, and linear magnification may be obtained from accommodating to a very near target.

Spasmus nutans This acquired disorder of unknown etiology consists of the triad of nystagmus, head nodding, and torticollis. The nystagmus is often asymmetric and 'shimmy like' in nature. It is self-limiting by the age of 4 years. Rarely, patients have an associated optic glioma.

Congenital motor nystagmus is pendular and usually horizontal, although torsional and vertical nystagmus are rarely seen. The eye movements continue throughout life but are typically less severe with maturation. The cause is unknown and a careful ocular examination must be performed to be certain the nystagmus is not secondary to poor vision. It is usually inherited as an autosomal dominant trait.

Latent nystagmus is a 'jerky' congenital fixation nystagmus that appears or is increased when one eye is covered. The slow phase of the nystagmus is always toward the covered eye. It is commonly associated with strabismus.

Monocular nystagmus Nystagmus confined to only one eye is rare. Usually the nystagmus is simply very asymmetrical in amplitude and frequency. Monocular nystagmus may occur with amblyopia, spasmus nutans, optic nerve gliomas, and multiple sclerosis.

Vertical nystagmus implies that nystagmus beats in a vertical direction and not that nystagmus is merely present in upward or downward gaze. It is unusual. Down beating nystagmus is virtually pathognomonic of disease at the cervico-medullary junction, particularly the Chiari malformation (see Chapter 2). Upbeat nystagmus may occur with lesions either in the low brain stem or cerebellum. Vertical nystagmus is commonly associated with administration of sedatives or anticonvulsant medication.

Special forms *See-saw nystagmus* is a peculiar type of dissociated vertical nystagmus that may be either congenital or acquired basis. Both eyes move as if a see-saw, one rising the other falling. Most cases of see-saw nystagmus are associated with temporal field defects. *Periodic alternating nystagmus* is a rare form of central vestibular nystagmus consisting of a rhythmic jerk type nystagmus that undergoes phasic or cyclic changes in amplitude and direction. Each cycle lasts from 60-180 seconds.

THE PUPILS AND LIDS

PUPILS

Anatomy The afferent limb of the pupillary arc is composed of the retino-mesencephalic neurons, those axons of the optic nerve destined for the pretectal area. Decussation of these fibers in the chiasm is similar to that of the visual fibers.

Efferent innervation is provided by two different systems, the parasympathetic and sympathetic. The sphincter of the pupil is innervated by the parasympathetic (third nerve) and dilated by the sympathetic. Parasympathetic fibers originate in the Edinger-Westphal nucleus in the midbrain, travel with other third-nerve fibers   to   the   ciliary   ganglion within the orbit, where postganglion fibers arise and travel with the short ciliary nerves to the pupil. Sympathetic neurons arise in the hypothalamus, course through midline of the brain stem to the high cervical cord and then travel to the superior cervical ganglion where third-order neurons originate. These accompany the internal carotid artery into the skull and then with branches of the trigeminal nerve, into the orbit. They reach the pupil via the nasociliary and long ciliary nerves.

Afferent defects In unilateral lesions of the macula and optic nerve a typical pupillary sign known as the Marcus Gunn pupil is seen. It is an invaluable objective sign of structural disease of the anterior visual pathways. Although both pupils are equal in size when a flashlight is used to test the pupillary response, the involved eye exhibits a decreased amplitude and prolonged latency in the reaction to light. This is best seen utilizing the so-called swinging flashlight test. A flashlight is swung back and forth from one eye to the other, illuminating each eye 5-10 seconds. The response of the affected eye is readily seen to be sluggish and in comparison with that of the good eye allows both pupils to dilate.

General defects Lesions affecting the intercalated neurons (those connecting the afferent fibers and the Edinger-Westphal nucleus) produce a specific disorder known as light-near dissociation. This means that pathologic changes in the rostral midbrain can produce defects of the light reflex while sparing the pupillary response to a near target. This is an essential component of the Argyll Robertson pupil; other features are small pupillary size and irregular shape. Although Argyll Robertson pupils are a classic sign of neurosyphilis, they also occur in diabetes. However, in children the most common causes of light-near dissociation of the pupillary response are midbrain mass lesions and hydrocephalus.

Efferent defects

Parasympathetic Lesions affecting the parasympathetic pupillo-motor outflow anywhere along its course from midbrain to the pupil may produce paralysis of pupillary constriction and dilation. The peripheral location of the pupillomotor fibers with the third nerve make them vulnerable to early damage in compressive lesions. A special type of efferent pupillomotor dysfunction due to postsynaptic denervation (probably at the ciliary ganglion) is known as Adie's pupil. The affected pupil is dilated and shows a slow response to light and equally slow redilation after relaxation of the near response. A distinctive feature of Adie's pupil is its sensitivity to very weak cholinergic medications. The condition may be associated with decreased deep tendon reflexes and it is thought to be viral in origin.

Sympathetic Interference with the sympathetic pupillary dilator fibers results in miosis with normal pupillary response to light and near but with failure to fully dilate in reduced illumination. It is usually part of the Horner's syndrome which consists of miosis, ptosis, and facial anhidrosis due to homolateral oculosympathetic paralysis. In children the etiology is usually congenital or traumatic, sometimes associated with brachial plexus injuries.

LIDS

Anatomy There are three separate systems serving lid function: the orbicularis oculi muscle innervated by the facial nerve (seventh) for lid closure; the levator muscle, innervated by the branches of the superior division of the third nerve, is the major elevator of the lid; and Muller's muscle innervated by the sympathetic system which adds additional elevation tone. Lesions within the brain stem, peripheral nerves, or muscles may affect lid position.

Ptosis

Parasympathetic Lesions of the third nerve or its superior division may produce severe ptosis with little or no evidence of levator function. It is usually accompanied by other signs of third-nerve dysfunction, such as a superior rectus paresis. Lesions of the third-nerve nucleus are uncommon and the resulting ptosis is bilateral since both levators are subserved by a single midline subnucleus.

Sympathetic The ptosis resulting from sympathetic dysfunction is usually no more than 2-3 mm and normal levator function is maintained. It is usually accompanied by miosis and facial anhidrosis (Horner's syndrome).

Congenital This is a relatively common condition and may be associated with a wide spectrum of lid dysfunction. It may be neural or muscular in origin.

Neuromuscular The two principal causes of neuromuscular ptosis are myasthenia gravis and progressive external ophthalmoplegia, which may have a myopathic or neuropathic basis. Some toxins, including botulism, diphtheria, tick paralysis, and some insecticides, may affect lid function and extraocular muscles.

Lid retraction When the upper lid is retracted above the limbus, allowing the sclera to be visible, patients have a typical facial expression of surprise or fear. This may occur with lesions around the aqueduct, primarily hydrocephalus, abnormalities of increased sympathetic tone as in thyroid ophthalmopathy, or as a result of certain drugs, such as edrophonium hydrochloride (Tensilon). A variable degree of lid retraction is a normal finding in the neonatal period.

Lagophthalmos refers to the inability to close the eyelids. It may result from structural lid abnormalities, mechanical restrictions, or paralysis of the orbicularis oculi.

Abnormal lid movements

Marcus-Gunn jaw winking refers to abnormal lid movement secondary to congenital synkinesia between the oculomotor and trigeminal neural pathways. It is characterized by variable ptosis and an involuntary spasmodic retraction of the upper lid with certain jaw movements. It is most often noted while the infant is sucking or swallowing.

Aberrant regeneration of the third nerve In cases of recovery of oculomotor nerve paralysis, especially that secondary to trauma or compression, misdirection of regenerating fibers may occur. Thus, the levator muscles may receive regenerating fibers originally destined for the extraocular muscles which would result in lid retraction with eye movement (especially adduction). Identification of this aberrant regeneration is sometimes of great importance for it does not occur in the presence of unresolved mass lesions.

Tics, hemifacial spasm, and myokymia Abnormal contractions of the eyelids usually consist of frequent blinking or tics. This is usually psychogenic in origin and resolves without therapy. Essential blepharospasm consists of repetitive uncontrolled spasms of the orbicularis oculi. Hemifacial spasm is a stereotyped simultaneous contraction of all facial muscles innervated by the seventh nerve but is rare in children. Facial myokymia is an apparent subcutaneous vermian movement from contraction of a few muscle units of the orbicularis oculi. It is a common occurrence particularly when one is fatigued; it rarely occurs in the presence of weakness of muscles innervated by the facial nerve and may then be a sign of a pontine lesion.

ABNORMALITIES OF THE OCULAR FUNDUS

PAPILLEDEMA

This term is reserved for elevation of the optic nerve resulting from increased intracranial pressure. It is characterized by edema of the optic nerve head, blurred margins of the disc, obliteration of the optic cup, hyperemia of the disc, engorgement of the veins, loss of venous pulsations, hemorrhages of superficial retinal layers, and peripapillary soft exudates. In incomplete forms, one may be required to periodically perform careful ophthalmoscopic examinations to determine whether changes of the nerve are consistent with papilledema. Characteristically, visual acuity remains unaffected until later in the course of long-standing papilledema, though transient visual obscurations may occur. Visual-field testing will document an enlarged blind spot and irregular constriction of the peripheral fields.

PSEUDOPAPILLEDEMA

Optic nerve head drusen, peripapillary inflammation, hyperopia, and papillitis may all mimic papilledema. The most common and important of these is optic nerve drusen which are deposits of hyaline material within the optic nerve of unknown etiology. The condition is inherited as an 'irregular' autosomal dominant trait. Both deep and superficial retinal bleeding may occur. Examination of both parents of a child with optic nerve 'edema' frequently establishes the correct diagnosis of pseudopapilledema with drusen bodies.

PAPILLITIS AND OPTIC NEURITIS

These conditions connote involvement of the optic nerve by inflammation, degeneration, or demyelination with secondary reduced visual function. If the process occurs near the surface of the optic nerve, visible swelling of the nerve is apparent. Commonly the process begins in the retrobulbar portion of the nerve and no morphologic changes occur in the ocular fundi until 6-8 weeks later when the first signs of optic atrophy become apparent. Optic neuritis and papillitis are often attended by severe visual loss, even to the point of no perception of light, but the prognosis for visual return is excellent. Unlike optic neuritis occurring in adults, childhood optic nerve inflammation is uncommonly a manifestation of diffuse demyelinating processes but is more often associated with previous viral infections.

OPTIC ATROPHY

When irreparable damage to optic nerve fibers has occurred, regardless of the nature of the initial insult, optic atrophy becomes apparent. Optic atrophy may occur as a primary abnormality; it may also be secondary to an adjacent retinal lesion or result from long-standing papilledema. Primary optic atrophy in children is usually inherited, secondary to compressive lesions, or metabolic in origin (see Table 13-2).

CONGENITAL ANOMALIES OF THE OPTIC NERVE

Optic nerve hypoplasia is an underdevelopment of optic nerve fibers within the setting of normal development of mesodermal elements and glial supporting tissues. It is probably the consequence of some intrauterine insult during the sixth to eighth weeks of gestation. The resulting nerve may be a small fraction of the normal size, or abnormal only in a small segment or sector. Lesions may be unilateral or bilateral and attended by visual acuities that range from normal to perception of hand motion only, depending on the extent of the defect. It may be an isolated defect or associated with midline intracranial defects, especially agenesis of the corpus callosum and septum pellucidum, endocrine abnormalities, and other ocular defects (aniridia). It is usually a sporadic anomaly without known etiology, although some cases have been attributed to maternal diabetes or maternal ingestion of quinine or phenytoin (septo-optic dysplasia).

Optic nerve colobomas are anomalies resulting from defective closure of the fetal cleft of the optic cup in its extreme posterior portion. It is associated with abnormal development of surrounding mesoblastic precursors of the choroid and sclera, with ectasia of the resulting tissue. The clinical appearance of colobomatous defects varies considerably. There may be deep colobomatous cupping of the disc with ectasia of tissue adjacent to the disc, or merely an irregularity or pit at the disc margin. Visual function may be severely affected or confined to a peripheral superior field loss. Although commonly a sporadic defect, several large families have been studied in which the abnormality was inherited as an autosomal dominant trait. It may also result from maternal LSD ingestion during pregnancy.

Tilting of the disc This anomaly usually presents as a nasal tilt of the disc and all retinal vessels emerging from the nasal aspect of the disc. It is commonly associated with errors of refraction, particularly myopia. The visual field defects resulting from this disc anomaly may mimic those associated with a chiasmal lesion namely bitemporal field defect.

LESIONS OF THE MACULA AND RETINA

Several types of inherited macular disorders occur in childhood. These are usually isolated anomalies, but in many instances retinal degeneration may signify systemic or neurologic disease.

Cherry-red spot This defect is seen as a bright or dull red area at the center of the macula, surrounded by a concentric white or yellow halo. It is caused by abnormal lipid deposition in the ganglion cells obscuring the choroidal vascular hue except in the area of the fovea which is free of ganglion cells. It has been reported in Tay-Sachs disease, Neimann-Pick disease, Sandhoff's disease, Farber's disease, and in Spranger's disease. A cherry-red spot is rarely seen in patients with infantile metachromatic leukodystrophy.

Ceroid lipofuscinoses These disorders, once referred to as cerebromacular degenerations, have different manifestations. In some forms, optic atrophy is a prominent feature (infantile forms) while in others, macular degeneration is apparent. In these latter forms, the macular area is grey with diffuse scattering of pigmentation and there is a poor foveal reflex. Electroretinography will aid in documenting retinal dysfunction. Although the biochemical defects in most of these disorders are not known, electron microscopic examination of biopsies of skin, conjunctiva, or lymphocytes may be useful in establishing the diagnosis.

Leber's amaurosis was originally described as a variant of retinitis pigmentosa. It is noteworthy because affected patients are blind or near-blind from birth or shortly thereafter. Pupillary reactions are sluggish; nystagmus and photophobia may occur. The ophthalmoscopic appearance is variable; the end-stage retinal appearance is similar to that of retinitis pigmentosa. Initially, however, a normal ophthalmoscopic appearance is

Table 13-2 Optic Atrophy in Childhood

Heritable disorders

Autosomal dominant trait
Optic atrophy inherited as an autosomal dominant trait is common. It is insidious in onset, and leads to mild or moderate visual loss in most cases. Its unique blue-yellow color loss distinguishes it from any other form of optic atrophy.

Autosomal recessive trait
If optic atrophy occurs at all as an isolated defect, it is very rare and leads to early and severe visual loss.

Leber's optic atrophy
Unique form characterized by sudden loss of central vision in the 2nd and 3rd decades of life with nondirect transmission and male preponderance. Although classified as an x-linked recessive it does not conform to rigid Mendelian rules. May be accompanied by other minor neurologic signs but is compatible with normal life expectancy.

Behr's optic atrophy
Inherited as an autosomal recessive trait, with onset before 10 years, and is associated with mental retardation, spasticity, and ataxia. Visual loss is significant but usually stabilizes in early adulthood.

Diabetes and optic atrophy
A distinct syndrome exists in which optic atrophy is associated with diabetes mellitus, diabetes insipidus, and nerve deafness. Inherited as an autosomal recessive trait and attended by severe visual loss.

Compressive lesions

Hydrocephalus
Optic atrophy may occur in hydrocephalus as the result of several different mechanisms. It may occur secondary to long-standing papilledema, as a consequence of compression of the chiasm by a dilated 3rd ventricle, or by stretching of the chiasm and its blood supply resulting from intracranial displacement of the brain stem to accommodate increasing cerebral volume. It may also represent cortical damage with transsynaptic degeneration through the lateral geniculate body in infants.

Optic nerve glioma

In children is considered by most authorities to be a congenital hamartoma. It can present as an orbital lesion with axial proptosis and unilateral visual loss, or as a chiasmal lesion with strabismus, and/or nystagmus, and visual loss. The chiasmal lesion may involve diencephalic structures or lead to hydrocephalus. Treatment is controversial but surgery is probably not indicated unless the proptosis is disfiguring. Irradiation of chiasmal lesions is carried out in some centers.

Craniopharyngioma

Most common intracranial tumor of nonglial origin in childhood, and arises from displaced squamous cells of the embryonic hypophysis. The tumor may be primarily intra- or suprasellar in location. Visual loss is one of the cardinal signs of a craniopharyngioma from compression of the chiasm or optic nerves. Papilledema is frequently evident indicating elevated intracranial pressure. Interference with pituitary function often leads to growth retardation in children with these tumors. Calcification within the tumor (not universally present) is easily seen on plain skull films. CT brain scan is the most useful diagnostic test. Although complete resection of these tumors has been advocated it is rarely accomplished.

Meningiomas and pituitary tumors

These are very rare childhood tumors but may present with unilateral or bilateral visual loss.

Metabolic causes

Most metabolic causes of optic atrophy interfere with the normal metabolism of glucose (the only energy source of the brain and optic nerve). Thus, hypoxia, hypoglycemia, and deficiencies of coenzymes, particularly water-soluble vitamins required for glucose metabolism, have been reported to cause optic atrophy. It is noteworthy that the optic nerve appears relatively resistant to these metabolic insults. Despite the frequency with which hypoxia and hypoglycemia occur in the perinatal period, optic atrophy is not a common sequela of metabolic disturbances.

common or there may be only slight granularity of the ocular fundus. Associated neurologic deficits include cerebellar dysfunction, mental retardation, and convulsive disorders.

Subacute sclerosing panencephalitis (SSPE) is known to be caused by reactivation of latent measles (rubeola) virus. It is characterized by progressive dementia, motor deterioration, and myoclonus. Focal areas of chorioretinitis may precede or accompany the progressive neurologic deterioration. Retinal hemorrhage is a prominent feature of these lesions.

REFERENCES

Harcourt B: Developmental abnormalities of the optic nerve. Trans Ophthalmol Soc UK 96:395, 1976

Hoff JT, Patterson RH: Craniopharyngiomas in children and adults. J Neurosurg 36: 299, 1972

Hoyt WF, Baghdassarian SA: Optic glioma of childhood: natural history and rationale for conservative management.Br J Ophthalmol 53:793, 1969

Jayalakshmi P, McNair-Scott TF, Tucker SH: Infantile nystagmus: a prospective study of spasmus nutans, congenital nystagmus, and unclassified nystagmus of infancy. J Pediatrics 77:177, 1970

Meadows SP: Retrobulbar and optic neuritis in childhood and adolescence. Trans ophthalmol Soc UK 89:603, 1969

Miller NR: Solitary oculomotor nerve palsy in childhood. Am J Ophthalmol 83:106, 1977

Norton EWD, Cogan DG: Spasmus nutans: a clinical study of twenty cases followed two years or more since onset. Arch Ophthalmol 52:442, 1954

14

Problems in Language Acquisition

Richard M. Flower, PhD

Problems in speech and language acquisition may be of twofold significance to physicians who care for children. First, speech and language play crucial roles in a child's development and learning. Not only is the mastery of language essential to the establishment of human relationships, it is also essential to concept development, to abstract thinking, and, eventually to academic success. Therefore, problems in speech and language acquisition may have far-reaching consequences.

Secondly, problems in speech and language acquisition are significant because they often comprise the most apparent manifestations of cognitive, sensory, and motor deficits — deficits that have implications well beyond their influence on speech and language. Therefore, delay in speech and language acquisition may denote the need for various diagnostic studies, or, at the very least, vigilant ongoing observation by the physician responsible for the child's care.

NORMAL SPEECH AND LANGUAGE ACQUISITION

Any discussion of deviant speech and language acquisition requires a definition of what constitutes normal speech and language acquisition. Readers who must reach conclusions regarding the relative normality of children's development should refer to more complete discussions (see references Prutting; Rees; Shriberg).

Language acquisition is currently viewed as a staged process, with each stage emerging in barely perceptible increments. Each stage is marked by specific characteristics, which appear to be universal. Therefore, although children differ substantially in the age at which the different stages of language acquisition emerge, the stages themselves are strikingly similar among virtually all children.

LANGUAGE BEHAVIORS

Language behaviors are usually classified into three categories, recognizing that each is by no means discrete or independent.

The **phonologic** aspects of language consist of the constituent speech sounds of the language and the systematized rules that govern the use of those speech sounds.

The **semantic/syntactic** aspects of language relate to meaning; to relationships between words and their referent concepts; to modifications in word forms effected to amplify meaning (e.g., changing word forms to denote pluralization, tense, etc.); and to ordering words into phrases and sentences.

The **pragmatic** aspects of language concern the rules that govern the operational use of language in social contexts. In developmental terms, this involves such factors as how children use language to accomplish various intentions, how they organize conversations, and how they vary their language usage according to what is socially appropriate in particular situations.

STAGES OF NORMAL LANGUAGE ACQUISITION

Prelinguistic stage (birth-9 months) The foundations of language acquisition are laid during this stage. Infants gradually establish themselves as individuals and begin to distinguish among people and objects. They respond with increasing discrimination to sounds around them, and ultimately respond appropriately to a few words. Although their vocal responses and vocal play contain an expanding repertoire of sounds, such sound-making may not relate directly to later phonologic development.

Stage I — the stage of first words (9-18 months) This stage is signaled by a child's first purposeful use of words. These words are usually names for people and objects or words that denote actions ('up,' 'bye-bye') or greetings ('hi'). The words rely on a limited phonology with many consisting of a consonant and a vowel ('no,' 'go,' 'ba' for ball, 'da' or 'ga' for dog, etc.) Two-syllable words may be produced as repetitions of the same syllable ('dada' for daddy, 'beebee' for baby, etc.) Toward the end of this stage, words may consist of consonant-vowel-consonant combinations ('hot,' 'moke' for milk, etc.) or of two different syllables ('cookie,' 'pitee' for pretty, etc.) During stage I, children begin to recognize the power of language as a tool for influencing other people's behavior.

Stage II — the stage of two-word combinations (1½-2 years) This stage begins when children combine two words to convey meanings that cannot be communicated with a single word. Such combinations represent rudimentary sentences. They may make actor-action statements ('daddy go,' 'baby cry'); specify location ('ball there,' 'where car'); indicate rejection ('no juice'); or define possession ('my book'). While children's phonology expands rapidly during this stage, more complex sounds are replaced by less complex sounds ('wight' for light, or 'dere' for there). These sound changes may render many words unintelligible to a listener who is unfamiliar with the child's speech.

Stage III — the stage of simple conversations (2-3½ years) is signaled by the emergence of verbal exchanges with another person. Children begin to ask questions and expect responses; they begin to respond to questions asked by other people, offering more detailed information than can be carried in one or two words. When two or more children are together, a remark from one child will elicit a response from another; that response will elicit a further response, and so on. Sometimes these conversations consist of the same responses repeated over and over again, but in the later portions of this stage conversations may involve sequences of several remarks. Yet, in these conversations, the same topic is maintained for a very brief time, with topics typically shifting rapidly during stage III discourse. Considerable refinement of the phonologic system is achieved during this stage, but sound changes still occur; therefore, some complex words may remain unintelligible to unfamiliar listeners.

Stage IV — the stage of rapidly increasing complexity (3½-8 years) provides the infinitely complex transition from child language to adult language. Advances occur so rapidly that they defy orderly analysis. Children now complete the mastery of the intricate rules that govern all aspects of language usage. Their vocabularies grow astronomically. Their sentences express more and more ideas, with each concept neatly embedded according to the forms of their language. Gradually, conversations with adults and with peers become longer and longer and, eventually the same topics are maintained throughout lengthy discourses. Early in stage IV, children may still encounter problems in the production of the most complex speech sounds, but these problems gradually diminish until, by the end of this stage, adult phonology is mastered. Midway in stage IV, the major milestone of school entrance occurs. With this event, many children experience for the first time the need to make themselves clearly understood by groups of strangers who are often impatient and unsympathetic. At this time, problems in language acquisition may suddenly become critical. School entrance introduces a new realm of language use, since a child must begin learning to read and write that language he has been speaking.

Stage V — adult language competence (8 years and over) By the time most children reach their eighth birthday, their language is essentially indistinguishable from adult language, in form if not in content. Cognition and language are intimately related throughout the early stages of language acquisition, but at stage V they become virtually inseparable. Throughout the remainder of life, vocabularies grow, sentence construction may be elaborated and polished, written language proficiencies improve, and sensitivity to social rules in language usage increases; but these are all refinements of a system that is essentially intact before stage V begins.

When we recognize that by their earliest school years children have already completed the major stages of language acquisition, the importance of early recognition of developmental problems becomes immediately apparent. Time lost in these critical years may never be regained.

DELAYED LANGUAGE ACQUISITION

Delayed language acquisition has been conventionally considered within a traditional medical diagnostic model. Delays have been viewed as manifestations of specific underlying pathologies. For example, profound hearing impairment impedes many aspects of language acquisition, and cleft palate interferes with the acquisition of phonology. In most instances, however, problems in language acquisition derive from many different factors. While some of these factors may be apparent in other functions (in eye-hand coordination, nonverbal reasoning, etc.) many may be uniquely manifested in language acquisition.

Classifications of complex factors are always hazardous because they necessitate oversimplification. For the sake of clarity, the principal factors associated with delayed and disordered speech and language acquisition are divided into five categories. It is important to remember that any single child may present problems in two or more categories.

PRIMARY LINGUISTIC AND COGNITIVE IMPAIRMENTS

There is something very special about speech and language. Many essential functions that subserve the processing and production of speech and language appear to be unique; the central nervous system probably has capacities that serve only speech and language behaviors. Hence, deficits and maturational lags in whatever subserves these capacities may be manifested only in speech and language acquisition. Problems may also be evident in other aspects of development, but they may be merely coincident rather than directly related to the speech and language deficits.

Some clinicians apply the diagnosis of **aphasia** to children whose developmental problems appear to be central in origin and primarily manifested in language acquisition. This diagnosis is generally inadvisable for two reasons. First, it implies more similarity to the acquired aphasias than actually exists. Second, in applying a single diagnosis to different children, one may incorrectly assume a common essential pathology when many different essential pathologies are probably present. At the current state of knowledge, it is probably best to use indefinite terminology such as 'children with specific deficits in language acquisition,' and then describe the particular manifestations of those deficits as accurately as possible.

Some children's developmental problems seem to focus primarily on the **acquisition of phonology**. Typically, these children persist in the use of the phonologic characteristics of earlier stages of language acquisition, characteristics that usually represent oversimplifications of adult phonology. Although phonologic disorders may sometimes symptomatize motor deficits, they may also be found in children with no obvious problems in motor coordination.

Another area of changing concepts about relationships between central factors and delayed acquisition concerns the interrelationships between cognitive development and language acquisition. Mental retardation has been considered among the 'causes' of language problems but this formulation is too simplistic. **Cognitive development and language acquisition are intimately related.** Certain steps in cognitive development probably must precede certain steps in language acquisition. On the other hand, language acquisition contributes to further cognitive development. Although cognitive deficits may underlie language deficits, language deficits may also underlie cognitive deficits. Therefore, interrelationships between cognition and language cannot be characterized on a simple cause-to-effect basis.

MOTOR IMPAIRMENT

Of all accomplishments of early childhood, speech development requires the most sophisticated neuromuscular control. Children with such obvious neuromuscular disorders as the static encephalopathies commonly encounter problems in speech acquisition. Less severe motor dysfunction, such as may be apparent among children described as presenting 'neurodevelopmental disorders' or 'minimal brain dysfunction,' can also interfere with speech acquisition.

Motor speech disorders are usually categorized as either dysarthrias or dyspraxias recognizing, nevertheless, that a single patient may have evidence of both conditions. **Dysarthria** results from disturbances in muscular control. Because of central or peripheral impairment in the neuromuscular system, speech movements are affected by some degree in weakness, slowness, incoordination, or loss of muscle tone. While these disturbances in neuromuscular control may sometimes be apparent in nonspeech movements as well, they are most apparent during speech production.

Dyspraxia, on the other hand, represents a disorder of programming or sequencing the intricate movements involved in speech production. Dysarthria may be differentiated from dyspraxia on the basis of the consistency of articulatory errors. The dysarthric speaker tends to make the same errors within the same phonetic contexts. The dyspraxic speaker shows greater inconsistencies, with predictable errors. Dyspraxic speech may be further characterized by frequent omissions of speech sounds, by much poorer intelligibility of connected speech than would be anticipated on the basis of single word productions, by misarticulations of vowels as well as consonants (dysarthric speech is primarily characterized by consonant misarticulations), and by disturbances in speech rate and stress patterns.

Children with apparently intact verbal comprehension but little or no spoken language were once described as presenting expressive aphasias. Currently, most clinicians describe these children as presenting severe speech dyspraxias or apraxias.

HEARING IMPAIRMENT

Presumably, every physician knows that children first learn speech and language by imitating the speech and language they hear. Nonetheless, there are far too many children with undiagnosed hearing impairments whose primary physicians have dismissed their speech and language problems with such conclusions as 'he'll grow out of it,' 'he's just stubborn,' or 'he's too young to evaluate.' These children may lose irretrievable time during the most crucial years of language acquisition because a physician failed to acknowledge the importance of their speech and language problems.

Although most physicians recognize the significance of chronic pervasive hearing impairments; i.e., reduced sensitivity affecting all frequencies, many overlook the importance of intermittent conductive hearing losses and sensorineural hearing losses characterized by normal low frequency sensitivity but markedly impaired sensitivity for the higher frequencies. There is growing and unassailable evidence showing the far-reaching consequences of the moderate conductive hearing impairments so frequently associated with otitis media, even when those hearing impairments are intermittent. While conservative management may be preferable from a medical standpoint, the longer an even moderate hearing impairment is present, the greater the likelihood of deficits in crucial aspects of learning and development.

Some hearing losses are characterized by different degrees of impairment within the frequency range that is critical for hearing speech; e.g., a child may have normal hearing at 500 Hz, a moderate impairment at 1000 Hz, and a severe impairment at 2000 Hz. These children hear speech in a grossly distorted manner; they may be able to differentiate among vowels, but be unable to differentiate among many consonants. Typically their speech is severely distorted, since, like all children, they learn to speak by imitating what they hear. Their problems are often further compounded by long delays in recognizing hearing impairment.

Families may ignore the hearing deficits because these children often respond normally to low-frequency environmental sounds. They may show normal awareness of even soft speech, although they are responding only to low-frequency elements and may not comprehend what is said. Physicians sometimes deduce normal hearing on the basis of responses to a 250 Hz tuning fork. Even 'tests' involving repetition of softly spoken digits can be misleading, since an alert youngster can sometimes recognize numerals merely on the basis of hearing their vowel sounds.

Unlike many factors that interfere with speech and language acquisition, some hearing impairments are reversible through skilled medical and surgical treatment. **It is essential that children with hearing impairments are identified at the earliest possible time.**

STRUCTURAL DEFICITS

Parents frequently search for structural deficits to account for children's problems in speech and language acquisition. In reality, speech problems are rarely accounted for by structural factors. Except for deficits that impede velopharyngeal closure, the human speech production mechanism seems capable of adapting to most individual differences in orofacial structures, or even to overt anomalies of those structures.

Tongue-tie or **ankyloglossia,** can limit elevation of the tongue required for production of certain speech sounds, but this condition is extremely rare. Neither micro- nor macroglossia is likely to seriously impede speech acquisition so long as normal mobility is maintained. However, in most instances, the tongue that appears structurally large is actually inordinately flaccid as the result of motor deficits which may have significant effects on speech production.

Dental malocclusions may interfere with the precise formation of a few sounds, but their influence tends to be specific and minimal. Although wide structural variations affecting the height of the palatal vault can be observed, none seems to have any influence on speech production.

On the other hand, **cleft palate** and other conditions that prevent isolation of the oral cavity from the nasal cavity virtually always interfere with speech production. While overt palatal clefts seldom escape early detection, submucous clefts, structural defects of the soft palate and pharynx, and neuromuscular dysfunction of the velopharyngeal sphincter may be less obvious. Early recognition and skilled intervention can, in most instances, eliminate or substantially reduce their devastating effects.

EMOTIONAL AND SOCIAL FACTORS

Psychiatric literature frequently implicates emotional factors as primary causes of delayed speech and language acquisition, applying such terms as 'elective mutism.' These attributions are probably simplistic. In most instances, closer scrutiny of children so described reveals other significant deterrents to speech and language acquisition.

Gross communication deficits usually characterize such conditions as infantile autism and childhood schizophrenia; but in these children, failures in speech and language acquisition are merely further manifestations of serious abnormalities in all aspects of interpersonal communication. Furthermore, there is growing evidence that these conditions are organic in origin.

Except for such rare situations as the total isolation of a child imprisoned by psychotic parents, it is also unwarranted to implicate social factors as sole deterrents to speech and language acquisition. On the other hand, social factors may determine the amount and kind of speech and language stimulation the child receives, and will exert substantial influences on his or her development. Parent-child and sibling relationships may particularly influence the quality and rate of speech and language acquisition. These relationships are probably even more influential when a child is already encountering developmental problems.

In considering social influences, it is important to recognize that children acquire the speech and language patterns of their communities. Although these patterns may appear aberrant according to the phonologic, syntactic, or pragmatic standards of other speech communities, they do not represent deviant development.

Some popular and even professional literature has identified bilingualism as a negative influence on speech and language acquisition. Yet all available evidence suggests that children with adequate potentials for language acquisition will learn two or more languages as easily as they learn one. On the other hand, when children encounter problems in the acquisition of one language, those problems seem to be compounded by simultaneous exposure to two languages.

EVALUATION

Before areas of evaluation that should be considered can be specified, those children who are at risk for significant developmental problems must be identified. There are general criteria which suggest those children who deserve careful scrutiny because of likely obstacles to speech and language acquisition.

Table 14-1 Risk Factors for Hearing Impairment in Infants*

1. Family history of childhood hearing impairment.
2. Congenital perinatal infection (e.g., cytomegalovirus, rubella, herpes, toxoplasmosis, syphilis).
3. Anatomic malformations involving the head or neck (e.g., dysmorphic appearance including syndromal or nonsyndromal abnormalities, overt or submucous cleft palate, or morphologic abnormalities of the pinna).
4. Birthweight less than 1500 gm.
5. Hyperbilirubinemia at level exceeding indications for exchange transfusion.
6. Bacterial meningitis, especially *Hemophilus influenzae.*
7. Severe asphyxia which may include infants with Apgar scores of 0 to 3 or who fail to institute spontaneous respiration by 10 minutes and those with hypotonia persisting to 2 hours of age.

* Joint Committee on Infant Hearing Screen (American Academy of Pediatrics, American Academy of Otolaryngology and Head and Neck Surgery, and the American Speech-Language-Hearing Association). Reproduced from Pediatrics 70:496-497, 1982.

Newborns at risk for later developmental problems can often be immediately identified. The Joint Committee on Infant Hearing Screening has defined factors that identify infants 'at risk' for hearing impairment (see Table 14-1). Most of these factors also identify infants at risk for other conditions that lead to delayed speech and language acquisition.

By age 10 months infants should respond consistently to sounds. They should recognize familiar people and respond appropriately to two or three words.

By age 18 months children should be using a few single words consistently and purposefully, not merely imitatively.

By age 30 months children should combine two or more words into simple sentences. Most of what they say should be understood by their families.

By age 4 years children should carry on short conversations with familiar adults and with other children. They should be able to express themselves with sufficient clarity so that most of what they say is understood by a sympathetic listener.

By age 5 years children should be able to carry on longer conversations, tell simple stories, and recount recent events and experiences. Most of what they say should be intelligible to any listener.

By age 6 years children should be able to function as independent communicators at school. While occasional errors may occur in the formation of complex sounds and in the pronunciation of difficult words, their speech should be completely intelligible to any listener.

By age 8 years children should be communicating in adult-like language. Occasional mispronunciations and grammatic errors may occur, but for all practical purposes, an 8 year old should be a proficient communicator.

Children at risk on the basis of these criteria do not necessarily require an immediate full-scale multidisciplinary evaluation. Nevertheless, some preliminary evaluation of the child's speech, language, and hearing is advisable. The need for further studies can be determined on the basis of this preliminary evaluation.

When comprehensive studies are in order, they are best carried out on a multidisciplinary basis, preferably by a group of specialists accustomed to working together. Such multidisciplinary 'teams' are found in most university medical centers, many community medical centers, and sometimes in public and private schools or other community agencies.

SPEECH AND LANGUAGE EVALUATION

The most efficient first step is to obtain a thorough speech and language evaluation by a competent speech pathologist. Such an evaluation will include assessment of all aspects of the child's communicative behaviors as well as descriptions of his phonologic, semantic/syntactic, and pragmatic development. Even when a child appears to use little or no expressive language, such an evaluation can document development in such important areas as language comprehension, nonverbal communication, and symbolic play.

Speech and language evaluations should determine whether or not significant delays in speech and language acquisition exist, define the severity of the delay, describe the child's other communicative and symbolic behaviors, and suggest additional areas for evaluation. It is most economical to delay formulation of a total diagnostic plan until after a speech and language evaluation has been completed.

HEARING EVALUATION

Although clinicians must be suspicious of absolute statements, one dictum can be presented without equivocation: **every child with apparent problems in speech and language acquisition should receive a careful hearing evaluation.** Hearing tests may be a routine component of the speech and language evaluation. Frequently, hearing screening tests are conducted, with further testing recommended when children fail to meet screening criteria. If such testing is not included, the child should be seen for evaluation by a competent audiologist.

Conventional hearing testing procedures have been refined to permit assessment of younger children. Although not a hearing testing procedure as such, **impedance measurement** can give helpful information about the middle-ear integrity of even very young children. The technology of **auditory brain-stem response measurement** is progressing rapidly toward effective hearing measurement even in early infancy. No longer does a child's age or general unresponsiveness justify delayed referral for hearing evaluation.

DEVELOPMENTAL EVALUATION

It is possible for developmental psychologists to inventory children's achievements in different aspects of cognitive, perceptual, and motor development. These evaluations will determine whether delays in speech and language acquisition are relatively specific or whether they are components of pervasive developmental deficits. A thorough developmental evaluation may not only make important contributions to the diagnosis of the speech and language problems, it may be essential for present and future educational planning.

The Denver Development Screening Test may provide some preliminary information. Under no circumstances, however, do such scales constitute an adequate developmental evaluation.

NEUROLOGIC EVALUATION

It is unlikely that any grave neurologic disorder would be manifested exclusively in delayed speech and language acquisition. Nevertheless, a complete neurologic evaluation may provide helpful information as to whether delays are accompanied by other neurodevelopmental lags. When parents are anxious about a child's developmental deficits, they may be reassured by ruling out gross CNS pathology. They may also gain helpful insights when other maturational lags are defined.

SOCIAL EVALUATION

Emotional and social factors have questionable significance as primary deterrents to speech and language acquisition; however, parent-child relationships and other intrafamilial relationships can be important in helping a child improve his communication. In other instances, referral for evaluation by a mental health professional may be advisable.

TREATMENT

Except for children with conductive hearing impairment or those with structural defects such as cleft palate, medical or surgical intervention has little effect on problems in speech and language acquisition. The physician's primary responsibilities with respect to these children include identification, referral for and coordination of evaluations, including integration and interpretation of their results to families, and referral for appropriate therapeutic and educational management.

Major responsibilities for treatment programs for children with delayed speech and language acquisition are usually assigned to speech pathologists. These programs have dual emphasis: the facilitation of speech and language acquisition, and obviation of such likely negative secondary consequences as unhealthy family and peer relationships and school problems.

INTERVENTION PROGRAMS FOR PRESCHOOLERS

During the preschool years, four different types of intervention programs may be available. The first program type emphasizes **counseling and instruction of parents,** helping them to understand the problems confronting their children and enabling them to carry out specific activities to facilitate speech and language development. Sometimes these services are provided through multidisciplinary programs for high risk infants and young children.

The second type of intervention involves **placement of these children in small groups with other children with delayed language acquisition and related developmental problems.** These programs are found in many speech and hearing clinics, community agencies, and some public school district programs for handicapped preschool children.

A third approach **enrolls children in regular nursery school programs** with the hope that the association with normal contemporaries will facilitate speech and language acquisition. This approach may suffice for children with uncomplicated delays in development, but is seldom sufficient for children with more serious delays.

The fourth alternative involves **regular individual sessions with a speech pathologist,** usually on a once or twice weekly basis. Most speech pathologists consider this pattern to be less desirable than programs involving small groups of children. The group programs offer real-life communication opportunities and provide greater stimulation. Sometimes individual instruction is used to supplement placement in either regular or special preschool group programs. Occasionally, it is used for children who are unduly upset or distracted by the presence of other children. Individual treatment programs are sometimes instituted because no other options are available.

INTERVENTION PROGRAMS FOR SCHOOL - AGE CHILDREN

After children with problems in speech and language acquisition enter school, other programs become available to them. Children with severe language disabilities may require placement in special classes, or rarely, in special schools where the major focus is on accommodation of their language disabilities. Less disabled children are usually enrolled in regular classrooms and attend special speech-language therapy sessions for a portion of the school day, usually on a twice or three times weekly basis. These services are available in most public school districts, but some families prefer to enroll their children in private or other community or medical center-based programs.

It must be remembered that children with problems in the acquisition of oral language are at great risk for failure in the mastery of written language skills after they enter school. This further underlines the essentiality of early recognition and treatment for children with problems in language acquisition.

REFERENCES

Miller JF: *Assessing Language Production in Children: Experimental Procedures.* University Park Press, Baltimore, 1980.

Naremore RC: Language disorders in children. *In* Hixon TJ, Shriberg LD, Saxman JH (eds) *Introduction to Communication Disorders.* Prentice-Hall, Englewood Cliffs, 1981, pp 137-175.

Northern J, Downs M: *Hearing in Children.* Williams & Wilkins, Baltimore, 1984.

Prutting C: Process: the action of moving progressively from one point to another on the way to completion. J Speech Hear Disord 44:3-30, 1979.

Rees NS: Learning to talk and understand. *In* Hixon TJ, Shriberg LD, Saxman JH (eds) *Introduction to Communication Disorders.* Prentice-Hall, Englewood Cliffs, 1981, pp 1-41.

Shriberg LD: Developmental phonological disorders. *In* Hixon TJ, Shriberg LD, Saxman JH (eds) *Introduction to Communication Disorders.* Prentice-Hall, Englewood Cliffs, 1981, pp 264-309.

Siegel G, Broen P: Language assessment. *In* Lloyd LL (ed) *Communication Assessment and Intervention Strategies.* University Park Press, Baltimore, 1976.

15

Headache

Bruce O. Berg, MD

The complaint of headache is common in children as well as adults and may be seen from infancy throughout adult life. Bille reported that 40% of children had experienced headache at some time before the age of 7 years and 75% by the age of 15 years. The very young, unable to adequately express their discomfort, may have an alteration in behavior and become unusually subdued, irritable, or irascible. Others may cry or hold their hand to their head, or press their head, usually forehead, against some cool firm surface. Anorexia or vomiting are often associated symptoms with these episodes.

Older children are better able to describe their discomfort from the headache. It is most important that examiners obtain the history as spontaneously related by the child without inadvertently suggesting to the patient what he thinks he means. Obviously, historical information must be obtained from the parents, usually the mother; again, one should be wary of historical details—obtaining information by asking questions from different perspectives. Some patients presume the term 'headache' conveys all necessary information and that no further characterization is required. It is not unusual that patients' or mothers' descriptions of the headache are not completely accurate.

NEUROANATOMICAL CONSIDERATIONS

Whether the origin of head pain is central or peripheral is not yet clear. The major pain-sensitive structures include the proximal portion of the cerebral arteries, the great venous sinuses and large venous tributaries. Other pain-sensitive structures include portions of the meninges, particularly in the basilar region, and scalp muscles. The cerebral substance, most of the meninges, the ventricular ependymal lining, and choroid plexuses are relatively pain-insensitive.

The intracranial pain-sensitive nerves include the trigeminal nerve which supplies the supratentorial regions of anterior and middle fossae, and the glossopharyngeal, vagus and the upper three cervical spinal nerves which supply the posterior fossa. Generally, when supratentorial pain-sensitive structures are stimulated, patients experience pain in the anterior half of the head; whereas, stimulation of infratentorial pain-sensitive structures results in pain in the posterior half of the head. Headaches may occur from abnormal vasoregulatory mechanisms, traction, and/or encroachment of any pain-sensitive structure.

Table 15-1 A Classification of Headache

I. Vascular headaches of the migraine type
A. Classic migraine
B. Common migraine
C. Complicated migraine
Hemiplegic
Ophthalmoplegic
Basilar artery migraine
Acute confusional state
Alice-in-wonderland syndrome
D. Cluster headache

II. Nonmigrainous vascular headaches
A. Systemic infection with fever
B. Convulsive states
C. Hypertension
D. Hypoxia
E. Miscellaneous

III. Muscular contraction headaches

IV. Psychogenic headaches

V. Traction headaches
A. Tumor
B. Hematoma
C. Abscess
D. Post lumbar puncture
E. Pseudotumor cerebri

VI. Headaches with cranial inflammation

VII. Headaches due to disease of other head or neck structures

Adapted and reproduced, with permission, from Dalessio DJ: Wolff's *Headache and Other Head Pain*. Oxford University Press, 1972.

CLASSIFICATION

The generally accepted classification of headache has merit but during the last decade there have been modifications of what truly represents migraine (see Table 15-1). For example, one can no longer presume that muscle contraction headache is typically 'tension headache' for migrainous patients may also complain of 'tightness, tension, aching' of cervico-occipital muscles and, further, some patients with continual headache of muscle contraction type have relief from vasoactive drugs rather than the usually administered analgesics. Again, the origin of these headaches is unclear but the current view of the pathogenesis of the migrainous headache is related to an unstable vasoregulatory mechanism.

PAIN OF OCULAR, AURAL, DENTAL, SINUS ORIGIN

Headaches may be related to visual problems, including decreased visual acuity, abnormalities of ocular motility, refractive errors, and astigmatism. Headaches in these cases are usually located in or about the orbit, forehead or temporal regions. They are usually steady, of mild to moderate intensity, and clearly related to activities where 'eye strain' could possibly be involved. The prevalence of ocular related headache is remarkably infrequent, much less than is commonly believed. Patients require a careful examination of ocular function, including determination of visual fields, acuity, ocular motility, and complete examination of ocular fundi. Therapeutic considerations are made only after complete examinations by a neurologist and/or ophthalmologist with recognized expertise in these matters.

Middle ear infections are occasionally a cause of headache, and dental inflammation, such as an abscess, can present as referred pain to the ear. Head pain localized to the temporomandibular joint seldom occurs in children; bilateral temporomandibular joint pain, however, is found in some patients with rheumatoid arthritis. Appropriate examination of the ears and teeth must be performed. Radiographic examination of the temporomandibular joints will usually demonstrate any significant changes.

Paranasal sinusitis may result in headache in children but, as in the case of adult patients, occurs with less frequency than commonly believed. Recurring sinus headache can present in childhood as pain over the maxillary antrum rather than the frontal or temporal regions because these sinuses only begin to develop in the latter part of the first decade. There is usually pain over the sinus when pressed firmly and radiographic confirmation of sinusitis is readily demonstrated.

INTRACRANIAL HYPERTENSION

Recurring headaches occur in the presence of intracranial hypertension. Tumors, chronic meningitis, or subarachnoid hemorrhage should be considered in the differential diagnosis. There are usually associated physical findings which point to the appropriate pathologic process. Recurring paroxysmal headaches are found in cases of intermittent flow of the CSF, as seen in the occasional chronic meningitides, or an intermittent obstruction of the third ventricle from a space-occupying lesion such as a colloid cyst. Traction or encroachment upon any pain-sensitive structure usually results in headache.

POST LUMBAR PUNCTURE HEADACHE

This is less common than believed and is characterized as bifrontal or occipital pain that is steady, usually appearing after the patient first sits up or stands following a lumbar puncture. The headache is thought to be secondary to a CSF leak through the meninges produced by the spinal needle and causing a dysequilibrium of CSF dynamics with subsequent distortion or traction of pain-sensitive structures. The headaches usually persist no more than 1 or 2 days but occasionally may persist several days; some patients may have nausea and/or vomiting. The treatment of choice includes bed rest, adequate fluid intake, either oral or parenteral fluids, and analgesics. The post lumbar puncture headache is not a major problem in children, presuming they remain supine for at least several hours following that lumbar puncture.

ALTITUDINAL HEADACHE

Altitudinal headaches are currently more frequently seen because of our population's interest in hiking and mountain climbing. When reaching an altitude of 6-8000 feet, some patients complain of generalized, throbbing headache. In addition, they may have other symptoms of shortness of breath, anorexia, and insomnia. The headache is made worse by jolting or vigorous activity, straining at stool, coughing or lying down. Symptoms usually abate spontaneously within several days remaining at the same altitude or more quickly if the patient descends to lower elevations. It has been suggested that Diamox administered several days before the mountain climbing may be of some protection.

ICE CREAM HEADACHE

One headache type that is quite common in children as well as adults is the 'ice cream headache.' This is characterized by a momentary 'sharp' midfrontal pain that occurs when some cold food or drink comes in contact with the palate or oropharynx. Rarely the pain is present in the temporal regions. Because this intense pain is so short-lived, there is no specific treatment other than swallowing some warm liquid. Interestingly, about 90% of patients with migraine have experienced the ice cream headache.

NECK - TONGUE SYNDROME

This is an unusual syndrome of head pain which occurs on sudden turning of the head. These patients have a unilateral cervical or occipital pain accompanied by ipsilateral numbness of the tongue. The pain usually occurs when patients sharply twist their head to one provocative position, presumably compressing the second cervical root in the atlantoaxial space. Afferent fibers from the lingual nerve projecting by way of hypoglossal nerve to the second cervical root, provide an interesting, though not unequivocally proven explanation. Treatment is implicit in that patients should avoid if possible, the one posture or activity which is associated with this momentary head pain and lingual numbness.

HEADACHE PROVOKED BY CHEMICAL AGENTS

There are known chemical agents recognized as provocators of headache in some persons. The notion that it is common for children to have headache because of 'food allergy' is often heard but there is little substantive evidence to support this view. Some of the known precipitating agents include phenylethylamine in chocolate, tyramine found in well-aged cheese, nitrites used as coloring agents in meats which may trigger the 'hot dog' headache, and monosodium glutamate associated with the 'Chinese restaurant syndrome.' This syndrome is characterized by headache, a feeling of facial tightness, occasional vertigo, nausea and/or vomiting, and diarrhea. Oxalates have also been implicated in recurring headache, abdominal pain and/or cyclical vomiting.

HYPERTENSION AND HEADACHE

Although a distinct relationship between hypertension and headache is generally accepted, details regarding such an association and its pathophysiology remain unclear. The problem is less notable in children than adults, probably because of the difference in prevalence rates of hypertension. There are no typical characteristics of the 'hypertensive headache,' for it may be localized or generalized, continual, dull, or throbbing. One must be ever mindful of the possibility of an existing pheochromocytoma, particularly if there are other signs consistent with neurofibromatosis or Hippel-Lindau disease (see Chapter 9).

POSTTRAUMATIC SYNDROME

Headache, a component of the posttraumatic syndrome, is relatively common in childhood. It usually appears within several days following the traumatic event; however, a smaller group of patients have onset of recurring headaches weeks later. There is no 'typical' quality of a posttraumatic headache.

Commonly, there is an increase in frequency and severity following the onset but there is generally an improvement over a period of weeks to months. As part of this syndrome, parents often complain of personality changes including hyperactivity, impaired judgement, impulsivity, and poor control of anger. It is most important to recognize the syndrome as quickly as possible and administer whatever therapeutic measures are indicated lest extraneous factors become interwoven in the primary symptom complex. An occasional patient has severe, frequent headaches and is best treated prophylactically, as in the case of frequent and severe migraine.

Some patients who are depressed either before or after the traumatic event find relief from administration of tricyclic antidepressants. As a general rule, firm, though gentle, supportive management is most effective.

CLUSTER HEADACHES

Cluster headaches usually occur in males over the age of 10 years. The headache starts in or around one eye and is intensely painful, spreading to the hemicranium. It is usually described as throbbing or pulsating. The headache commonly occurs at night, usually occurring once daily, for weeks to several months. Occasionally, a patient will have several episodes in one day.

There is conjunctival hyperemia with ocular tearing, nasal stuffiness, sweating, facial flush and Horner's syndrome. The duration of the headache is usually up to several hours. Once the cluster of headaches has ceased, the patient is headache free until the next cluster of headache recurs.

PSYCHOGENIC HEADACHES

The occurrence of headaches which have a psychogenic basis are not uncommon in childhood. The headache is commonly described as continual and having a dull quality. The duration of headache may range from many hours to weeks, frequently precluding the child's attendance at school or other regularly scheduled activities. It is not uncommon for the child to describe the headache as being 'severe,' 'can't stand it,' 'excruciating' while manifesting a calm, serene facial expression.

The clinician must carefully determine the quality of the headache while remaining ever mindful of potential problems at home, school, and other patient interpersonal relationships. It is of great benefit to obtain complete psychological testing followed by a family interview and possibly family therapy.

MIGRAINE

Migraine is an inherited disorder characterized by paroxysmal episodes of vasoregulatory instability. During the episodes, there is vasoconstriction of intracerebral vessels, which precipitates the neurologic signs and symptoms, followed by extracerebral and probably intracerebral vasodilation, thought to be the cause of the headache. Both phases may occur simultaneously. The pathophysiology of this unstable vasoregulation is not known.

The vascular changes of migraine are believed not to be secondary to abnormal neural discharges. Hence, a variety of vasoactive substances in the plasma, including acetylcholine, bradykinin, histamine, norepinephrine, prostaglandins, and serotonin have been implicated.

Most studies have demonstrated decreased plasma levels of serotonin during the attack, while urinary excretion of free serotonin is increased. Approximately 90% of serotonin is carried by the platelets and a plasma-releasing factor has been implicated.

Migraine affects patients of all ages. Bille found 2.5% of children under 7 years and 4% of children 7-15 years old are affected by migraine. It is thought that the prevalence of migraine in the general population is about 20%. About 75% of adult patients with migraine have onset of symptoms before the age of 10 years and 20% before the age of 5 years.

Though the acute attack of migraine in the child is similar to the adult there is a greater variability of symptoms. Children usually have shorter migrainous attacks and they are more often associated with nausea and/or vomiting. About 60% of child patients are male; whereas, females comprise about 75% of adult migrainous patients. Children more commonly have recurring abdominal pain, cyclical vomiting, or vertiginous episodes as manifestations of migraine, and there is a higher incidence of sleep disorders.

Recognized factors that commonly provoke migraine in children include changes of lighting, as in the case of leaving a dark room and walking into the daylight, physical exertion, hunger, or automobile travel.

CLASSIC MIGRAINE

This variety of migraine is often accompanied by visual phenomena including 'sparklers, colored spots, visual obscurations, distortions, and/or hallucinations.' Though adults more readily describe such visual phenomena, small children, if carefully questioned, may describe unusual 'scary' things they have perceived before the headache.

It is thought that about 10-40% of children with migraine recount some associated manifestation of visual abberation. Occasionally, a child will describe visual distortions with misperceptions of space and time. Others may spontaneously note 'funny feelings' (dysesthesiae) in their extremities or about their face.

The symptoms generally progress to headache which may be localized or generalized and characterized by a continual or throbbing headache. There is commonly anorexia, nausea and/or vomiting and most children, because of photophobia, prefer a darkened room. Duration of headache is usually several hours but may last the entire day. As the headache lessens, the patient is usually rather tired and may fall into a deep sleep. Commonly, the child is quite well the next morning.

COMMON MIGRAINE

This type of migraine is notable for its lack of readily recognized prodrome. Visual aberrations are less likely to occur. Rather, the patient may demonstrate behavioral changes, lethargy, vertigo and/or vomiting. The headache is not well localized and may last for a few hours to several days. The child may have a continual dull headache with superimposed paroxysms of severe headache.

COMPLICATED MIGRAINE

Hemiplegic migraine, an uncommon phenomenon, is more common in children than adults and is characterized by an abrupt onset of hemiparesis that is usually followed by headache. The weakness may last for several hours to days. Another subset of patients with hemiplegic migraine usually have the weakness affecting the same side, lasting from hours to days, even after the headache has disappeared. This latter group has a strong family history of similar attacks. Hemianesthesia may occur in both types but is more common in the latter type.

Ophthalmoplegic migraine The typical features of this form of migraine include orbital or periorbital pain which may migrate to one side of the head, followed by an ipsilateral ophthalmoplegia, usually affecting the third nerve. The fourth and sixth cranial nerves may also be involved. The headache disappears within a few hours but the ophthalmoplegia may last for days to weeks. Ophthalmoplegic migraine may occur any time throughout childhood and has been reported in infant patients.

Basilar artery migraine is more common in females and may occur at any age. It is characterized by a variety of brain stem and/or cerebellar signs including transient visual loss, vertigo, tinnitus, ataxia, and some patients have a transient hemiparesis. These findings are usually followed by a severe occipital headache with concomitant vomiting. An association of basilar migraine and convulsive activity has been suggested by some authors, and some patients may significantly improve following prophylactic administration of anticonvulsant medication.

Acute confusional state Recurring episodes of confusion on a migrainous basis is rare, but does affect some juvenile patients. The episodes are characterized by impairment of sensorium, agitation, lethargy, and dysarthria, sometimes progressing to stupor. Headaches, nausea, and vomiting may not be present; the duration of episode may last for a matter of hours. The age of affected children has ranged from mid-childhood throughout adolescence. The clinician must be particularly careful not to overlook the possibility of hypoglycemia, toxic states, or an infectious process.

Alice-in-wonderland syndrome This is a rare form of migraine in childhood, characterized by distortions of vision, space, and time. Some patients note micropsia and/or metamorphosia, in addition to other sensory hallucinations. These symptoms may either precede or are associated with headache, but they may occur unaccompanied by headache.

Benign paroxysmal vertigo These are recurring episodes of vertigo and ataxia in young children, usually 2-3 years of age, without known alteration of consciousness. The neurologic examination is normal although there are usually abnormal oculovestibular responses. The hearing is normal and there is no known tinnitus reported. Some patients may have nystagmus during the episode. Others may have torticollis during the attack which may last for hours. There is a high incidence of migraine in children who have had benign paroxysmal vertigo at an earlier age.

Paroxysmal leg pain There are rare child patients who complain of paroxysmal leg pain that is thought to have a migrainous basis. Duration of pain lasts from minutes to several hours and is usually nocturnal.

Cyclical vomiting was considered several decades ago as a 'convulsive equivalent' or 'abdominal epilepsy.' The disorder is characterized by recurring episodes of nausea and vomiting and sometimes associated with recurring abdominal pain. The mother often describes the child as 'not looking right' for hours before the onset of recurring vomiting episodes, which may continue throughout the day, often leaving the child dehydrated and lethargic. Patients commonly fall into a deep sleep and wake feeling refreshed although dry. About 75% of these patients develop typical symptoms of migraine in later childhood and adult life.

TREATMENT

If the basis of the child's headache is other than migraine, such as infectious processes of the teeth, ear, or ocular abnormalities, appropriate specific therapy must be administered. Children with occasional migraine of mild to moderate severity may be effectively treated with Tylenol and bed rest. Fiorinal is also an effective drug for the occasional episode of migraine, particularly if the onset is not abrupt.

Though ergot compounds have been frequently used for adult patients with migraine, they are of lesser value for the child patient because they must be administered as quickly as possible after the onset of symptoms. Childhood migraine usually has an abrupt onset and the patient is unable to take medication quickly enough for relief of symptoms. Further, The child cannot carry the medication on his person. If the child is old enough, at least 10 years or older, ergot preparations may be used.

For those uncommon child patients who have migraine at such frequency and severity that their normal life's activities are significantly altered, prophylactic therapy is recommended. Propranolol is an effective medication in this regard with infrequent side-effects that may include fatigue, nausea, and hypotension. This medication blocks β-adrenergic vascular receptors and prevents vasodilation. The drug should not be administered to asthmatics, patients with sinus bradycardia, or congestive heart failure.

Phenobarbital, and less commonly phenytoin, have also been used prophylactically, administered in anticonvulsant doses. The serum levels must be monitored, as in the case of patients treated for seizure disorders.

Other drugs that have been considered include amitriptyline, cyproheptadine, and clonidine. Methysergide has been used in those patients who have been recalcitrant to other treatment modalities. There is a high incidence of adverse side-effects, however, including pulmonary and retroperitoneal fibrosis. Although rarely used in adult patients for limited periods of time, it is less frequently used in child patients and only when the administration is meticulously controlled.

REFERENCES

Bille B: Migraine in school children. Acta Paediatr Scand 51:(Suppl 136):1, 1962.

Dalessio DJ: *Wolff's Headache and Other Head Pain,* 3rd Ed. Oxford University Press, Oxford, 1972.

Golden GS, French JH: Basilar migraine in children. Pediatrics 56:722, 1975.

Prensky AL: Migraine and migrainous variants in pediatric patients. Pediatr Clin North America 23:461, 1976.

Raskin NH, Appenzeller O: *Headache.* Saunders, Philadelphia, 1980.

16

The Hypotonic Infant

Bruce O. Berg, MD

GENERAL CONSIDERATIONS

Muscle tone refers to the resistance of muscle to passive stretch, and its evaluation is a major component of the motor system examination. **Hypertonia** is usually found in upper motor neuron or corticospinal tract dysfunction, and although uncommon in the newborn, may be observed in some infants who have experienced a severe hypoxic insult, marked intraventricular hemorrhage, or bacterial meningitis. **Hypotonia** is more common and may be seen in a variety of abnormal processes which affect the brain or any part of the motor unit. Hypotonia must be distinguished from weakness, as demonstrated in some cerebellar lesions where hypotonia is present but muscle power is normal. It should be recognized, however, that hypotonia of the newborn and young infant is usually accompanied by some loss of muscle power.

Since clinicians are frequently called to evaluate the hypotonic neonate or infant, it is important to be familiar with the assessment of muscle tone and underlying regulatory mechanisms. The importance of this evaluation is apparent when considering the changes in tone that normally occur during maturation of the infant and the major role muscle tone plays in determining the Apgar score.

REGULATORY MECHANISMS OF MUSCLE TONE

Muscle tone is regulated by several mechanisms: physical characteristics of muscle and associated connective tissue structures; and a neural regulatory system which includes the sensory end-organs (receptors) and related neural pathways.

SENSORY END - ORGANS

The principal receptors are the muscle spindles found in virtually all skeletal muscles, and the Golgi tendon organs which, when compared to muscle spindles, are present in slightly decreased numbers within the tendons. There are more spindles in muscles that participate in rapid or finely coordinated movements than in the larger, postural sustaining muscles.

Muscle spindles are fusiform structures about 4-7 mm long, 80-200 μ in diameter, and are embedded within the muscle substance. They are composed of thin striated muscle (intrafusal) fibers which have connective tissue in their mid or equatorial regions and are attached at each end to the

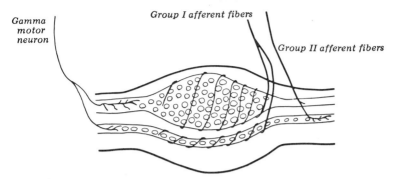

Fig. 16-1 Nuclear bag and nuclear chain intrafusal fibers within a muscle spindle. Group I fibers, the primary afferents, innervate both the nuclear bag and nuclear chain fibers. Group II fibers, the secondary afferents, innervate primarily nuclear chain fibers but may innervate nuclear bag fibers.

encapsulating connective tissue sheath which surrounds them. The capsule appears swollen in midportion, giving the receptor a spindle-like appearance (see Figure 16-1).

There are two types of intrafusal muscle fibers, called nuclear bag and nuclear chain fibers. The nuclear bag fibers are relatively long and wide and contain aggregations of central nuclei; nuclear chain fibers are comparatively short and thin and contain serially arranged nuclei. Within each spindle are usually two nuclear bag fibers and four to five nuclear chain fibers.

The myelinated afferent fibers from muscle are classified by their diameter size with largest fibers in group I and fibers of smaller diameter in groups II and III. The primary afferent Ia fibers of muscle spindles, a sub-population of group I, coil about the noncontractile portion of the nuclear bag and nuclear chain fibers. Group II fibers, the secondary afferent neural fibers, terminate in flower spray endings at the ends of nuclear chain fibers.

Golgi tendon organs are structurally more simple and are found in the muscle-tendon junctions or buried within the tendon. They are approximately 700 μ long, 200 μ wide, and are contained within a delicate connective tissue capsule made up of several longitudinal compartments derived from that capsule. The ends of the Golgi tendon organs are continuous with connective tissue of muscle and/or tendon. This receptor is innervated by Ib afferent fibers which do not branch until they reach the receptor capsule and, after penetration of the capsule, arborize into secondary and tertiary myelinated branches. Physical distortion of these terminal rami results in the discharge of the afferent fibers. The Golgi tendon organ has a protective function for extrafusal fibers as well as relaying proprioceptive information to the central nervous system.

The efferent fibers innervating the skeletomotor (extrafusal) fibers arise from the large alpha motoneuron pool within the ventral horn of the spinal cord; smaller gamma motoneurons within that same neuronal pool innervate the intrafusal fibers of muscle spindles at the polar, contractile regions. Activation of the gamma motoneurons results in contraction of the intrafusal fibers (see Figure 16-2).

Any stretch of extrafusal fibers will stretch the intrafusal fibers, initiating an afferent discharge from both the muscle spindles and Golgi tendon organs. If there is continued muscle stretch, the Golgi tendon organs will continue or increase their rate of discharge, suggesting that Golgi tendon organs are arranged in series with the extrafusal fibers.

Because the spindles are arranged in parallel with the extrafusal muscle fibers, contraction of extrafusal fibers reduces the stretch on the spindle intrafusal fibers and afferent discharge activity decreases. In contrast, extrafusal muscle contraction increases the discharge of the Golgi tendon organ. These neural interrelationships maintain control of muscle spindle and Golgi tendon organ afferent discharges and, hence, the length of extrafusal fibers. The primary Ia nerve fibers are sensitive to changes of both muscle fiber length and velocity of stretch; secondary endings are sensitive primarily to the length of the fibers. A suprasegmental input from the cerebral cortex, cerebellum, basal ganglia, reticular formation, and other areas of the spinal cord coactivates both alpha and gamma motoneurons.

DEVELOPMENTAL ASPECTS OF MUSCLE TONE

When considering the embryological development of neural receptors and the progressive myelination of peripheral nerves it is reasonable that changes of muscle tone occur. Muscle spindles are recognized in the human embryo as early as 11 weeks' gestation. The capsule is formed by 12 weeks and the spindle appears mature between 20 and 31 weeks' gestation. Muscle spindles are not functionally mature until later. As the receptors develop and myelination of peripheral nerves continues, there is an increase in discharge activity of the receptors, motor nerve conduction velocities, and muscle tone (see Table 5-2).

The changes of muscle tone that occur with increasing maturation of the central and peripheral nervous systems have been used as the basis for assessing the gestational age of the newborn infant. Such methods have not been universally accepted in their entirety and other physical findings including characteristics of ear cartilage, external genitalia, amount of breast tissue, and plantar cutaneous creases have been found to be as valuable in determining gestational age. The evaluation of muscle tone does play an important role, however, in assessing the neurologic maturation of the infant.

CLINICAL EXAMINATION

The evaluation is subjective at best, and requires some experience in the interpretation of normal ranges of tone found at different chronological ages. The infant should be at rest with the head in midline position and the limbs moved passively. Truncal tone is assessed by suspending the infant with the abdomen held on the examiner's hand. Normal full-term infants assume a posture with straightened back, flexed limbs, and the head held straight ahead or extended. Hypotonic infants held in a similar manner are truly limp, draping over the examiner's hand. The tone of shoulder girdle

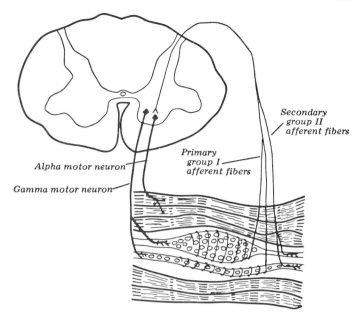

Fig. 16-2 Stimulation of the alpha motor neurons through mechanism of the gamma loop system.

muscles is demonstrated by suspending the infant vertically while supporting the infant's axillae. Full-term infants will adduct their arms with the shoulder girdle fixed, whereas hypotonic infants tend to 'slip through' the examiner's hands.

There is progressive increase in muscle tone from lower to upper limbs. At 28 weeks' gestation there is little or no resistance of the limbs to passive muscle stretch, but by 32 weeks, flexor tone is apparent in the lower limbs. By 36 weeks muscle tone has further increased in the legs and is now apparent in the arms. At term, the normal infant has flexor tone in all limbs (see Figure 16-3).

DIFFERENTIAL DIAGNOSIS

Patients may have hypotonia of one limb or of all muscle groups. Generalized hypotonia is usually secondary to a process which adversely affects the central nervous system. The axial musculature is affected more than the limbs. In such cases hypotonia is usually more prominent than weakness, stretch reflexes are preserved, if not brisk, and there are commonly other indications of central involvement. A variety of metabolic abnormalities may result in central hypotonia, including hypoxia, hypoglycemia, or the toxic effects of medication administered prenatally to mother or newborn. Myasthenia gravis or the myasthenic syndrome affect neuromuscular transmission and may also result in generalized hypotonia. Infant botulism must always be considered in early infancy as a cause of generalized hypotonia (see Table 5-1).

	6 months 28 weeks	6½ months 30 weeks	7 months 32 weeks	7½ months 34 weeks	8 months 36 weeks	8½ months 38 weeks	9 months 40 weeks
1. POSTURE	Completely hypotonic	Beginning of flexion of thigh at hip	Stronger flexion	Frog-like attitude	Flexion of the four limbs	Hypertonic	Very hypertonic
2. HEEL TO EAR MANOEUVRE							
3. POPLITEAL ANGLE	150°		110°	100°	100°	90°	80°
4. DORSI-FLEXION ANGLE OF FOOT			40-50°		40-50°		Premature reached 40 wk 40° / Full term
5. 'SCARF' SIGN	'Scarf' sign complete with no resistance			'Scarf' sign more limited		Elbow slightly passes midline	Elbow almost reaches midline
6. RETURN TO FLEXION OF FOREARM	Upper limbs very hypotonic lying in extension			Flexion of forearms begins to appear, but very weak	Strong 'return to flexion'. Flexion tone inhibited if forearm maintained 30 sec in extension	Strong 'return to flexion' Forearm returns very promptly to flexion after being extended for 30 sec.	

Fig. 16-3 Increase of muscle tone with increasing maturity. (Reproduced with permission from: Amiel-Tison C: Neurological evaluation of the maturity of newborn infants. Arch Dis Childh 43:89, 1968.)

When one limb is affected there is an abnormality of the reflex arc. Examples of limb hypotonia include traumatic neuropathy or, more commonly, congenital brachial plexus palsy. One must not overlook the possibility of clavicular or humeral fractures mimicking or occurring simultaneously with brachial plexus palsies.

Hypotonia is found in a wide variety of pathophysiologic processes (see Table 16-1). It is essential to carefully document the history of the infant as well as the mother with particular regard to administration of drugs such as barbiturates or other sedatives, and magnesium sulfate. A methodical examination is imperative. Most biochemical abnormalities are quickly identified or eliminated by the determination of serum electrolytes, assay for amino acids and organic acids. Structural abnormalities are demonstrated by computerized brain tomography.

The explanation for hypotonia in some infants is not readily determined, despite an extensive evaluation. Commonly, as the patient matures other abnormal neurologic findings become apparent including chorea, athetosis, or ataxia. These syndromes are generally considered as static encephalopathies. A few syndromes are not readily classified and deserve some comment for although they could be considered as having a cerebral basis, it is more prudent to be less specific until more clinical information regarding their etiology is available.

Table 16-1 Hypotonia and Associated Conditions

I. Cerebral	
Chromosomal abnormalities	Down's syndrome, Turner's syndrome, etc.
Congenital malformations	(See Chapter 2).
Developmental	Short gestational age.
Infection	Sepsis, meningitis, encephalitis.
Metabolic	Aminoacidurias. Drug intoxication (e.g., barbiturates). Fucosidosis. Hyperammonemia. Hypertilirubinemia. Hypermagnesemia. Hypocalcemia. Hypoglycemia. Hypothyroidism. Leigh disease. Leukodystrophies (Canavan's disease, acute infantile leukodystrophy, metachromatic leukodystrophy, infantile neuroaxonal dystrophy). Mannosidosis. Organic acidemias. Sphingolipidoses (gangliosidoses — Gm1, Gm2; Niemann-Pick).
Perinatal trauma	Ischemia/hypoxia. Intracerebral hemorrhage.
II. Brain stem/spinal cord	
Arthrogryposis	
Congenital malformations	
Degenerative diseases	Progressive spinal muscular atrophy. Progressive bulbar palsy (Fazio-Londe syndrome)
Glycogen storage disease, type II	
Infection	Poliomyelitis; other enteroviruses.
Vascular	Angiomas, intraspinal hemorrhage.
III. Peripheral nerve	
Congenital polyneuropathy	Polyneuropathies of any cause.
Familial dysautonomia (HSN III)	
Giant axonal neuropathy	
Guillain-Barre syndrome	
IV. Myoneural junction	
Myasthenia gravis	Associated with hyper- hypothyroidism, lupus erythematosus; adverse effect of some antibiotics (kanamycin, colistin, neomycin).
Myasthenic syndrome	
Infant botulism	
V. Muscle	Muscular dystrophies. Congenital myopathies. Inflammatory disease of muscle.
VI. Others	Prader-Willi syndrome. Benign congenital hypotonia. Sensory deprivation.

Patients with **Prader-Willi syndrome** commonly have low birth weights, early feeding difficulties with feeble suck, or problems with swallowing. Hypotonia persists and within several years they become remarkably obese and commonly have voracious appetites. Other typical features include 'almond-shaped' palpebral fissures, small hands and feet, hypogonadism, and mental retardation.

Benign congenital hypotonia is a diagnosis of exclusion and should be considered only after all other diagnostic possibilities have been carefully eliminated. These children have normal neurologic examinations with the exception of hypotonia. Serum enzyme assays, electrophysiological evaluations, and muscle biopsies are normal. Prognosis for this group of children is uniformly good.

Children who have been subjected to marked **sensory deprivation** in one way or another are commonly hypotonic. Examples of this include congenital blindness or infants who have been deprived of normal human relationships. Some patients within this group may have lessening of symptoms when environmental and/or interpersonal relationships are improved.

REFERENCES

Amiel-Tison C: Neurological evaluation of the maturity of newborn infants. Arch Dis Childhood. 43:89, 1968.

Boyd IA, et al: *The Role of the Gamma System in Movement and Posture.* Association for the Aid of Crippled Children, New York, 1964.

Cuajunco F: Development of the neuromuscular spindle in human fetuses. Contrib Embryol 28(173):97. 1940.

Cuajunco F: Development of the human motor end plate. Contrib Embryol 30(195): 129, 1942.

Dubowitz LMS, Dubowitz V, Goldberg C: Clinical assessment of gestational age in the newborn infant. J Pediatrics 77:1, 1970.

Dubowitz V: *The Floppy Infant,* 2nd Ed. (Clinics in Developmental Medicine, vol 76). Spastics International, London, England, Heinemann, 1980.

Granit R: The functional role of the muscle spindles — facts and hypotheses. Brain 98:531, 1975.

17

Ataxia of Childhood

Thomas K. Koch, MD and Bruce O. Berg, MD

Ataxia (Gr. *ataktos* = lack of order) refers to any incoordination of movement manifested by dysmetria and decomposition of the normal fluidity of movement. Ataxia of central origin is secondary to abnormalities of afferent and/or efferent cerebellar neural pathways.

Sensory ataxia results from impairment of proprioception as seen in diseases affecting the posterior columns of the spinal cord, such as pernicious anemia or tabes dorsalis, and/or sensory neuropathies affecting nerve fibers of large diameter. Patients with sensory ataxia rely on visual information to facilitate their orientation in space; when visual clues are not present, truncal instability is increased and patients may fall (positive Romberg sign). (See Tables 17-1, 17-2).

NEUROANATOMIC CONSIDERATIONS

The cerebellum develops from thickening of the dorsal alar plates of the metencephalon. During the first 2 months of gestation, symmetrical swellings on the dorsal brain stem protrude largely into the fourth ventricle; because of a rapid proliferation of neuroblasts during the third month there is midline fusion and dorsal enlargement to such extent that the cerebellum overlies the fourth ventricle, part of the pons, and medulla. Portions of neuroblasts of the alar plates migrate to the marginal zone, ultimately becoming the cerebellar cortex and cerebellar nuclei (the dentate, emboliform, globose, and fastigial nuclei). The fissures and lobules of the vermis, as well as the flocculonodular lobes are developed 30-60 days earlier than the hemispheres. At birth, however, the cerebellum appears very much like that of the adult; cerebellar differentiation and migration, in addition to myelination, account for its postnatal increase in size.

The flocculonodular lobe, the **archicerebellum,** is phylogenetically the oldest part of the cerebellum. The **paleocerebellum,** the next oldest component, denotes the anterior lobe and posterior part of the vermis (pyramis and uvula). The newest phylogenetic cerebellar structure, the **neocerebellum,** includes the lateral hemispheres and the mid-vermis.

The cerebellar cortex overlies the medullary white matter which consists of nerve fibers that project to and from the cerebellar cortex. Deep in the medullary core are four pairs of nuclei. The cerebellum itself is attached to the brain stem by three peduncles: inferior peduncle (restiform body), middle peduncle (brachium pontis), and the superior peduncle (brachium conjunctivum). The flocculonodular lobe, uvula, and

257

Table 17-1   Clinical Signs of Cerebellar Dysfunction

Midline structures (vermis, flocculonodular lobe, fastigial nucleus)
    Abnormal extraocular motility (see Chapter 13)
        Gaze evoked nystagmus
        Ocular dysmetria
        Optokinetic nystagmus abnormalities
    Head tilt
    Titubation

Lateral structures (cerebellar hemispheres, dentate, emboliform
        and globose nuclei)
    Abnormal extraocular motility
        Gaze apraxia
        Gaze evoked nystagmus
        Ocular bobbing
        Ocular dysmetria
        Ocular flutter
        Opsoclonus
        Optokinetic nystagmus abnormalities
    Abnormal rebound (see Chapter 1)
    Tremor (resting and action or intention tremor)

nodulus, the vestibular part of the cerebellum, are concerned with maintenance of equilibrium. Reciprocal neural connections of the vestibular nuclei and the cerebellum traverse the inferior cerebellar peduncle.

The anterior lobe and portions of the cerebellar posterior lobe have neural connections with the spinal cord in which information from the torso and limbs is transmitted via the dorsal and ventral spinocerebellar tracts to the cerebellar cortex. The paleocerebellum projects to the lateral vestibular nucleus and influences the spinal cord via the reticulospinal and vestibulospinal pathways, regulating posture and muscle tone through connections with the alpha and gamma efferent cells of the spinal cord.

The neocerebellum has a relationship with the cerebral cortex wherein afferent fibers from the cerebral cortex are projected to the contralateral cerebellar cortex through pontine nuclei. Efferent fibers from the neocerebellum course primarily to the dentate nucleus, then to the red nucleus and reticular formation; impulses are then relayed to the thalamus and ultimately the motor cortex. *The cerebellum serves as an elegant modulator of descending motor activity* (Figure 17-1).

CEREBELLAR ANOMALIES

It is not surprising, when considering the orderly and interrelated progression of embryologic development of the nervous system, that isolated cerebellar anomalies are rare. Complete cerebellar agenesis probably does not occur; however, a wide variety of other structural abnormalities are occasionally seen such as the absence of one cerebellar hemisphere, vermis or

Table 17-2 Clinical Features of Cerebellar Component Dysfunction

Archicerebellum	Gait ataxia; nystagmus; vertigo; wide-based station.
Paleocerebellum	Gait ataxia; incoordination of lower limb movement; wide-based station.
Neocerebellum	Gait ataxia/patient falls to side of lesion; dyssynergia; dysmetria; hypotonia; intention tremor; nystagmus.

a diffuse cerebellar hypoplasia. Generalized hypoplasia may be sporadic or familial and is found in Down's syndrome as well as in trisomy 5, 13, and 18.

Complete or partial absence of the vermis is secondary to the failure of midline fusion of the two dorsal alar plates of the developing metencephalon. A wide range of associated cerebellar and/or cerebral anomalies have been reported such as Dandy-Walker syndrome (see Chapter 2). One syndrome of familial agenesis of the vermis is associated with episodic hyperpnea (Joubert syndrome) and is characterized by periods of hyperpnea occasionally alternating with apneic spells. Other manifestations of this syndrome include mental retardation, a pendular or rotary nystagmus with conjugate, irregular eye movements; CNS malformations including encephaloceles and heterotopia have been reported.

Chiari malformations are a relatively commonly encountered anomaly and include varying degrees of hind-brain malformations with protrusion of the cerebellar tonsils below the level of the foramen magnum.

Platybasia, sometimes associated with Chiari malformations, is defined as a condition where, on lateral skull roentgenogram, the odontoid process extends above Chamberlain's line, an imaginary line drawn from the dorsal aspect of the hard palate to the posterior margin of the foramen magnum. It is inherited as an autosomal dominant trait with variable penetrance and is characterized by flattening and upward displacement of the floor of the posterior fossa. There is compression of posterior fossa structures, and stretching of the lower cranial nerves may occur.

Patients usually have symptom onset during the second or third decades of life and are manifested by head tilt, nystagmus, ataxia, lower cranial nerve palsies, and progressive spasticity. Patients usually have a short neck with a low hair-line. Recommended treatment is the surgical decompression of the posterior fossa.

It is remarkable that many patients with significant cerebellar malformations demonstrate only mild signs of cerebellar dysfunction. Hypotonia is usually present during the early years of life, the acquisition of milestones may be delayed, and the child may be inordinately clumsy; however, their coordination may improve remarkably with time.

HYSTERIA

Signs and symptoms resembling those of cerebellar dysfunction may have an hysterical basis; they are usually present after the first decade but may occur earlier.

260

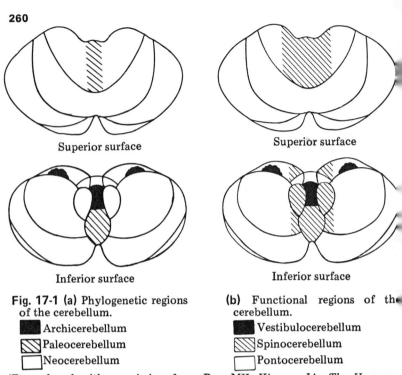

Superior surface

Superior surface

Inferior surface

Inferior surface

Fig. 17-1 (a) Phylogenetic regions of the cerebellum.

- Archicerebellum
- Paleocerebellum
- Neocerebellum

(b) Functional regions of the cerebellum.

- Vestibulocerebellum
- Spinocerebellum
- Pontocerebellum

(Reproduced with permission from Barr MK, Kiernan JA: *The Human Nervous System,* Harper & Row, Philadelphia, 1983.)

The etiology is commonly apparent to an experienced clinician for the 'incoordinate' movements and dysequilibrium are usually florid, often having a bizarre quality, and are not associated with valid signs of cerebellar dysfunction.

Commonly, if the patient is assisted by the examiner, or the incoordinate movements are restrained, that incoordination becomes more exaggerated and, in fact, requires an admirably functioning nervous system to carry out the movements. As a rule, the younger the patient, the more primitive or elemental are the findings. Often the symptoms will disappear with firm but gentle supportive measures; however, the basic problem(s) can be uncovered only with common-sense psychotherapy.

INFECTION

An acute cerebellar ataxia may result from bacterial, viral, fungal, or parasitic infections, either by direct local inflammatory process or a para- or postinfectious process. An acute cerebellar syndrome may occur in some systemic infections that do not directly affect the nervous system such as diphtheria, leptospirosis, scarlet fever, and typhoid fever. Rarely, *Mycoplasma pneumoniae* has been implicated. In these cases the pathophysiology has not been clearly established.

An acute ataxic syndrome has also been reported to be associated with coxsackievirus, echovirus, infectious mononucleosis, Japanese B encephalitis, mumps, pertussis, polio, rubeola, rubella, typhoid, and varicella. In varicella infection, probably the most commonly associated virus with this syndrome, ataxia ordinarily occurs about 1 week after onset of symptoms but may also occur before the varicelliform eruption has appeared. Generally, in these circumstances, the prognosis is quite good.

An unusual variant of Guillain-Barre syndrome, first described by Fisher, is also characterized by ataxia, ophthalmoplegia, weakness, and hyporeflexia. It is uncommon in childhood and the outlook is generally good. The specific pathophysiology is unknown.

One syndrome of **acute cerebellar ataxia** is characterized by its sudden onset with about one-half of patients having had some nonspecific illness several weeks earlier. Usually it occurs during the first several years of life and is characterized by truncal and limb ataxia often with striking tremors of the limbs, trunk, and head. On occasion, the tremors may be quite marked and interfere not only with intentional movement but also while the patient attempts to be quietly supine. Nystagmus occurs in about one-half of patients with some ocular movements that may appear chaotic. There are few other associated neurologic signs or symptoms, although some patients complain of headache and/or photophobia. They are not febrile and there is no nuchal rigidity. The CSF is, for the most part, normal although mild pleocytosis and elevation of protein have been reported.

The diagnosis of acute cerebellar ataxia is one of exclusion and the clinical course is variable. Usually, improvement occurs over a period of several months but may be longer. Occasionally, the patient has complete recovery within several weeks. Some patients will have a temporary regression during their recovery which seems to be associated with a respiratory or gastrointestinal infection, but then resume their neurologic improvement following the resolution of the infection.

About one-third of patients have complete recovery, one-third have mild residual clumsiness, and about one-third have permanent sequelae including ataxia, dysarthria, personality and behavioral abnormalities, and mental subnormality.

As noted earlier, an acute ataxic syndrome has been associated with a variety of viral agents. Whether the inability to identify an etiologic agent sets the syndrome of acute cerebellar ataxia apart from other ataxic syndromes in which an apparent etiologic agent has been identified remains speculative.

There is one ataxic syndrome, similar in many ways to those noted above, except that patients have opsoclonus (see Chapter 13), myoclonus, and an occult neuroblastoma. The symptoms and signs precede the detection of the tumor. Patients have an acute onset of symptoms that are remarkably striking. Administration of ACTH or prednisone may be of great benefit in lessening those symptoms.

Since the tumor is not apparent when the patient is first seen, the clinician must diligently seek out its presence. In some cases, the tumor has been first detected months after the symptom onset.

Echinococcosis Intracerebral hydatid cysts of echinococcosis are uncommon except in certain countries including Argentina, Australia, New Zealand, and particularly Uruguay. The condition does exist in the USA and should always be considered in the differential diagnosis of any patient with symptoms of ataxia and other signs of CNS dysfunction, particularly if that patient has been exposed to dogs or related species, and grazing animals. The dog is the definitive host, sheep or other grazing animals are the intermediate hosts, and man is accidentally infected.

Echinococcosis is more common in children than adults and neurologic symptoms and signs include fits, intermittent headache, signs of intracranial hypertension, ataxia, and long tract signs.

A remarkable characteristic of this disease is that in the presence of extensive involvement of the brain by large hydatid cysts, the manifestations of cerebral dysfunction may appear relatively minor.

Intracerebral hydatid cysts can be surgically removed but this should only be attempted by neurosurgeons with particular expertise in these techniques. Neurosurgical removal of echinococcal cysts combined with the administration of mebendazole has been described but there are no significant numbers of patients reported who have received combined neurosurgical and medical treatment from which reliable conclusions can be derived.

TOXINS

Ataxia may result from the toxic effects of certain drugs. Children are most commonly affected by drug ingestion and if ataxia occurs, it is usually transient, and may or may not be dose-related. **Anticonvulsants** are the most frequent offenders, particularly barbiturates, phenytoin, and carbamazepine (see Table 17-3).

In the case of phenobarbital and phenytoin, ataxia may appear with serum levels greater than 40 μg/dl and 20μg/dl respectively, and will disappear with reduction in serum levels to therapeutic range. However, primidone, a barbiturate that is largely metabolized to phenobarbital, may also produce ataxia and nystagmus unrelated to serum phenobarbital levels.

Signs of cerebellar dysfunction are usually transient and include truncal and/or limb involvement, dysarthria, tremor, and occasionally nystagmus. Although nystagmus is often first to appear before the ataxia, this is not always the case. Whether there are structural changes of cerebellar histology following long-term anticonvulsant administration, particularly in the case of phenytoin, is yet controversial.

Table 17-3   Ataxia Secondary to Toxins

Anticonvulsant medication	Alcohol
Bromides	
Carbamazepine	**Organic chemical agents**
Clonazepam	Ethyl chloride
Phenobarbital	Toluene
Phenytoin	
Primidone	
Tumor chemotherapeutic agents	**Heavy metals**
5-fluorouracil	Lead
Methotrexate	Mercury
Procarbazine	Thallium
Phencyclidine	

When carbamazepine is the drug in question, ataxia may be observed with toxic serum levels of the drug but there is considerable individual variation in the relationship of serum drug levels and ataxic manifestations of toxicity. Clonazepam may also be a cause of ataxia.

Alcohol ingestion may result in cerebellar dysfunction in children as well as adults. Signs and symptoms of intoxication are generally transient, but permanent truncal ataxia may result from chronic alcohol abuse. Usually a problem of adults, it is, unfortunately, increasingly becoming a pediatric problem as well.

Intoxication from **heavy metals** is relatively uncommon in the USA but must always be considered in the differential diagnosis of ataxia. Lead poisoning in children is usually manifested as an encephalopathy with signs of intracranial hypertension and cerebellar dysfunction including limb tremor and wide-based gait. Neuropathologic studies of rat pups intoxicated from lead have shown an interstitial cerebellar edema with particular damage to capillaries. The reason for these changes remains unknown.

Thallium intoxication is rare and usually is secondary to ingestion of pesticides or other industrial products. Acute symptoms include vomiting and diarrhea, ataxia, tremors, choreoathetosis; some patients have signs of cranial nerve palsies and polyneuropathy. Intoxication over a period of weeks is characterized by alopecia with central and peripheral nervous system dysfunction. Some patients become stuporous or comatose. Whenever alopecia is associated with progressive neurologic signs and symptoms, thallium intoxication should always be considered. Thallium levels can be determined from blood, urine, and specimens of hair.

Both **inorganic and organic mercury** are occasionally responsible for neurologic symptoms including confusion, convulsions, ataxia, tremor, choreoathetosis, and signs of polyneuropathy. Mercury can be detected in blood, urine, and hair.

TRAUMA

Both open and closed head injuries may cause disruptions of cerebellar function. The bulk of pediatric head injuries result in concussion with a transient impairment of consciousness but no focal deficit. Occasionally, signs and symptoms of a posttraumatic syndrome are apparent with irritability, recurring headache, vertigo, and attentional deficit, and in young children behavioral changes. Ataxia sometimes occurs.

Posterior fossa subdural or epidural hematomas and cerebellar parenchymatous damage results in progressive obtundation, intractable vomiting, vertigo, and truncal and/or limb ataxia. Immediate surgical intervention is required in these cases.

TUMOR

About 60% of intracranial tumors of children 2 years and older are below the tentorium cerebelli. Intracranial tumors of infancy, however, are primarily supratentorial (see Chapter 8).

Signs of intracranial hypertension include headache, nuchal rigidity, vomiting, impaired vision either secondary to papilledema or cranial nerve dysfunction, and macrocephaly in infant patients. Signs of cerebellar dysfunction may be manifested only by truncal ataxia, as in the case of med-

Table 17-4 Spinocerebellar Degenerative Diseases

Disease type	Clinical characteristics
Friedreich's ataxia (autosomal recessive) (autosomal dominant)	Both types of inherited traits have similar clinical features with the onset of signs and symptoms commonly occurring from mid 1st to 2nd decades. Pes cavus usually with hammer toes occurs in the majority of patients. Ataxia is striking abnormality, usually present in latter part of 1st decade but may occur earlier. There is loss of posterior column function (impaired perception of vibration and position sense). Dysarthria is usually present with ataxic respirations. Nystagmus is commonly observed and occasional patients have retinal pigmentary degeneration and later in the disease course optic atrophy may be present. Episodic vertigo and rarely deafness reported. Stretch reflexes are significantly decreased to absent, particularly in the lower limbs, and plantar responses are usually extensor. Kyphoscoliosis commonly occurs and impairment of bowel and bladder function is frequent. ECG abnormalities are found in most patients including decreased amplitude of QRS complex and T wave abnormalities. Average age at death in autosomal recessive and dominant traits is 26.5 and 39.5 years.
Roussy-Levy syndrome (autosomal dominant)	Slowly progressive disease in which signs and symptoms, primarily a gait disturbance, usually begin in childhood. Ataxia is associated with polyneuropathy and has clinical features similar to both Friedreich's ataxia and Charcot-Marie-Tooth disease. In addition to ataxia, patients have nystagmus, hypotonia with significantly decreased to absent stretch reflexes and atrophy of distal muscles. Impaired to loss of posterior column function. As disease progresses, there is loss of peripheral sensation. It is undetermined whether this is truly a distinct clinicopathologic entity.
Olivopontocerebellar atrophy (autosomal recessive and dominant traits reported)	A rare disease characterized by loss of neurons in the cerebellar cortex, pons, and inferior olivary nuclei. There is variable neuronal loss in spinal cord and basal ganglia. Categorized into 5 types on basis of clinicopathologic findings and hereditary transmission (Konigsmark and Weiner). Although usual onset of ataxia is in adult life, it may occur during 1st decade. Other findings include visual loss, tremors of limbs and head, and impairment of posterior column function.
Olivocerebellar degeneration	Kindred described by Gordon Holmes with degeneration of cerebellum and inferior olives. Additional families have been reported. Onset almost always in adults but rarely occurs in adolescence. Striking feature is ataxia in limb and trunk with dysarthria. Course is slowly progressive.
Dentatorubral atrophy (heritability ?)	An uncommon disorder affecting both sexes and characterized by ataxia and myoclonus. Gradual dementia is not uncommon. Dysarthria of at least mild degree is present.
Familial spastic paraplegia (autosomal dominant and recessive)	Disorder affects both sexes. Attainment of developmental milestones commonly delayed. Gradual increase of muscle tone in lower limbs with hyperreflexia and extensor plantar responses. Usually no loss of muscle bulk and no impairment of posterior column function. Arms usually remain unaffected until late in the course of the disease. No impairment of bowel or bladder function. Patients with dominant form of disease appear to progress more slowly than those with recessive trait.

ulloblastomas located in the midline. More commonly, the mass lesion affects more extensive portions of the cerebellum and results in hypotonia, truncal and/or limb ataxia, and nystagmus.

Remote effects of neoplasms are more commonly seen in adult patients with nonmetastatic carcinomatous cerebellar degenerations. Primary tumors are most often found in the lung, breast, ovary or uterus, and bowel. Lymphomas also have been implicated. Children may have a cerebellar syndrome with leukemia, Hodgkin's disease, the reticuloendothelioses and most notably, occult neuroblastomas.

VASCULAR LESIONS

Children who have symptomatic vascular lesions within the posterior fossa are relatively uncommon. The onset of symptoms is acute, following hemorrhage from either an aneurysm or AVM, or subacute should the vascular lesion present as a space-occupying mass of increasing dimensions. The quality of the history points to the cerebellum and other structures within the posterior fossa, and CT head scans and/or cerebral angiography should establish the diagnosis.

Vertebrobasilar occlusive disease is a well recognized, though uncommon, cause of ataxia associated with hemiparesis and occasional abnormalities of extraocular motility. Symptoms may be recurrent and transient or result in permanent stroke. The pathophysiology has included abnormalities of cervical vertebrae, trauma, or congenital cyanotic heart disease.

Basilar migraine may occur in children, manifested by recurring transient episodes of ataxia, vertigo, and alternating hemiplegia (see Chapter 15). A family history of migraine and the transient recurring nature of the attacks support a diagnosis of migraine.

SPINOCEREBELLAR DEGENERATIVE DISEASES

It has been difficult to adequately classify the wide range of degenerative diseases which affect the spinal cord and/or cerebellum, primarily because of the tendency to classify clinical phenomena on a descriptive basis but also because of the lack of understanding of their neurochemical mechanisms. Neuropathologic studies have not provided definitive information.

These diseases are generally slowly progressive and familial wherein other involved family members tend to have a similar clinical course. Diseases considered within this broad category are distinct clinicopathologic entities while, at the same time, may share similar features with other diseases, suggesting there is some neurochemical common denominator.

The disease prototype is Friedreich's ataxia, characterized by ataxia, nystagmus, pes cavus, and kyphoscoliosis. It is inherited as an autosomal recessive or dominant trait. Other major diseases considered within this disease category are listed in Table 17-4.

REFERENCES

Gilman S, Bloedel JR, Lechtenberg R: *Disorders of the Cerebellum.* Davis, Philadelphia, 1981.

Greenfield JG: *The Spinocerebellar Degenerations.* Blackwell, Oxford, 1954.

Konigsmark BW, Weiner LP: The olivopontocerebellar atrophies: a review. Medicine 49:227, 1970.

Weiss S, Carter S: Course and prognosis of acute cerebellar ataxia in children. Neurology 9:711, 1959.

18

Movement Disorders

Bruce O. Berg, MD

GENERAL CONSIDERATIONS

Unusual movements are common in children and one must be able to distinguish an involuntary movement disorder from the fidgetiness of an otherwise normal child. Nose rubbing, scratching, or a 'nasal salute' may be secondary to an allergic process or a tic, while similar recurring episodic movements such as brushing hair from the forehead or eyebrow could be a manifestation of a photic fit. Recurring nasopharyngeal noises may be secondary to an allergy, convulsive disorder, or a tic.

Disorders of movement are less common in children than adults; it is not always easy to determine if the movements are truly abnormal. Anxiety and stress tend to increase their frequency and severity and, except for ballism and some patients with severe torsion dystonia, movement disorders disappear during sleep. Involuntary movements that occur during sleep, however, may be a manifestation of convulsive activity.

Movement disorders may have an insidious onset and are often initially overlooked by parents and even the critical eye of teachers and physicians. Occasionally, the child is thought to be simply clumsy but sooner or later it becomes apparent that the recurring movements are involuntary. Patients may have other alterations of their neurologic status, including changes of posture, muscle tone, and stretch reflexes. It is common to have associated behavioral changes such as irritability, irascibility, forgetfulness, or apathy; some patients are dysarthric or anarthric.

NEUROANATOMIC CONSIDERATIONS

Clinicopathologic studies have associated movement disorders with the extrapyramidal system. Although not specifically neuroanatomically defined, it is traditionally accepted that the extrapyramidal system includes the basal ganglia, the subthalamic nuclei (Luys bodies) found in the basilar portion of the diencephalon, and the substantia nigra, the largest nuclear mass in the mesencephalon. The caudate nucleus, the putamen, and the pallidum comprise the basal ganglia. The claustrum is also sometimes included.

The term **corpus striatum** is sometimes used synonymously for the basal ganglia. Other related terms used frequently are **neostriatum** (caudate and putamen), the most recent structures to appear phylogenically; the paleostriatum, referring to the pallidum (globus pallidus); and the **archi-striatum** (amygdaloid nucleus), the oldest of the large subcortical nuclear masses. The principal afferent fibers to the basal ganglia terminate in the caudate and putamen and come primarily from three sources; namely, virtually all major cortical areas, fibers from the intralaminar thalamic nuclei, and the substantia nigra. Fibers from the caudate nucleus and putamen then proceed to the pallidum.

The internal component of the pallidum directs major efferent fibers to the thalamus (ventral lateral, ventral anterior, and intralaminar nuclei) and to the substantia nigra in the mesencephalon. The thalamic fibers are carried by the ansa lenticularis and lenticular fasciculus which later join the thalamic fasciculus. Thalamic nuclei also receive fibers from the cerebellum.

The ventral lateral and ventral anterior nuclei direct their efferent fibers to the prefrontal and precentral cortex. These efferent neural pathways are important for they ultimately influence the corticospinal and corticobulbar tracts. There are other projections from the basal ganglia to the substantia nigra. The basal ganglia receive their main input from the cortex and thalamus and project back to the thalamus, but they have no efferent fiber tracts that course directly to the spinal cord. The thalamus has the important function of integrating information from the basal ganglia and cerebellum en route to the cerebral motor cortex.

CLINICAL SYNDROMES WITH ASSOCIATED MOVEMENT DISORDERS

ATHETOSIS

Athetosis may be present in patients who have sustained some perinatal insult. These patients are commonly hypotonic during infancy though stretch reflexes are brisk; the athetotic movements may not be apparent until after 12-36 months of age.

Other causes of athetosis include prenatal injury, developmental anomalies, kernicterus, abnormalities of uric acid metabolism, Leigh's disease, juvenile Niemann-Pick disease, ataxia-telangiectasia, Wilson's disease, Hallervorden-Spatz syndrome, Pelizaeus-Merzbacher disease, adverse effects of neuroleptic drugs (levodopa and phenothiazines), postencephalitis or posttraumatic states.

There is no one specific pathologic lesion associated with this movement disorder. If secondary to perinatal hypoxia, a neuronal loss is most prominent in the caudate nucleus, putamen, and globus pallidus, but may also be demonstrated in the thalamus, amygdala, and portions of the hippocampus. There is commonly hypermyelination of the putamen and globus pallidus with coarse bundles of myelinated fibers lending a 'marbled' appearance (status marmoratus) to these structures.

Although there is no specific **treatment** for athetosis at this time, physical therapy may be of some usefulness in maintaining joint mobility and gait training. Administration of levodopa with a decarboxylase inhibitor has resulted in some symptomatic improvement, especially in lessening muscular rigidity. Surgical procedures including stereotactic thalamotomy and, more recently, cervical spinal cord electrode implantation and stimulation have been reported to be of some benefit in the occasional patient, particularly those without corticospinal tract involvement.

BALLISM

Ballism, uncommon at any age, is rare in children. It is characterized by violent flailing of one limb (monoballismus) ipsilateral arm and leg (hemiballismus), or bilateral limbs (biballismus) and may be so severe that the patient is thrown from the bed to the floor. This florid movement disorder is associated with lesions, usually secondary to vascular occlusion, involving the contralateral subthalamic nucleus. It is seen rarely as a transient stage in the progressive deterioration of patients with subacute sclerosing panencephalitis and, rarely, other viral encephalitides.

Patients may die from exhaustion, and meticulous supportive medical care is essential. Current **treatment** to lessen the severity of this movement disorder consists of administration of barbiturates or phenothiazines. There is usually a gradual reduction of the ballismic movements, but some patients have residual athetosis and/or chorea. In those patients who do not respond to medication, surgical lesions have been made in the globus pallidus or thalamus with varying results.

CHOREA

Chorea is usually thought to be secondary to perinatal trauma or a manifestation of Sydenham's or Huntington's disease. This movement disorder occurs, however, in many other pathophysiologic processes (see Table 18-1).

Sydenham's chorea commonly has an insidious onset; typical clinical features include chorea, incoordination, and weakness. Often the child appears restless or fidgety, and becomes emotionally labile. It is not unusual that parents do not know when the process actually began; and when first evaluated by physicians, the child may be thought to have an emotional problem or ataxia. Facial grimacing, dysarthria and, rarely, anarthria may be present. Voluntary movements and muscle power can be mildly to severely impaired and hypotonia is commonly found. Stretch reflexes are often pendular as seen in the knee jerk. Plantar responses are flexor. The sensory system is normal.

Because of the association with rheumatic fever, a search for streptococcal infection must be made; however, throat cultures have not been particularly reliable in identifying the organism. Anti-streptolysin-O titers, though widely used, are often of little diagnostic help, for they rise early and decline quickly. Other antibody tests include anti-desoxyribonuclease B (anti-DNase B) antihyaluronidase (AH), antistreptokinase (ASK), and antinicotinamide-adenine dinucleotidase (anti-NADase). A twofold titer increase is present if samples are obtained within 2 months of the streptococcal infection.

Table 18-1 Medical Conditions in which Chorea has been Reported

Cerebral degenerative diseases

Hallervorden-Spatz syndrome; Lesch-Nyhan syndrome; cerebral lipidoses; presenile dementia; 'senile' chorea.

Infectious diseases

Diphtheria; St. Louis encephalitis; SSPE; postencephalitic syndrome; lues; mumps; pertussis; rubeola; scarlet fever; typhoid; varicella.

Metabolic diseases

Addison's disease; ataxia-telangiectasia; beriberi; burns; hypocalcemia; hypoglycemia; hypomagnesemia; hypoparathyroidism; phenylketonuria; porphyria; pregnancy; thyrotoxicosis; vitamin B_{12} deficiency; Wilson's disease.

Toxic disorders

Carbon monoxide; fenfluramine; hyoscine; INH; kernicterus; levodopa; lithium; mercury; metoclopramide; phenothiazines; phenytoin; reserpine.

Trauma

Posttraumatic syndrome.

Tumor

Brain tumors.

Vascular diseases

Cerebrovascular disease; Henoch-Schonlein purpura; lupus erythematosus; polycythemia vera.

Adapted from Greenhouse AH: On chorea, lupus erythematosus, and cerebral arteritis. Arch Intern Med 117:389-393, 1966.

Valvular heart disease is found in about one-third of patients with Sydenham's chorea; other manifestations of rheumatic fever include polyarthritis, erythema marginatum, and subcutaneous nodules. If there is no clinical or laboratory evidence upon which to establish a rheumatic basis for patients with 'pure' chorea, only later manifestations of arthritis and/or carditis will lend retrospective evidence of the disease. It is recomended, therefore, that all patients with Sydenham's chorea and chorea of unknown cause should be treated with continual antibiotic prophylaxis, consisting of either monthly injections of 1.2 million units of benzathine penicillin G or the oral administration of 200,000 units of penicillin given twice daily. The duration of prophylaxis should be continued at least until the end of the second decade; however, it is prudent to continue the treatment indefinitely.

Patients should be as quiet as reasonable for the family setting. This may require bed rest and administration of barbiturates, chlorpromazine or haloperidol. Usually, the choreic movements lessen within several days following the start of medication and are completely controlled within days to several weeks. Medication can gradually be withdrawn after a period of several months although occasional patients require a longer period of treatment. If there are recurrences of chorea following drug withdrawal, the medication may have to be reinstituted. The duration of Sydenham's chorea varies from about 1 month to several years; about two-thirds of patients have recurrence of chorea. There is usually complete recovery but mild incoordination or tremor may persist.

Neuropathologic studies have shown only nonspecific findings including arteritis with some neuronal loss in the caudate nucleus, putamen, and multiple diffuse areas of neuronal loss in the cerebral cortex and cerebellum.

Huntington's chorea is a progressive degenerative disease, inherited as an autosomal dominant trait, characterized by chorea, dementia, and hypotonia. Some patients have bradykinesia or rigidity, tremors and, rarely, convulsions. The disease usually affects adults, but about 5% of patients are less than 14 years old and infants may be affected. It is more commonly inherited from the father than the mother. The clinical presentation in children is different from the adult and is characterized by early onset of dementia, hypokinesia, and rigidity. Convulsions occur in about one-half of child patients. The seizures are usually generalized with tonic/clonic activity, myoclonic or akinetic spells. Occasionally, ataxia and tremors are present. The average survival is 8-10 years.

If convulsions are present, anticonvulsant medication should be administered (see Chapter 10). Unfortunately, there is no effective medication to adequately control the movement disorder although phenothiazines are sometimes of temporary usefulness. Children with rigidity may have some improvement with antiparkinsonism drugs.

Neuropathologic findings include marked neuronal loss in the caudate nucleus and putamen. Similar changes may also be found in the thalamus, cerebellum, and subthalamic nuclei. Cortical atrophy with ventriculomegaly are present.

Benign familial chorea is a nonprogressive, though persistent, chorea that begins during childhood; it is not associated with mental deterioration This movement disorder is inherited as an autosomal dominant trait. There is no treatment of significant benefit.

Familial paroxysmal choreoathetosis is a condition characterized by paroxysmal episodes of choreoathetosis and/or dystonia. There are at least two syndromes included within this category. The more common type, *paroxysmal kinesigenic choreoathetosis,* is notable for recurring paroxysmal episodes of choreoathetosis that are usually precipitated by startle or initiation of movement and occur particularly after rest. The duration of the episodes is less than 5 minutes. Symptoms are usually controlled by administration of barbiturates or phenytoin.

A second, apparently related syndrome, *paroxysmal dystonic choreoathetosis,* is often precipitated by emotional stress, fatigue, or following consumption of alcohol. The episodes may persist up to several hours and have been identified as early as the first year of life. These patients have had symptomatic improvement with administration of clonazepam but have responded poorly to barbiturates or phenytoin.

DYSTONIA

Dystonia refers to abnormal involuntary twisting movements or postures. Because of the twisting quality of movement, the term **torsion dystonia** is appropriate.

Dystonic movements may be segmental, focal, or generalized, involving trunk and/or limb. Segmental or focal dystonia is usually seen in adult patients and include writer's cramp, spasmodic tortocollis, spasmodic dysphonia, oral-mandibular dystonia and blepharospasm. Generally, the younger the patient at onset of symptoms, the more likely those symptoms will become generalized.

There are variable forms of inheritance (see Table 18-2). The recessive form, seen predominantly in Ashkenazim, tends to be progressive; whereas, the dominant form may have exacerbations and remissions.

Commonly, torsion dystonia starts as an abnormal movement or posture that becomes apparent at the initiation of movement — 'action dystonia.' Children typically have onset of action dystonia affecting one leg, usually a twisting or turning in of the foot and leg. Adults more often have dystonia first affecting the upper limbs. Fatigue often increases the severity of movement.

The diagnosis of **idiopathic torsion dystonia** requires that, in addition to dystonia, the patient has a normal perinatal and developmental history, there has been no antecedent disease or drug consumption that could possibly result in dystonia, there is no impairment of intellectual function, motor or sensory symptoms, and there is no abnormality of copper metabolism.

Treatment A variety of medical and surgical procedures have been attempted to treat dystonia but there is no one therapy of particular benefit. Administration of diazepam, haloperidol, and numerous other drugs have been of limited usefulness. Levodopa has been of some benefit in about 20% of patients and, more recently, it has been demonstrated that high doses of trihexyphenidyl has resulted in significant improvement in an even greater number of patients. The production of lesions in the ventral lateral thalamic nucleus by a variety of neurosurgical methods, particularly cryothalamotomy, may result in significant reduction of symptoms; however, the risks of relapse are high. Bilateral thalamotomies can be carried out, but there is an even greater risk of either hemiparesis or loss of speech and language.

Torsion dystonia may be a devastating disease and physicians should enlist all supportive facilities available to assist the patient and family. About one-third of patients become bedbound or confined to a chair, one-third remain moderately disabled and the remaining one-third remain mildly disabled yet independent.

Table 18-2   Classification of Dystonic States

I. Primary
   A. *Hereditary*
      Autosomal dominant
      Autosomal recessive
      X-linked recessive
      Paroxysmal dystonic choreoathetosis.

   B. *Idiopathic*
      Generalized, segmental, focal.

II. Secondary
   A. *Associated with other hereditary neurologic disorders*
      Wilson's disease
      Huntington's disease
      Hallervorden-Spatz syndrome
      Juvenile neuronal ceroid-lipofuscinosis
      Glutaric acidemia.

   B. *Environmental*
      Perinatal cerebral trauma
      Infection
      Postinfectious states
      Reye's syndrome
      Head trauma
      Focal cerebral vascular injury
      Brain tumor
      Toxins: levodopa, antipsychotic drugs, metoclo-
         pramide, fenfluramine, anticonvulsants.

III. Psychological

Adapted from Fahn S, Eldredge R: Definition of dystonia and
   classification of the dystonic states. *In* Eldridge R, Fahn S
   (Eds) Dystonia. *Advances in Neurology,* Vol. 14, Raven
   Press, New York, 1976, pp. 1-5.

BOBBLE-HEAD DOLL SYNDROME

This is an intermittent 'bobbing' movement of the head and neck with a
frequency of 2-5 Hz, appearing much like a doll's head supported by a
spring wire. Often the head movements can be voluntarily stopped on
command, only to reappear when the child's attention is directed to other
stimuli. Most reported patients have cysts or other obstructive space-
occupying lesions in the region of the third ventricle or aqueduct of Sylvius.

CHIN QUIVERING

This is an unusual, benign, involuntary movement of chin muscles, inherited as an autosomal dominant trait, with symptom onset at birth or early

life. The chin trembling is rhythmical, varying from fine to coarse, with a rate of about 3 Hz. Emotional stress or startle may provoke the chin quivering; but it may be unprovoked, with episodes lasting up to 30 minutes. There are no other known associated neurologic abnormalities and there is no known relationship to the palmomental reflex.

SPASMUS NUTANS

This is a self-limiting condition of unknown origin occurring in infants, usually between 4 and 12 months of age, as an episodic abnormal posturing of the head, and intermittent head nodding which may be in any direction, lasting only a matter of seconds. There is associated nystagmus which can be horizontal, vertical, or rotary, and while usually bilateral may be monocular. The head nodding and nystagmus disappear without treatment within a period of a few months to no longer than 1 or 2 years. There are virtually no sequelae, although rare cases of persistent nystagmus are reported. Optic gliomas are occasionally present.

TICS

Tics are involuntary, stereotyped, quick purposeless movements that usually involve the same muscle or muscle groups. Facial, neck and /or shoulder muscles are most often involved as in eye blinking, widening of the palpebral fissure, dilation of nares with facial grimacing, head movements, or shoulder shrugging. Whether a simple movement or variations on a theme, they are repetitive and generally affect the same anatomical region, as compared with chorea in which muscle jerks move unpredictably from place to place. Myoclonus, a paroxysmal brief, rapid contraction of part of a muscle, muscle, or group of muscles, must be considered in the differential diagnosis.

As in the case of specific disorders of movement, tics are usually increased in frequency and severity when the patient is under stress; they disappear during sleep. They are common in childhood with a reported incidence ranging from 4-23% of children; boys are affected three times more commonly than girls. The age of symptom onset ranges from 3-15 years with a mean age of 7 years. (See Table 18-3.)

A **simple, transient tic,** commonly called a 'habit pattern,' has been reported to affect up to one-fourth of children at one time or another. They are rarely first noted before school age or in adolescence. Simple tics usually persist weeks to no longer than 6 months; however, other simple tics may appear.

The pathophysiology of tics is not understood and there is no unequivocal evidence to presume the simple tic has a psychogenic basis. The traditional recommendation is to quietly observe and support the child rather than 'reminding' or 'correcting' him. There is merit, however, in understanding areas of stress for the child at home and school. This may require psychological testing, a family interview, and possibly family therapy by those with specific expertise in child behavior.

Treatment   Occasionally, the simple tic may severely disrupt a child's activities at home and school. These patients may benefit from daily administration of low doses (1-2 mg/day) of haloperidol; the administration of drugs should be reserved only for those occasional patients who are

Table 18-3 Tics

	Simple tic of childhood	Complex (motor) tics	Tourette's syndrome
Onset	3-15 years	Up to 15 years	2-15 years
Duration	Weeks to months	Intermittent; may be lifelong	Lifelong
Quality of tic	Motor tics	Motor tics, occasional vocal tics	Multiple motor & vocal tics
Clinical course	Generally good	Variable	Variable learning disability is common, compulsive behavior, obsessive thoughts, coprolalia, echolalia, palilalia.

severely incapacitated by the tic. Duration of therapy should be no longer than several months, for simple tics are generally a self-limiting phenomenon. Should the tic persist longer than 6 months, one must consider the possibility that the patient has a complex, chronic tic and provide careful long-term follow-up evaluations.

Complex tics are characterized by varying multiple tics that are motor and/or vocal; they tend to be chronic. The mean age of onset is about 7 years of age although the history is generally established at a mean age of 11 years. There is a range of variability of complex tics, with Tourette's syndrome representing the most severe form. The tics commonly begin as eye blinking, twisting or turning of the head and/or neck, shoulder shrugging, or any variation thereof.

Some patients with **Tourette's syndrome** have complex, stereotyped movements including hopping, jumping, truncal or pelvic gyrations, thigh tapping, repetitive twisting or turning around. There may be compulsive touching or hitting other persons, biting, or smelling objects within the immediate environment. There is a ritualistic quality to some activities such as rearranging objects in the immediate environment, foot stamping, or assuming unusual postures.

Vocalizations may also be present and include grunting, clucking sounds, repetitive sounds of swallowing, or as if clearing the throat, nasal snuffing, screams, shrieks, and occasional animal sounds such as barking or growling.

Some patients with Tourette's syndrome will explosively utter the usually well recognized obscenities (coprolalia). Others will repeat a word or phrase over and over that has been said to them (echolalia), and some will repeat a word or phrase with increasing rapidity (palilalia).

The commonly held view that Tourette's syndrome is primarily found in Ashkenazim and other Central Europeans is probably a reflection of an initially skewed population data base rather than epidemiologic fact. Males are affected about four times more frequently than females and there appears to be a significant number of patients with positive family histories. An autosomal dominant mode of inheritance, with variable clinical expression has been suggested, but a polygenic inheritance cannot be excluded.

Learning disabilities have been found in about one-third of patients with Tourette's syndrome. Areas of cognitive dysfunction are variable and attentional deficit disorders are common. There is persuasive evidence that the central nervous system stimulants (methylphenidate, dextroamphetamine, or pemoline) commonly used for treatment of attentional deficit disorders may precipitate the first symptoms of Tourette's syndrome, or exacerbate tics and vocalizations during the course of treatment. Should tics appear under these circumstances the drug should be discontinued in most cases.

The clinical problem must be tactfully and completely discussed with the parents and child for there is no easy solution. The physician should never underestimate the potential for intrafamilial disruption that so frequently occurs when one family member has Tourette's syndrome. The therapeutic goal is the elimination of tics and maintenance of the family's normal activities as much as possible. This usually requires combined administration of medication and on-going family therapy.

Treatment Haloperidol appears to be the most consistently useful drug, providing relief from tics in at least 50-75% of patients. It should be started at low doses of 0.5 mg daily to be increased by another 0.5 mg each week until the patient receives a total daily dose of 2-3 mg. Generally patients who have a good response require no higher drug dosage. If they have not had a good response with doses up to 6-8 mg/day there is little chance the drug will be of any usefulness.

Extrapyramidal reactions may occur following administration of haloperidol and include dystonia, akathisia, hyperreflexia, opisthotonus, or oculogyric crises. The severity of the abnormal signs and symptoms are usually dose related and tend to disappear or become less severe when the dosage is reduced. In these cases, 25-50 mg of diphenhydramine should be given IV, to be followed by daily administration of benzotropine mesylate at a dosage of 0.5 mg bid.

In cases where haloperidol has provided no relief from symptoms, other drugs have been used including pimozide, penfluridol, and clonidine. These drugs have been found to reduce symptoms in less than 25% of patients. Carbamazepine and clonazepam have also been reported to be of benefit to the occasional patient. The treatment of patients with complex, chronic tics, and particularly Tourette's syndrome, is difficult and frustrating not only for the patient and family but also for the physician. Family therapy and patient support groups are most important and should be an integral part of the treatment plan.

TREMORS

Tremors are rhythmic oscillations of variable frequency that usually affect only the hands, although the head and torso are occasionally involved. Some tremors are present when the patient is not otherwise moving (resting tremor) as seen in parkinsonism; whereas, others occur only when a limb is moved or while maintaining a posture (action tremor). The frequency of the tremor may be of assistance in establishing the diagnosis for those of 3-7 Hz are seen in conditions such as Parkinson's syndrome and more rapid tremors of 8-9 Hz are found in some toxic states.

A **familial tremor (essential tremor)**, inherited as an autosomal dominant trait, may appear early in childhood. The tremor is usually bilateral, affecting the hands first at a frequency of about 8 Hz. The tremor may be slowly progressive until early adult life, when it often tends to stabilize, and then with aging tends to decrease in severity. However, some older patients have progression of symptoms affecting the head, neck, mouth, and tongue. Commonly, rapid tremors do not interfere with fine motor coordination but coarse tremors may preclude any coordinated movement. Adult patients may have lessening of symptoms from daily administration of propanolol or for a short period after a drink or two of spirits. Children with familial tremor rarely need any treatment.

In rare instances, tremor is a manifestation of **hysteria,** and is observed primarily in adolescents. In these cases, the tremor is usually coarse, of variable frequency, and often has a bizarre quality. Commonly, when attempts are made to restrain the affected limb, the tremor may move to other limbs.

Iatrogenic tremor, usually of rapid frequency, may occur as an adverse effect of certain drugs including the CNS stimulants, some antihistamines, and psychotropic drugs including phenothiazines, tricyclics, or lithium

Occasionally, tremors are present in **metabolic abnormalities** such as thyrotoxicosis in which patients may have a rapid, fine tremor of fingers and hands, best observed when the arms are outstretched. Other metabolic disorders in which tremors may be present include hypocalcemia, hypomagnesemia, and uremia. Tremors may also be present in patients with Hallervorden-Spatz syndrome and juvenile Huntington's chorea.

REFERENCES

Aron MA, Freeman JM, Carter S: The natural history of Sydenham's chorea. Am J Med 38:83, 1965.

Denny-Brown D: *The Basal Ganglia and their Relation to Disorders of Movement.* Oxford University Press, 1962.

Eldredge R, Fahn S (Eds): Dystonia. *Advances in Neurology,* Vol 14. Raven Press, New York, 1976.

Fahn S, Calne D, Shoulson I (Eds): Experimental therapeutics of movement disorders *Advances in Neurology,* Vol 37. Raven Press, New York, 1983.

Golden GS: Tics and related disorders in childhood. *In* Moss AJ (Ed), *Pediatrics Update, Reviews for Physicians.* Elsevier, New York, 1981.

Marsden CD, Harrison MJG: Idiopathic torsion dystonia (dystonia musculorum deformans). Brain 97:793, 1974.

Martin JP: *The Basal Ganglia and Posture.* Pitman Medical Publishing, London, 1967.

19

Intracranial Hypertension

Lawrence H. Pitts, MD and Michael S. B. Edwards, MD

As intensive monitoring of critically ill patients has become safer and more routine, there has been a growing interest in the monitoring of a variety of brain-related phenomena in pediatric patients who have central nervous system pathology. Intracranial pressure (ICP) has become prominent in this field as a parameter that can be readily monitored, and it is now considered an important diagnostic, therapeutic, and prognostic adjunct to the neurologic examination and radiologic procedures.

There is no evidence that monitoring and treatment of intracranial hypertension have improved the outcome in any specific class of CNS disorder. However, anecdotal examples abound in which the development of intracranial hypertension closely parallels deterioration of the patient, and in which successful management of increased ICP has been attended by a good outcome.

Without question, raised ICP can cause focal or diffuse brain dysfunction in a variety of disorders such as hydrocephalus, brain abscess, intracranial tumor, head injury, and encephalopathy; in some instances, it may kill the patient. For these reasons, the monitoring of ICP and treatment of intracranial hypertension in both pediatric and adult populations with CNS pathology have received increasing attention over the past 10 years. Because of this trend, a framework for the rational treatment of intracranial hypertension in the pediatric population must be provided.

INDICATIONS FOR ICP MONITORING

HEAD INJURY

ICP monitoring is routine in most trauma centers that treat pediatric head injury. Although head injury in children is less frequently complicated by intracranial hematoma formation than is head injury in adults, diffuse brain swelling and elevated ICP are seen commonly in children and young adults after coma-producing craniocerebral trauma. CT scans can document the presence of small ventricles and the absence of cortical sulci and cerebrospinal fluid cisterns at the base of the brain and around the brain stem. This loss of CSF-containing intracranial space compensates for the increased volume of other intracranial components. A previous assumption

Table 19-1 Lovejoy Criteria — Clinical Staging in Reye's Syndrome

Stage I	Vomiting, lethargy, and sleepiness. Laboratory evidence of liver dysfunction. Type I EEG.
Stage II	Disorientation, delirium, combativeness, hyperventilation, hyperactive reflexes, appropriate response to noxious stimuli. Liver dysfunction. Type II EEG.
Stage III	Obtundent, coma, hyperventilation, decorticate rigidity, preservation of pupillary light reaction and oculovestibular reflexes. Laboratory evidence of liver dysfunction. Type II EEG.
Stage IV	Deepening coma, decerebrate rigidity, loss of oculocephalic reflexes, large fixed pupils (occasionally with hippus), disconjugate eye movements in response to caloric stimulation of the oculovestibular reflex. Minimal liver dysfunction. Type III EEG.
Stage V	Seizures, loss of stretch reflexes, respiratory arrest, and flaccidity. Type IV EEG.

Adapted and reproduced with permission from: Lovejoy FH, et al: Clinical staging in Reye's syndrome. Am J Dis Childh 36:128, 1974.

was that increased brain volume after head injury resulted from increased brain water; and, indeed, traumatic cerebral edema is a concomitant of severe head injury. In pediatric head injury, however, there is evidence that increased brain volume is due to an increased cerebrovascular volume and in some cases, to increased cerebral blood flow (CBF). Although initial cerebrovascular engorgement can be offset by a commensurate decrease in CSF volume, this compensating mechanism may be inadequate to offset large changes in cerebral blood volume or other increases in intracranial volume, such as hematoma or edema formation. Therefore, when the brain's intrinsic compensatory mechanisms have been exhausted, additional therapeutic measures may be required to restore ICP to normal.

ICP should be monitored when children are in traumatic coma. Using Glasgow Coma Score (GSC) criteria, traumatic coma is defined as the absence of eye-opening to any stimulus, of verbalizing, and of the ability to follow commands (GSC 3-8). In addition, ICP monitoring should be considered in patients who, although they have an occasional eye-opening response or speak an occasional word (GSC 9-10), fail to improve within 12-24 hours of injury. (See Table 7-1.)

Patients with consciousness impaired to this degree have an increased risk of intracranial hypertension. We believe that the relatively small risk of ICP monitoring is outweighed by the benefit gained from control of the raised ICP. While there is no uniform correlation between ICP and outcome (e.g., that normal ICP always results in a good outcome, or intracranial hypertension a bad outcome) there is, in general, a correlation between ICP changes and outcome.

The ICP monitoring should be continued until ICP values remain below 20 mm Hg for at least 24 hours without specific therapy. In general,

ICP elevations are most pronounced in the several days immediately following head injury, and tend to return to normal within 3-5 days. However, in rare instances, there is a more prolonged period of ICP elevation of up to 2-3 weeks. Although intracranial infection rates increase with prolonged ICP monitoring, there are generally few infections when monitoring is discontinued within a week of injury.

REYE'S SYNDROME

One major complication of Reye's syndrome is an encephalopathy with severe cerebral swelling; this leads to intracranial hypertension, and that, if not controlled, leads to cerebral infarction, and death. Conversely, when this intracranial hypertension can be controlled or prevented, complete recovery with intact cerebral function is now regularly achieved.

Institution of ICP monitoring in all patients in stage IV or V (Lovejoy classification) (see Table 19-1) is recommended, and patients who progress rapidly from stage II to stage III should also be considered strongly as candidates for ICP monitoring. ICP monitoring can be discontinued on the basis of the criterion for head injury: ICP of less than 20 mm Hg for 24 hours without treatment. Most patients whose ICP remains below 20 mm Hg will improve neurologically up to stage II.

HYDROCEPHALUS

The management of hydrocephalus in pediatric patients occasionally may warrant ICP monitoring. ICP can be determined intermittently by placing a needle into a shunt reservoir or, in cases of communicating hydrocephalus, by a needle in the lumbar subarachnoid space; pressures are determined manometrically or by a strain gauge transducer. When the clinician is uncertain about a child's CSF dynamics on purely clinical or radiologic grounds these pressure measurements sometimes correlate deterioration with intracranial hypertension and confirm the impression of clinically significant hydrocephalus.

In some patients, longer periods of ICP monitoring may be helpful. Children with obstructive or communicating hydrocephalus from intraventricular bleeding may require treatment by ventriculostomy. If ventricular blood or elevated protein preclude shunt placement, external drainage by ventriculostomy will normalize ICP. ICP monitoring can be used to dictate the frequency of CSF drainage, as there may be some advantage in maintaining ICP slightly above the normal range to facilitate reopening of CSF absorptive pathways.

In a few patients who have a suspected shunt malfunction, and in whom other tests of shunt function are indeterminate, ICP monitoring for 1-2 days may help to establish the presence of intermittent or sustained intracranial hypertension and the need for revision of the CSF shunt. Conversely, in these hydrocephalic patients, ICP monitoring may demonstrate that no ICP elevation is present and that placement or revision of a CSF shunt is not necessary. However, since ICP monitoring carries at least some risk of infection, particularly when a CSF shunt is in place, it should be limited to only those patients in whom more standard tests of CSF shunt function are inconclusive or unsatisfactory.

POSTOPERATIVE MONITORING

Some children undergoing intracranial surgery may benefit from early postoperative monitoring of ICP. Surgery for brain tumors, particularly malignant tumors, may be attended by postoperative cerebral swelling. Knowledge of ICP will allow judicious use of fluid restriction and ventilatory control in the first few postoperative days. Temporary postoperative hydrocephalus is not uncommon, particularly after posterior fossa and intraventricular surgery, and ICP monitoring may direct CSF withdrawal for control of ICP until normal CSF pathways are reestablished.

If the postoperative neurologic evaluation is difficult because of sedation or anticipated postoperative neurologic impairment, ICP monitoring can be used until the neurologic status improves sufficiently to allow clinical assessment of brain function.

PRESUMED INTRACRANIAL HYPERTENSION

It is generally unwise to treat patients for presumed intracranial hypertension by the various methods discussed later in this chapter, except temporarily while ICP monitoring is being established. Each of the therapies for raised ICP carries some inherent risk, and the therapy should be applied only as specifically needed. In particular, sedation or the induction of iatrogenic coma (e.g., barbiturate coma) should be employed only in conjunction with ICP monitoring. ICP monitoring is recommended for children who are comatose after any insult that may produce intracranial hypertension, such as encephalitis or near-drowning.

SIGNIFICANCE OF INTRACRANIAL HYPERTENSION

ICP is chosen as a parameter for monitoring because it is a critical component of cerebral perfusion and because it is relatively easily and safely measured.

Cerebral perfusion pressure (CPP) is defined as the mean systemic arterial pressure (SAP) minus the mean ICP (CPP = SAP − ICP). Figure 19-1 shows curves for CBF as a function of CPP in normal and hypertensive patients. In normal humans and experimental animals, CBF diminishes linearly with CPP falling below 50 mm Hg; in hypertensive humans and experimental animals, CBF falls linearly with CPP below about 75 mm Hg. The relatively horizontal portion of the CBF curve, where CBF remains constant despite increasing blood pressure, is due to autoregulation: changes in cerebral arteriolar diameter cause a higher or lower cerebrovascular resistance, such that flow remains constant with changing pressures. Thus, by knowing SAP and ICP, we have considerable information regarding mean CBF.

When there is a brain injury and abnormal ICP, CBF may not follow the curves shown in Figure 19-1. If cerebrovascular resistance cannot change in response to changing CPP, then autoregulation is lost and CBF

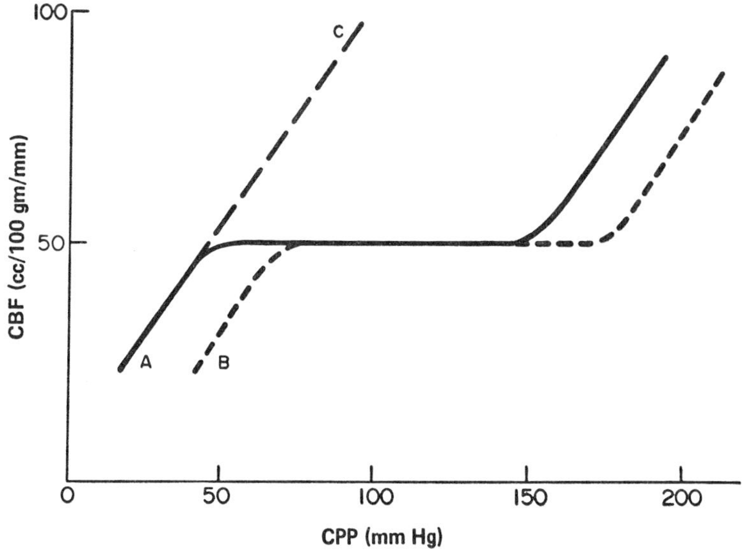

Fig. 19-1 Cerebral blood flow (CBF) as a function of cerebral perfusion pressure (CPP = mean arterial pressure minus intracranial pressure). Curve A depicts CBF for normotensive humans, and curve B for hypertensive humans. Curve C shows a linear rise in CBF with rising CPP, seen with loss of autoregulation.

passively drifts up or down with CPP. This loss of autoregulation can be global (affecting all regions of the brain) or focal (affecting areas of injury).

The question of focality is important to ICP considerations. Whereas some pathologic processes involve the entire brain diffusely, in which case ICP elevations are due to widespread increased cerebral tissue or fluid volume, more commonly ICP elevations arise from focal brain abnormalities. Since brain is viscoelastic and does not act as an ideal fluid, 'whole-head' ICP often will be lower than focal ICP. Lesions such as an intracerebral hematoma or a 'trapped ventricle' may cause quite high local ICPs, while mean ICPs measured at some point remote from the focal pathology are much lower.

This concept of focality is very important when considering therapy of intracranial hypertension. In particular, as is suggested in Figure 19-1, ICP must be lowered well below the level of 40-50 mm Hg that, with normal blood pressures, should give satisfactory CBF. ICP in the region of focal neurologic damage and increased mass could be considerably higher than a 'whole-head' ICP of 50 mm Hg. Focality must also be considered in relation to blood gas requirements for the injured brain. While an arterial pO_2 of 60 mm Hg will give greater than 95% oxygen saturation, focal cerebral injury with marked local increases in ICP, and local relative hypoperfusion can result in an unusually high oxygen extraction from cerebral blood; a higher PaO_2 will provide some, if only slight, increase in oxygen-carrying capacity of blood. This small additional amount of available oxygen may make the difference in viability or nonviability of marginally perfused injured brain tissue. For these reasons it is recommended to treat patients with raised ICP to achieve a considerable safety margin of CPP above 55 mm Hg and PaO_2 above 80 mm Hg.

While CBF directly measures brain tissue perfusion, CBF technically is difficult to determine. In addition, current techniques for CBF determination often will not reflect areas of focal ischemia — the most dangerous perfusion abnormality seen in CNS disorders. Cerebral metabolic studies are also technically difficult to perform. Positron emission scanning can examine focal cerebral metabolism, but it is a research tool at this time, not readily applicable in critically ill patients. Cerebral metabolic rate of oxygen can be determined by the Fick principle if arterial and jugular venous blood samples are available; however, repeated use of this method is not feasible, nor is the method sufficiently sensitive to determine ongoing brain damage.

Thus, ICP monitoring is important, achievable, and of major potential benefit to the patient with significant intracranial pathology.

TREATMENT OF INTRACRANIAL HYPERTENSION

The treatment of raised ICP requires monitoring of a valid ICP to dictate the specific appropriate therapy, as well as its quantity and duration. We treat ICP presumptively only in the emergency room setting, before ICP monitoring can be established. As soon as is practicable, either in the operating room or at the bedside, and then the monitoring data are used as the basis for subsequent therapy.

Treatment of ICP without the knowledge of specific ICP levels can lead to overtreatment or undertreatment and to potentially dangerous errors. There is a wealth of clinical material indicating that ICP changes cannot be predicted accurately on the basis of changes in the neurologic examination. In comatose patients, ICP variations are common — sometimes with little change in the neurologic examination or vital signs. Although CT scans can suggest the presence or absence of intracranial hypertension, the correlation between a given CT scan and level of ICP often is poor. One must, therefore, rely heavily on ICP monitoring and the knowledge of specific ICP values.

EMERGENCY TREATMENT
OF PRESUMED INTRACRANIAL HYPERTENSION

Metabolic abnormalities or intracranial infection that cause altered levels of consciousness are discussed in Chapters 3 and 6, respectively. Patients who are comatose after head injury are presumed to have raised ICP, which should be treated immediately. These children are intubated by the most experienced physician available, preferably an anesthesiologist, and are ventilated either by AMBU-bag or by a volume ventilator. Ventilation parameters are chosen to produce moderate hyperventilation with result-ant arterial pCO_2 of between 25 and 30 mm Hg. Inspired oxygen levels should be adjusted to achieve PaO_2 greater than 80 mm Hg. Mannitol (1.5 gm/kg) is routinely given as a rapid IV bolus. Normal blood pressures must be established promptly, and initial fluid resuscitation is carried out with-out regard to possible intracranial hypertension. After a satisfactory blood pressure level is established, maintenance crystalloid fluids are adminis-tered at a rate calculated to be 60-70% of normal maintenance fluid re-quirements.

If the patient has a history or external evidence of head injury, and if brain stem compression is evident from the physical examination, the patient should immediately be taken to the operating room for explora-tory trephination. If brain stem compression is not evident, the comatose patient is taken immediately for CT scanning. Subsequent management is based on the findings of these early diagnostic tests. ICP monitoring by intraventricular or subdural catheter or by subarachnoid bolt is established as early as is feasible within the overall resuscitation management require-ments of the individual patient. Subsequent ICP control is outlined in the following sections.

OPERATIVE MANAGEMENT OF INTRACRANIAL HYPERTENSION

When intracranial studies disclose mass lesions, operative removal is an essential factor in controlling raised ICP. Such masses can range from intra-cerebral hematomas or abscesses to subdural collections of blood, pus, or effusion fluid. In infants, chronic subdural effusions sometimes can be removed percutaneously via an open anterior fontanelle. Brain abscesses and primary and metastatic tumors can grow very large in children, and can cause a markedly increased ICP. Most pediatric brain tumors occur in the posterior fossa, and such masses, even when quite small, can raise ICP if they impede CSF drainage and cause obstructive hydrocephalus. Both obstructive and communicating hydrocephalus can cause marked elevation in ICP, and may require an operation to divert the CSF.

In rare circumstances, when all other measures fail to control intra-cranial hypertension, cranial decompression with removal of portions of the bony calvarium and subjacent dura has been employed. Although some good results have been reported with this management, it is consid-ered a last resort, and can be avoided almost universally by the judicious application of the other therapies described in the following sections.

NONOPERATIVE MANAGEMENT OF RAISED ICP

Medical control of intracranial hypertension is best considered as a bal-anced application of a number of therapies: sedation; head elevation; in-tubation and ventilation control; hyperosmolar therapy; diuretics; CSF drainage; paralysis; temperature control; and barbiturate coma (unproven).

The simplest, safest, and most reversible methods are employed first. If these are not successful, then therapies with associated greater risks are used to maintain optimal ICP and cerebral perfusion.

Sedation is a cornerstone of ICP control. Struggling or agitation causes increases in intrathoracic pressure and increased venous pressure so that cerebral venous drainage is impaired. For sedation, IV morphine sulfate (0.05-0.1 mg/kg) should be given hourly. Narcotics have the advantage of being readily reversible by narcotic antagonists should there be concern about a deteriorating level of consciousness from the neurologic disorder, as opposed to depression by the narcotic itself. In some instances, when it is started as prophylaxis against seizures, IV phenobarbital (1-3 mg/kg, initial dose; 1-1.5 mg/kg twice daily, maintenance dose) will effectively sedate a patient.

The risk of sedative use is directly related to respiratory depression, and respiratory depression can be extremely dangerous if it is not recognized and treated. In addition, sedation depresses consciousness, so that it may be difficult to distinguish between changes in level of consciousness related to medication only and changes related to neurologic deterioration from the underlying cerebral disorder. ICP monitoring gives added assurance of a stable intracranial situation, and some depressed consciousness can be accepted.

Head elevation is generally employed when intracranial hypertension is or may be present, as long as elevation does not lower SAP substantially. Elevation of 20-30 degrees above the horizontal will facilitate cerebral venous drainage. Although elevation also diminishes the arterial pressure by placing the head above the heart, the autoregulation mechanism (by which the cerebral vascular resistance is lowered and CBF is maintained, despite small decrements of systemic blood pressure) should compensate for this effect, at least in areas where autoregulation is preserved.

Intubation and ventilatory control are mainstays of control of intracranial hypertension. For adequate tissue oxygenation in regions where cerebral perfusion may be diminished, oxygen levels in the blood should be maintained in the 80-100 mm Hg range. Of equal importance is the maintenance of normal arterial CO_2 pressures. Even small increases in pCO_2 can cause cerebral vasodilation with a resultant increase in cerebral blood volume and raised ICP. Conversely, modest hyperventilation will cause vasoconstriction and lower ICP in most individuals. Cerebral vasoconstriction to hypocarbia is a robust response and generally persists despite considerable brain damage. In a patient with modest ICP elevation, arterial pCO_2 should be controlled within the range of 25-30 mm Hg. If ICP becomes elevated acutely, the patient should be further hyperventilated as necessary. Because the choroid plexus regulatory mechanism restores a normal CSF pH over 8-12 hours following an increase in ventilation, prolonged hyperventilation at a given level eventually ceases to cause cerebral vasoconstriction. Therefore, hyperventilation is best used as an adjunct to other methods of ICP control.

Typically, the respiratory minute volume should be increased to lower ICP acutely while other therapies are begun to achieve satisfactory ICP levels. As ICP falls, minute volumes are reduced so that the CO_2 rises toward 30 mm Hg; thus, hyperventilation can be reapplied, should ICP rise acutely again. In most instances, since the patient can develop intracranial hypertension while being weaned from a ventilator, ICP monitors are left in place until after the patient is extubated. The ICP monitor can reassure the physician that a return to a normal ventilatory status is not adversely affecting ICP and cerebral perfusion.

Hyperosmolar therapy is also a modality that is frequently employed for controlling intracranial hypertension. Mannitol is given as a single dose IV bolus (0.25-1 gm/kg; 0.5 gm/kg is usually effective). Typically, mannitol will exert its effect over a period of 10-20 minutes; after that time, hyperventilation often can be diminished as ICP control becomes satisfactory. Serum sodium and osmolality should be monitored routinely in patients undergoing ICP monitoring, particularly when mannitol or other diuretics are used. Administration of mannitol is continued for control of ICP up to serum osmolalities of 330 mOsm/liter. Above this level, there is intrinsic dysfunction due to hyperosmolality; therefore, higher levels should be avoided.

One problem that arises when large amounts of mannitol are used is that of dehydration and arterial hypotension. In this circumstance, administration of mannitol is supplemented with plasmanate or serum albumin, which are hyperosmolar but not diuretic. These colloid solutions are effective only for 6-8 hours and, therefore, must be used intermittently. Although this is an expensive form of therapy, it allows maintenance of a high serum osmolality without the potential dangers of shock and diminished CPP.

Diuretics also are used to dehydrate the patient so that elevated serum osmolality is maintained and the available free water that contributes to brain edema is diminished. 'Loop' diuretics such as furosemide (Lasix) and ethacrinic acid are preferred since these affect the distal renal tubule and increase free water loss more than salt loss. In addition, Lasix appears to diminish CSF production, and experimental evidence suggests that ethacrinic acid may have a direct effect on brain cells to diminish brain edema.

CSF drainage can be employed if an intraventricular catheter is used to monitor ICP. Drainage is particularly beneficial in cases in which some form of increased CSF is contributing to the intracranial hypertension. Hydrocephalus often accompanies intraventricular hemorrhage or posterior fossa tumors, which can occlude the aqueduct or other CSF pathways. If the ventricles are quite small, however, CSF drainage can collapse a ventricle entirely and allow brain tissue to occlude the monitoring catheter. Thus, CSF drainage is recommended only when hydrocephalus is part of the clinical picture, or under unusual circumstances, such as when the removal of even a very small amount of CSF will reduce intracranial hypertension that is refractory to other therapies.

Paralysis with long-acting muscle relaxants (pancuronium 0.05 mg/kg, IV, as needed) can dramatically lower ICP, particularly in patients who remain agitated despite attempts at sedation. Muscle relaxation can effectively lower ICP at times, even in patients in whom no muscle movement is apparent — presumably by preventing thoracic muscular contraction, increased intrathoracic pressure, and diminished cerebral venous return. Paralysis adds the significant risk of the patient's being unable to breathe spontaneously, should the ventilator malfunction or become disconnected. However, alarm systems currently are available in most intensive care units and should provide a sufficient margin of safety.

Temperature control should be employed routinely in managing the patient with raised ICP. In febrile patients, normothermia can be achieved, under most circumstances, with cooling blankets and aspirin. In some patients, hypothermia to 33-34C has helped to control intracranial hypertension. Cooling often will cause a patient to shiver, which can increase ICP; shivering, however, can be controlled with paralyzing agents. Cooling blankets are used to produce any desired level of hypothermia, but care should be taken to protect the skin from local damage due to pressure and low temperatures.

Barbiturate coma is an experimental method for control of intracranial hypertension, and is currently being evaluated in several prospective trials. Preliminary data suggest that it might be useful in cases of diffuse head injury and possibly in Reye's syndrome; however, no conclusive data have yet been presented.

Barbiturates have been employed in a number of cases, but anecdotal reports leave the efficacy of this treatment uncertain and the optimum dosage quite undefined. Doses of pentobarbital (Nembutal) that have been used are 5-7 mg/kg given as an IV loading dose, followed by 1-3 mg/kg hourly. Dosages are modified to achieve electroencephalographic silence for 30-60 seconds (so-called burst suppression) or continued electrocerebral silence. As long as ICP control is achieved, serum levels of up to 15 mg% pentobarbital have been recommended.

Barbiturate use entails a number of risks, most notably hypotension. This risk can be countered by slow drug administration and by the appropriate use of a Swan-Ganz catheter for pulmonary artery and wedge pressure monitoring to direct fluid administration. A number of infections in these critically ill patients in barbiturate coma have been reported, although they may or may not have been related to the barbiturate therapy. Extreme caution must be employed if barbiturates are used in the management of intracranial hypertension. Optimally, since barbiturates are still of unproven value in this area, they should be used only in the setting of a well-defined and approved study.

REFERENCES

Bruce DA, et al: Diffuse cerebral swelling following head injuries in children: the syndrome of 'malignant brain edema.' J Neurosurg 54:170-178, 1981.

Bruce DA, et al: The effectiveness of iatrogenic barbiturate coma in controlling increased ICP in 61 children. *In* Shulman K, et al (Eds): *Intracranial Pressure IV.* Springer-Verlag, New York, 1980, pp. 630-632.

Silverman D, et al: Irreversible coma associated with electrocerebral silence. Neurology. 20:525, 1970.

Venes J: Intracranial pressure monitoring in perspective. Child's Brain. 7:236-251, 1960.

Venes JL, Shaywitz BA, SpencerDD: Management of severe cerebral edema in the metabolic encephalopathy of Reye-Johnson syndrome. J Neurosurg 48:903-915, 1978.

20

Coma

Roger P. Simon, MD

Coma is not a diagnosis but rather the product of a wide spectrum of life-threatening conditions that damage the central nervous system or depress its function. Appropriate therapy is dependent upon an accurate analysis of the underlying etiology and pathophysiology of the unconscious state.

Coma refers to a sleep-like state from which the patient cannot be aroused; the eyes do not open, there is no speech, and extremities move neither to command, nor to appropriately ward off noxious stimuli. Non-purposeful reflex movements may be retained, however.

Stupor resembles coma except that the stuporous patient is arousable with vigorous stimulation; when that stimulation is removed, the stuporous state quickly supervenes.

EMERGENCY EVALUATION

At the time of initial evaluation, it is critical to take certain emergency steps to prevent further, possibly permanent, brain damage (see Table 20-1). Providing sufficient oxygen and ventilation are the initial critical issues. Deeply comatose patients should be intubated immediately to assure adequate ventilatory support.

The possibility of **reversible hypoglycemic encephalopathy** should also be addressed immediately by obtaining blood for serum glucose determination and then administering 1 mg/kg of concentrated glucose solution (50% dextrose) without waiting for the laboratory report of serum glucose concentration. At the stage of flaccid coma, a delay of greater than 15 minutes in treating the hypoglycemia will result in permanent CNS damage.

Repetitive seizures can produce brain damage. **Paralysis and ventilation do not protect against this CNS injury.** Status epilepticus may manifest itself only by recurrent or continual focal motor activity in a single limb, digit, or side of the face. These subtle signs of status epilepticus have the same implications for emergency treatment as more florid manifestations of generalized seizures. Parenteral diazepam is usually administered, followed by a longer-acting anticonvulsant drug such as phenytoin. A small but clear risk of precipitating cardiorespiratory arrest following IV administration of diazepam must be realized, especially if other drugs have been previously given (see Chapter 10).

Table 20-1 Emergency Management of the Comatose Patient

Immediately	Next	Later
Assure adequacy of oxygenation and ventilation.	Obtain the history	Determine serum cium, liver and renal function tests, and Cl
	Determine serum electrolytes and arterial blood gases. Correct severe acid-base and/or electrolyte abnormalities.	
Draw blood for serum glucose determination and then administer 1 mg/kg D50W.	Consider lumbar puncture for diagnosis of meningitis or subarachnoid hemorrhage.	Blood and urine evalution for toxicological studies.
Control seizures.	Obtain an ECG.	Chest x-ray.
Rapid physical examination to determine major abnormalities, particularly signs of trauma.	Control body temperature.	
	Neurologic examination and possible treatment of increased ICP.	EEG for diagnosis

Arterial blood gas acid-base abnormalities are frequent in coma (see Table 20-2). Respiratory acidosis is a warning of impending respiratory failure, and acidosis or alkalosis of any cause may result in electrolyte shifts and cardiovascular abnormalities.

Signs of **meningeal irritation** such as nuchal rigidity or Brudzinski's sign may be seen in infectious meningitis, subarachnoid hemorrhage, or herniation of cerebellar tonsils. However, signs of meningeal irritation may not be present in children under two years of age and particularly in early infancy.

Funduscopic examination may reveal evidence of **increased intracranial pressure;** however, papilledema may not be apparent for hours following the onset of that increased pressure. If intracranial hypertension is present, immediate therapy with hyperventilation will probably be effective in reducing pCO_2 to 25-30 mm Hg. Other therapeutic measures are listed in Table 20-3 (see also Chapter 19).

Body temperature must also be controlled. While hypothermia poses no risk to the nervous system except for the risk of ventricular arrhythmia during rewarming, hyperthermia ($\sim$42C) of any cause may result in irreversible damage to the nervous system.

ANATOMY OF CONSCIOUSNESS

Consciousness requires the function of both the cerebral hemispheres and the brain stem reticular activating system (RAS). Unconsciousness requires that one or both of these structures (RAS or both cerebral hemispheres) are compromised. The reticular formation, responsible for consciousness, occupies the paramedial brain stem from the level of the midpons to rostral midbrain. Its function is the production of arousal, or simply, wakefulness, apparent clinically by spontaneous or stimulus-induced eye opening. The cerebral hemispheres, on the other hand, produce higher functions of awareness which are manifested clinically by goal directed or purposeful motor behavior, or by the use of language.

Awareness, the function of the cerebral hemispheres, is not possible without stimulation from the reticular formation to produce arousal and wakefulness. Therefore, coma can be produced by a brain stem lesion, even in the absence of hemispheric pathology. On the other hand, bilateral hemispheric impairment may occur following cardiac arrest, for example, with sparing of the brain stem. After a few days such patients will manifest arousal with eye opening, and ultimately sleep-wake cycles. but they may never regain intellectual functions of awareness. These patients are in a functionally decorticate state, distinct from coma. This state of wakefulness without awareness may persist indefinitely with supportive care and has been termed a **persistent vegetative state.**

Table 20-2   Metabolic Coma:
Differential Diagnosis by Acid-Base Abnormalities

Respiratory alkalosis	Metabolic acidosis
Hepatic encephalopathy	Hyperosmolar coma
Psychogenic coma	Diabetic ketoacidosis
Salicylate intoxication	Uremic encephalopathy
Sepsis	Lactic acidosis
Hypoxia	Paraldehyde ingestion
(pulmonary edema)	Methyl alcohol ingestion
	Ethylene glycol ingestion
	Isoniazid ingestion
	Sepsis (terminally)
Respiratory acidosis	**Metabolic alkalosis**
Respiratory depressant drugs (e.g., bromides, ethanol, barbiturates, or other sedative-hypnotic drugs)	Coma unusual
Acute or chronic pulmonary failure	

Reproduced with permission from: Plum F, Posner J: *Diagnosis of Stupor and Coma,* 3rd ed. Davis, Philadelphia, 1980.

Table 20-3 Therapy for Cerebral Edema

Drug	Dose	Route	Indications/comments
Glucocorticoids			
Dexamethasone (Decadron)	1 mg/kg, then 0.25 mg qid	IV or PO	Dexamethasone preferred for at least miner-
Prednisone	6 mg/kg, then 2.5 mg qid	PO	alocorticoid effect; effective for 6-12 hours;
Methylprednisolone	6 mg/kg, then 2.5 mg qid	IV or PO	concomitant antacid treatment probably
Hydrocortisone	30 mg/kg, then 10 mg qid	IV or PO	indicated.
Dehydrating agents			
Mannitol	0.25-1 gm/kg/dose	20% IV solution	Effective immediately; major dehydrating effect is short-lived, and more than two IV doses rarely of value. Causes osmotic diuresis
Urea	1-5 gm/kg	IV	and electrolyte imbalance. Not effective with
Glycerol	1.5-4 gm/kg/day	PO	serum osmols above 320. Glycerol effective PO; nausea and vomiting common.
Avoid salt free intravenous fluids			
Hyperventilation	to pCO$_2$ 25-30		ICP reduction of 10-80% within 2-30 minutes; return to baseline in 5 minutes following discontinuation.
Hypothermia	32-36 C		ICP reduction by 50% over 4-12 hours.

APPROACH TO THE DIAGNOSIS

There are only three pathophysiologic mechanisms which may produce coma: mass lesion, metabolic encephalopathy, or seizures (ongoing seizure activity or the postictal state). The goal in evaluating the comatose patient is to select the correct etiologic category and proceed with appropriate diagnostic and therapeutic measures.

Mass lesion To fulfill the anatomic criteria for unconsciousness, a supratentorial (hemispheric) mass lesion producing coma must expand and either compress the contralateral hemisphere to cause bilateral hemispheric dysfunction or, more commonly, produce pressure on the rostral brain stem to affect the normal function of the reticular formation.

A **supratentorial mass lesion** producing coma will initially produce unilateral hemispheric signs or symptoms; e.g., hemiparesis, hemisensory deficit, or aphasia, if the dominant hemisphere is involved. Coma supervenes as the brain becomes progressively compromised. Deterioration occurs in a characteristic rostral-caudal manner, as manifested by hemispheric dysfunction followed by impaired function of the thalamus, the midbrain, pons, and then the medulla. This predictable progression of signs and symptoms produced by transtentorial herniation of the brain across the cerebellar tentorium is the hallmark of an expanding supratentorial mass (see Figure 20-1).

A **subtentorial (brain stem) lesion,** on the other hand, will alter consciousness early, occasionally suddenly, by directly involving the reticular activating system. The orderly rostral to caudal progression of signs, typical of supratentorial masses, will not be seen. Since the ocular motor pathways traverse the paramedial reticular formation responsible for consciousness, evaluation of lateral eye movements is most useful in assessing brain stem function. The finding of preserved eye movements essentially excludes the diagnosis of a brain stem lesion as the cause for coma.

Metabolic encephalopathy Metabolic abnormalities diffusely affect the nervous system. The history is usually one of progressive somnolence, often preceded by intoxication or delirium. Neurologic findings are usually symmetrical. If motor signs are asymmetrical, as occasionally occur in hypoglycemia and hepatic encephalopathy, the asymmetry is never prominent and may alternate from side to side. The pupillary light reflex is preserved, with only rare exceptions, including glutethimide intoxication, anoxia, profound hypothermia, atropine intoxication, or with barbiturate levels beyond those necessary to produce apnea. Children who have ingested drugs often have markedly miotic pupils; this is found in about 88% of children given narcotics, 72% with phenothiazines, 35% with alcohol, and 31% with barbiturates. In contrast, miotic pupils are found in only 3% of children in coma secondary to trauma.

The metabolic encephalopathies of purulent meningitis or subarachnoid hemorrhage are associated with prominent meningeal signs, except in infants, but these signs are lost in deep coma.

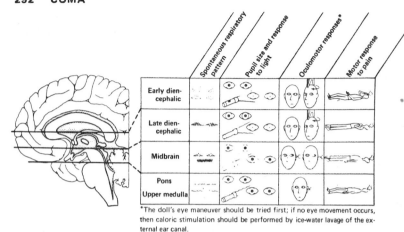

*The doll's eye maneuver should be tried first; if no eye movement occurs,
then caloric stimulation should be performed by ice-water lavage of the external ear canal.

Fig. 20-1　Symptoms at various levels of anatomic involvement of the brain.
(Adapted and reproduced with permission from Plum F, Posner JB:
The Diagnosis of Stupor and Coma, 3rd ed. Davis, 1980.)

Seizures as a cause of coma are usually readily apparent since recovery
of consciousness is rapid, following cessation of the convulsive activity.
There is an abrupt onset of unconsciousness followed by postictal confusion. Prolonged postictal coma may occur following status epilepticus and
in some patients whose seizures are associated with abnormal state of the
central nervous system, such as metabolic encephalopathies including
hyponatremia, hypoglycemia, or acute or chronic structural abnormalities
such as congenital malformations, head trauma, or encephalitis. In the absence of focal brain disease, the neurologic examination following a seizure
is usually symmetrical; bilateral extensor plantar responses may be present.

PHYSICAL EXAMINATION

The most helpful features of the **general physical examination** include
signs of trauma and/or elevation of blood pressure. The latter may be an
indication of acute intracerebral hemorrhage or a posterior fossa mass
lesion. In the rare condition of hypertensive encephalopathy, the blood
pressure is usually greater than 250/150, but in children this subacute symmetrical encephalopathy may occur with blood pressures as low as 160/
100 mm Hg.

The **neurologic examination** is the keystone of diagnosis in the
comatose patient. Funduscopic evaluation may reveal papilledema or retinal hemorrhages compatible with acute hypertension or increased intracranial pressure. Subhyaloid (preretinal) hemorrhages in adult patients
strongly suggest subarachnoid hemorrhage and, in the child patient, also suggest subdural hematoma and trauma, particularly child abuse. Respiratory
rate and pattern, pupillary size and reactivity, ocular motility, and the
motor response to pain must be evaluated in detail.

Respiration Normal respiration implies a high level of neurologic function with an intact brain stem to the thalamic level. Bilateral cortical damage may result in periodic respiration (Cheyne-Stokes) in which hyperventilation rhythmically alternates with apnea. Rapid regular breathing suggests systemic acid-base abnormalities (respiratory alkalosis or metabolic acidosis), pulmonary edema, or a midbrain lesion causing central neurogenic hyperventilation. Ataxic, or irregular respiration, implies pontomedullary damage. Marked hypoventilation progressing to apnea in comatose patients is commonly due to sedative drug overdose.

Pupils Normal pupils are usually 3-4 mm in diameter but may be larger in young children. They are equal bilaterally and constrict briskly and symmetrically in response to light stimulus. Slightly smaller, reactive pupils are present in metabolic coma, or in the early stages of rostral-caudal herniation due to thalamic and hypothalamic compression, probably because of interruption of descending sympathetic pathways. Midposition or slightly dilated pupils, 5-7 mm, which are nonreactive to light result from damage at midbrain level or below. Small pupils, 1-1.5 mm in diameter, may indicate focal damage at the pontine or cerebellar level; such lesions in childhood are rare. Other common causes of miosis, pupils less than 2 mm, in children include poisoning by opiates, phenothiazines, or organophosphates.

Asymmetric pupillary size is a normal finding in about 20% of the population. Differentiation from early oculomotor nerve dysfunction is most important, especially after head injury. In physiological anisocoria, both pupils respond to light with the same degree of briskness; further, ocular motility reveals no evidence of third nerve abnormality. Asymmetry of pupillary size accompanied by sluggish reactivity of the larger pupil implies a structural lesion of the midbrain or oculomotor nerve.

Extraocular motility In awake patients, eye movements are controlled by volitional direction from the cerebral hemispheres. Ocular motility in comatose patients with an intact brain stem can be tested on a reflex level. Full reflex eye movements in a comatose patient attest to the integrity of the brain stem and essentially exclude a posterior fossa lesion as cause for the coma.

The oculocephalic reflex, or doll's head-eye phenomenon, is performed by holding the patient's eyes open and rocking the head from side to side multiple times. If full gaze to the left and right are induced, the brain stem is intact. If the eyes remain 'locked' in primary position, or straight ahead, there is compromise of brain stem function (see p. 292).

The oculovestibular reflex (caloric stimulation) is performed only after first assuring the tympanic membrane is intact, and then positioning the head in midline and raised 30 degrees from the horizontal. The lateral semicircular canals, now in vertical plane, will respond maximally to stimulation. About 50 cc of ice water are injected into the external auditory canal, against the tympanic membrane. If the brain stem is intact there is tonic deviation of the eyes to the side of ice water irrigation. As with the doll's head-eye maneuver, an asymmetry or absence of eye deviation implies a structural or metabolic brain stem lesion.

Motor response   Evaluation of the highest level of motor response in a comatose patient is one of the most helpful aspects of the examination. Although motor movements in comatose patients are occasionally spontaneous or secondary to manipulation such as endotracheal suctioning, their elicitation usually requires introduction of a painful stimulus to induce the motor movement. *Failure to include a painful stimulus in evaluation of a comatose patient is perhaps the most common and most costly mistake in the diagnostic evaluation.* Strong pressure applied to the supraorbital ridge by the examiner's thumb or to the patient's nail beds are effective painful stimuli. The stimulus should be applied alternately to each side of the body to avoid misinterpreting a negative response that may actually be secondary to a hemisensory defect. Asymmetry of the elicited motor responses is evidence of hemiparesis.

The quality of motor response also requires attention. The highest level of response is localization of an offending stimulus by the patient; that is, the patient attempts to reach toward the site of induced pain. Such purposeful movement suggests a high level of retained brain function.

The **decorticate response** to pain (flexion of upper extremities at the elbow and extension with internal rotation of lower extremities) suggests a lesion compressing brain at the thalamic level. The **decerebrate response** to pain (extension and internal rotation of both upper and lower extremities) most often occurs with midbrain lesions. In cases of pontomedullary lesions, there is usually no response to pain, though flexion of the knees is sometimes seen (see Figure 20-1).

INTERPRETATION OF NEUROLOGIC FINDINGS

The central issue in evaluating the comatose child is to determine whether coma is the result of an intracranial mass lesion for which neurosurgical intervention may be critical, or a metabolic encephalopathy or postictal state for which medical management is the treatment of choice.

INTRACRANIAL MASS LESION

This critical differentiation between an expanding intracranial mass lesion and a metabolic encephalopathy can be made with a high degree of certainty based upon features of the neurologic examination. *Four neurologic parameters are of particular importance: respiratory pattern, pupillary size and reactivity, reflex eye movements, and motor responses to pain.*

The history and early neurologic findings of **supratentorial mass lesions** (see Table 20-4) are suggestive of hemispheric dysfunction. Hemiparesis is typical and language abnormalities may be present with lesions affecting the left hemisphere. As the mass expands, there is increasing somnolence from compression of the contralateral hemisphere or rostral thalamus. Stupor progresses to coma, although the examination may continue to show prominent asymmetry of motor responses or reflexes, re-

Table 20-4   Supratentorial Mass Lesions

Intracerebral hemorrhage	Epidural abscess
Subdural hematoma	Massive cerebral infarction with edema
Epidural hematoma	(occurring 24-48 hours after onset)
Brain abscess	Brain tumor (rarely causes rapidly progressive coma)

flecting the hemispheric origin of the lesion. Rostral-caudal compromise of the brain continues.

Recognition of this segmental compromise of brain function points to a hemispheric mass lesion with transtentorial herniation as the appropriate diagnosis, and dictates the urgency of neurosurgical intervention. Once the pontine level of function is reached, a fatal outcome is virtually inevitable, but even at midbrain stage with nonreactive pupils, the chance of a meaningful survival is significantly lessened.

Should the supratentorial lesion be so placed that it can cause herniation of the medial portion of the temporal lobe, the uncus, and produce direct pressure on the midbrain, signs of midbrain compromise with pupillary dilation can occur before coma. In this **uncal syndrome,** the patient is lethargic but arousable; the ipsilateral pupil is large and sluggishly reactive to light. It is critical to recognize this pupillary evidence of midbrain compromise for, with little additional warning, consciousness may be lost rapidly and progression to full midbrain stage with its associated poor prognosis may occur.

Subtentorial mass lesions, including those of the brain stem and/or cerebellum, in adults are most often the result of basilar artery embolus or thrombosis, or from hemorrhage into the brain stem or cerebellum. These lesions are rare in childhood; however, tumors affecting these structures are more common.

Midbrain lesions will impair pupillary function, producing midposition pupils that are nonreactive to light stimulus. Tiny, or 'pinpoint,' pupils may be present in patients in early stages of coma secondary to compromise at the pontine level (pontine or cerebellar hemorrhage). Conjugate deviation of the eyes secondary to subtentorial lesions results in direction of gaze away from the side of the lesion and toward the side of hemiparesis. Disconjugate eye movements, especially an internuclear ophthalmoplegia, strongly suggests a subtentorial lesion. Motor responses to pain do not differentiate subtentorial from supratentorial lesions since decerebrate, decorticate, or flaccid responses to noxious stimuli may occur with lesions at either site.

Respiratory patterns observed in subtentorial lesions are invariably abnormal but of little usefulness in localizing the lesion. Later in the course of transtentorial herniation from a supratentorial lesion, differentiation from a subtentorial lesion is not possible, for signs of pontomedullary dysfunction can be produced by either.

METABOLIC COMA

The history of patients with metabolic coma is different from those with intracranial mass lesions, for there is no suggestion of focal hemispheric dysfunction. Loss of consciousness is rarely sudden, as compared with subarachnoid hemorrhage, seizure, or brain stem stroke. There is usually a history of increasing intoxication, somnolence, delirium, or agitation, progressing gradually to stupor and finally coma. In contrast to mass lesions, headache is not an initial symptom of metabolic coma, except in the case of carbon monoxide poisoning.

Symmetrical neurologic findings are characteristically found, though fluctuating hemiparesis is occasionally seen in hypoglycemic or hepatic encephalopathy. Decorticate or decerebrate posturing is uncommon in metabolic coma but may occasionally occur in hepatic, uremic, anoxic, hypoglycemic or early sedative drug-induced coma; it is the rule in Reye's syndrome. Myoclonus is also suggestive of metabolic coma.

Neurologic findings of particular importance in metabolic encephalopathy include the retention of reactive pupils and symmetrical motor examination. Except for rare exceptions, retained pupillary reactivity to light stimulus is the hallmark of metabolic coma. These exceptions include those patients comatose from glutethimide (Doriden) overdose, massive barbiturate overdose with apnea requiring ventilatory support, acute anoxia-ischemia, hypothermia to the point of coma, and atropine poisoning. The respiratory pattern in metabolic coma may provide further help in establishing a specific diagnosis. A categorization based upon arterial blood gas abnormalities is presented in Table 20-2.

Probably the most common cause of metabolic coma is **sedative drug overdose**. Barbiturates are the prototypical drug group but identical syndromes may be produced by any sedative hypnotic including meprobamate, chlordiazepoxide, diazepam, glutethimide, ethchlorvynol, methaqualone. One feature of sedative drug-induced coma that distinguishes it from metabolic encephalopathy of endogenous organ failure is reduced to absent oculocephalic responses. Further, cold caloric stimulation may show reduced to absent eye movements or a skew deviation, commonly with the eye ipsilateral to the otic canal being irrigated, showing a forced downward deviation. These ocular findings are present even in early stages of coma, when painful stimuli induce writhing or thrashing about. Spontaneous eye movements are retained in metabolic coma of endogenous organ failure.

The EEG of patients who are comatose from sedative drugs may be isoelectric, and in the case of long-acting barbiturates may remain isoelectric for over 24 hours.

Full recovery from drug-induced coma occurs with supportive care alone. Treatment should consist of ventilatory support and hydration. **Analeptic drugs should never be used.** Although barbiturates are dialyzable the morbidity and mortality of coma secondary to short-acting barbiturates are clearly lower in conservatively managed patients.

Alcohol produces a syndrome similar to the sedative drugs but impairment of lateral eye movement is uncommon. Peripheral vasodilation is prominent, producing tachycardia, hypotension, and hypothermia. Stupor is found with blood alcohol levels ranging from 250-300 mg/dl, and coma occurs with levels of 300-400 mg/dl.

Narcotic overdose is characterized by hypoventilation and pinpoint pupillary constriction that is mimicked in children only following administration of miotic eye drops or organophosphate poisoning. Diagnosis is confirmed by rapid pupillary dilation and awakening after intravenous administration of the narcotic antagonist, naloxone hydrochloride (Narcan), 0.01 mg/kg to be repeated 1-3 times in 2-3 minute intervals. The duration of action of Narcan is only 2-3 hours and the repeat doses are frequently necessary, especially following intoxication with long-acting narcotics such as methadone hydrochloride.

Disorders of electrolytes and serum osmolarity are common causes of coma in childhood. Although measured osmoles can be obtained in many laboratories by freezing point depression technique, a rapid and accurate quantitation of effective serum osmoles can be obtained by the following equation:

$$mOsm/kg = 2(Na + K) + (glucose/18) + (BUN/2.8)$$

Consciousness is altered if serum osmolality is less than 260 mOsm/kg or greater than 330-350 mOsm/kg. Coma with focal seizures is common in the hyperosmolar state. Hyponatremia may often cause neurologic dysfunction with serum sodium levels below 120 mEq/liter and more commonly with levels less than 100 mEq/liter. When serum sodium levels fall rapidly, symptoms occur at higher serum levels of sodium; delirium and seizures are commonly presenting features.

Meningitis and encephalitis may be manifested by signs of metabolic encephalopathy such as confusion, somnolence, or delirium, in addition to signs and symptoms of systemic infection. Neurologic findings are usually symmetrical; approximately 20% of patients are comatose when first seen. Headache is common and an attempt should be made to arouse stuporous patients to determine its presence.

Signs of meningeal irritation must be carefully assessed to avoid delay in performing a lumbar puncture. These signs may not be present in infant patients and up to 20% of adults. The diagnosis of CNS infection is established by examining the CSF. Opening pressure at lumbar puncture may be as high as 600 mm H_2O. Cell counts range from 10 mononuclear WBC/mm^3 in patients with viral encephalitis, to over 10,000 WBC/mm^3, primarily polymorphonuclear leucocytes, in patients with purulent meningitis. Only rarely will patients with encephalitis or meningitis have no cells in the CSF at the first lumbar puncture. In cases of bacterial meningitis, the CSF glucose is commonly reduced to levels below 40 mg% with simultaneous normal blood glucose levels; the CSF glucose is almost always normal in viral encephalitis. The CSF protein is often elevated in both meningitis and encephalitis.

Subarachnoid hemorrhage may also present as a metabolic encephalopathy. Blood within the subarachnoid space of children is most commonly due to head trauma or ruptured arteriovenous malformations. Ruptured aneurysms are uncommon before the age of 30 years, although mycotic aneurysms secondary to subacute bacterial endocarditis can be seen at any age. Onset of subarachnoid hemorrhage is sudden and always includes headache which is typically, but not necessarily, severe. Fifty percent of patients will have hypertension as a result of subarachnoid hemorrhage. Consciousness is frequently lost transiently or permanently at onset of hemorrhage. Decerebrate posturing or, rarely, seizures may occur at this time. If the patient is conscious, moderate to marked confusion is common.

Funduscopic examination may show acute hemorrhages in the nerve fiber layer secondary to sudden increased intracranial pressure, or the typical subhyaloid (preretinal) hemorrhages. Signs of meningeal irritation are not demonstrable for at least several hours after the hemorrhage and are absent in deep coma.

The ECG may reveal a number of abnormalities that are presumably adrenergically mediated such as peaked P waves, short PR interval, tall U waves, or deeply inverted T waves. The peripheral WBC is modestly elevated but rarely above 15,000/mm^3.

Although clear evidence of subarachnoid blood on CT scan may obviate the need for spinal fluid examination, the CSF findings are diagnostic, usually with marked elevation of the opening pressure at lumbar puncture, often above maximal recordable pressures, using standard CSF manometers; that is, greater than 600 mmH_2O. The fluid is grossly bloody and contains 100,000 to over 1 million RBCs/mm^3.

White blood cells enter the subarachnoid space as a normal component of peripheral blood and are, therefore, in the same proportion as the white cell count of the peripheral blood. Chemical meningitis caused by blood in the subarachnoid space may, however, produce a pleocytosis of several thousand white blood cells during the first 48 hours and a reduction of CSF glucose between the fourth and eighth days after the hemorrhage. Hypoglycorrhachia is also seen in 5-15 days following neonatal intracranial hemorrhage. With this exception, the CSF glucose in the subarachnoid hemorrhage is normal. *A major error is to attribute the blood from subarachnoid hemorrhage to a traumatic spinal puncture* (see p. 301).

In cases of subarachnoid bleeding, the supernatant of the centrifuged CSF will be a yellow color (xanthochromia) within several hours following the hemorrhage, because of hemoglobin breakdown from red blood cells (see Table 20-5). This is critical to the diagnosis and requires appropriate handling of the CSF (see p. 301).

Reye's syndrome, an encephalopathy associated with fatty degeneration of liver, is a major cause of delirium progressing to coma in infants and children. There is a seasonal increased incidence from November to April with a peak incidence in February. Commonly, patients have had a preceding viral illness, often varicella or influenza B. The syndrome may be heralded by protracted vomiting and a delirious state that progresses to coma within 2 days (see Table 19-2). Seizures are common, but usually self-limited. When coma ensues, decerebrate posturing is common and focal neurologic signs are rare. Sustained hyperventilation and hepatomegaly are usually noted. Examination of the CSF reveals a normal protein and cell count. The blood sugar is frequently reduced because of hepatic failure and this may be reflected in a low CSF glucose. Serum SGOT and arterial ammonia levels are characteristically elevated, the prothrombin time is prolonged, but serum bilirubin is normal. The presence of icterus makes the diagnosis of Reye's syndrome doubtful. CNS impairment is not well correlated with the degree of hepatic dysfunction.

Table 20-5   CSF Pigmentation Following Intracranial Hemorrhage

	Onset	Peak	Clearance
Oxyhemoglobin (pink)	½-4 hours	24-35 hours	7-10 days
Bilirubin (yellow)	8-12 hours	2-4 days	2-3 weeks

Treatment is directed to control increased intracranial pressure and maintain a cerebral perfusion pressure (systemic arterial pressure minus intracranial pressure) greater than 50 mm Hg. This requires early placement of an intracranial pressure monitor and intubation with controlled ventilation maintaining pCO_2 below 22 mm Hg (see Chapter 19). Additional therapeutic measures include the maintenance of normal body temperature, the serum glucose at 150-200 mg/dl and serum osmolality below 320 mOsm/liter. Sterilization of the gastrointestinal tract with enemas and administration of neomycin are sometimes of value.

HYSTERICAL COMA

Hysterical coma is rare in young children but more commonly seen in the adolescent. The neurologic examination is normal. Pupils constrict briskly to light but lateral eye movements following oculocephalic testing may or may not be present since visual fixation can suppress this reflex. There are several findings, however, that cannot be voluntarily mimicked and their presence excludes the diagnosis of hysteria. These include the slow regular conjugate 'roving eye movements,' commonly seen in endogenous coma; slow, often asymmetric and incomplete eye closure following passive elevation of the lids by the examiner (voluntary closure of the eyelids during passive opening is nearly universal in fictitious unresponsiveness); and no nystagmus following caloric stimulation. *The presence of nystagmus after caloric stimulation virtually establishes the diagnosis of hysteria.*

PROGNOSIS IN COMA

Determination of the etiology of coma is essential in order to reasonably consider prognosis. Patients unconscious from sedative drug overdose usually have a prompt and complete recovery; whereas, comatose patients following cerebrovascular or other forms of hypoxic-ischemic insult have a rather poor outlook. It is commonly believed that recovery from coma in childhood is vastly superior to that of adult patients. This is undoubtedly true in coma secondary to head injury where reported 'recovery' of patients under the age of 10 years is about 70%; whereas, in patients over 60 years of age, recovery from posttraumatic coma may be prolonged. Statements regarding the permanence of neurologic deficits in the latter group should probably be made not earlier than 1 year after the injury.

The prognosis for children who are comatose following cardiac arrest is less encouraging; in one series of 26 patients, 69% died and only 3 were normal at discharge.

BRAIN DEATH

No specific criteria for brain death in the pediatric age group have been adopted. Legal definitions vary from one state to another. In the State of California, the pertinent statute notes in part that 'a person shall be pronounced dead if it is determined by a physician that the person has suffered a total and irreversible cessation of brain function. There shall be an independent confirmation of the death by another physician.'

The most stringent criteria are those published by the Harvard ad hoc committee. No person satisfying these criteria has regained consciousness. The criteria include no response to external stimuli; no spontaneous movements during 1 hour of observation; no spontaneous respiration for 3 minutes off a respirator if the pCO_2 is normal at the start (blood oxygenation should be normally maintained during the absence of ventilatory effort by delivering 100% oxygen at high flow through a cannula placed in the endotracheal tube); no brain stem or spinal reflexes; an isoelectric EEG using maximal gains and widely spaced electrodes with two tracings obtained 24 hours apart; no hypothermia (less than 32.2C or 93F) or sedative hypnotic drugs can be present.

The isoelectric EEG is thought to be a 'helpful confirmatory test' but is the one criterion not mandated for diagnosis of brain death. Though the EEG is not necessary for diagnosis of brain death, an isoelectric EEG confirms death in children as well as adults when head trauma and poisoning have been excluded.

LUMBAR PUNCTURE

Any suspicion of infectious meningitis is an absolute indication for lumbar puncture. Another indication is for documentation of intracranial or subarachnoid blood. The major hazard associated with this procedure is the possibility of precipitating or hastening transtentorial herniation. Reported studies document an incidence of deterioration following lumbar puncture, even in high risk groups with known intracranial masses, that varies widely from 1-2% to 30%. The risk is not well correlated with the presence of papilledema or elevation of CSF opening pressure at the time of the procedure. Many reports note a particular risk of herniation following lumbar puncture in patients with brain abscess.

Differentiation of blood secondary to a traumatic lumbar puncture and that originating from hemorrhage within the central nervous system is

Table 20-6   CSF in Full-term and Premature Neonates

CSF	Full-term	Premature
WBC count (cells/mm³)	0-32 (mean 8.2)	0-29 (mean 9)
Protein (mg/dl)	20-170 (mean 90)	65-150 (mean 115)
Glucose (mg/dl)	34-119 (mean 52)	24-63 (mean 50)
CSF/blood glucose ratio	0.44-2.48 (mean 0.81)	0.55-1.55 (mean 0.74)

Modified and reproduced with permission from Fishman RA: *Cerebrospinal Fluid in Diseases of the Nervous System.* Saunders, 1980.

often critical. Clearing of blood as additional CSF leaves the needle, or a decrease in the red cell count from the first to third tubes, are helpful indications of traumatic tap. Examination of the supernatant of the centrifuged specimen will always make this differentiation, since the enzyme for converting hemoglobin to bilirubin, heme oxygenase, is necessary for production of xanthochromia. Production of xanthochromia requires hours and then clears over days. The supernatant fluid from a traumatic lumbar puncture is, therefore, clear. The time course of the color changes of CSF following subarachnoid bleeding is summarized in Table 20-5.

In cases of traumatic lumbar puncture, white blood cells and protein enter the CSF with the red blood cells. Assuming the peripheral blood values are normal, 1 mg% of CSF protein and one white cell can be accounted for every 1000 RBCs in the CSF. Normal CSF values for the newborn are found in Table 20-6.

REFERENCES

Bruce DA, et al: Pathophysiology, treatment and outcome following severe head injury in children. Child's Brain 5:174-191, 1979.

Johnston RB, Mellits ED: Pediatric coma: prognosis and outcome. Develop Med Child Neurol 22:3-12, 1980.

Margolis LH, Shaywitz BA: The outcome of prolonged coma in childhood. Pediatrics 65(3): 477-483, 1980.

Posner J: *Diagnosis of Stupor and Coma,* 3rd Ed. Davis, Philadelphia, 1980.

Seshia SS, Seshia MMK, Sankaran K: Coma following cardiorespiratory arrest in childhood. Develop Med Child Neurol 21:143-153, 1979.

Seshia SS, Seshia MMK, Sachdeva RK: Coma in childhood. Develop Med Child Neurol 19:614-628, 1977.

Appendix

Growth Record for Infants
in relation to gestational age and fetal and infant norms (combined sexes)

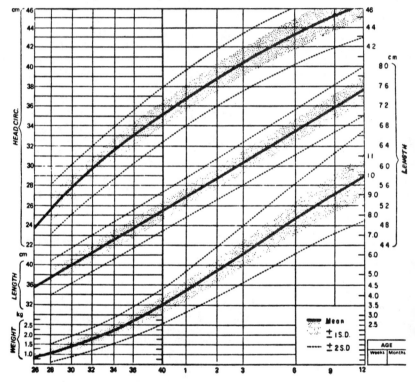

Reproduced with permission from Babson SG, Benda GI: Growth graphs
for the clinical assessment of infants of varying gestational age. J
Pediatr 89:814, 1976.

303

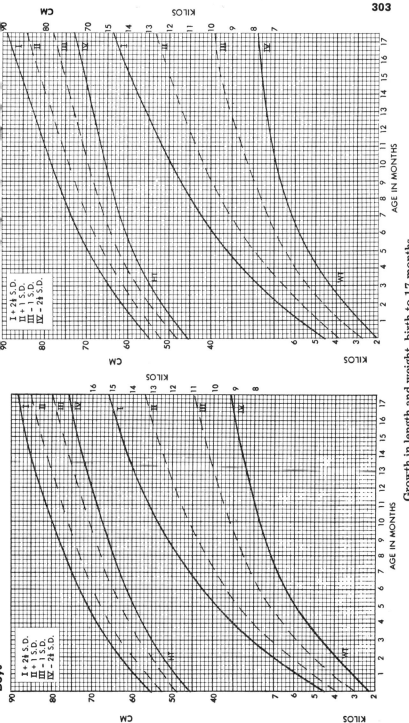

Growth in length and weight, birth to 17 months

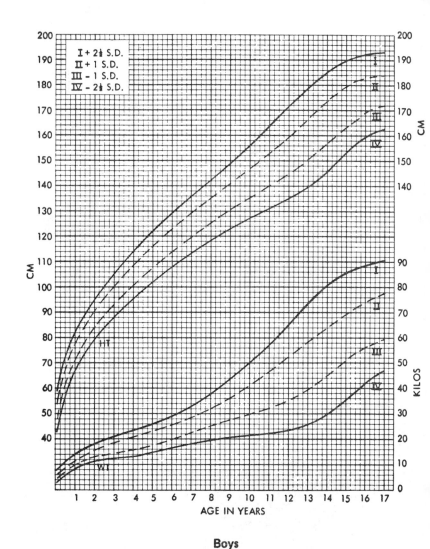

Boys

Growth in height and weight, birth to 17 years

Courtesy of Neonatology Division, Department of Pediatrics,
University of California, San Francisco

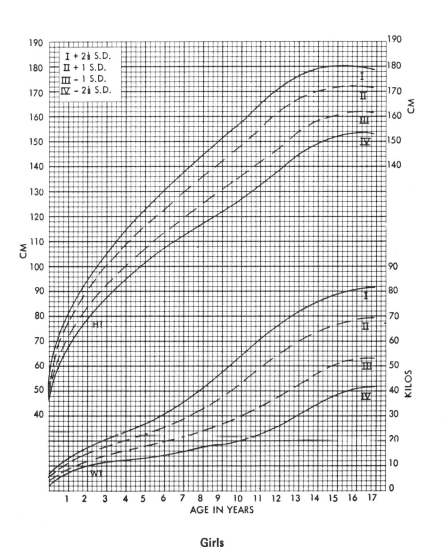

Girls

Growth in height and weight, birth to 17 years
Courtesy of Neonatology Division, Department of Pediatrics,
University of California, San Francisco

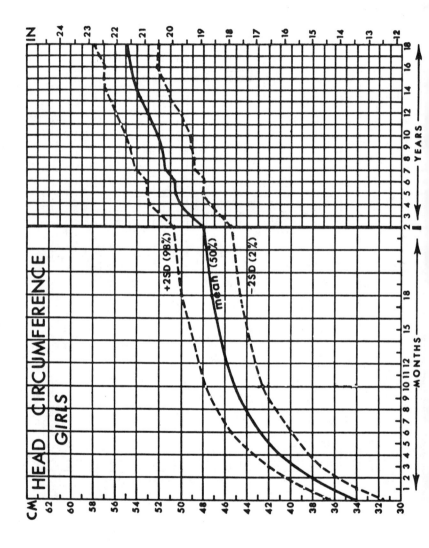

Reproduced with permission from Nellhaus G: Head circumference from birth to eighteen years. Practical composite international and interracial graphs. Pediatrics 41:106, 1968.

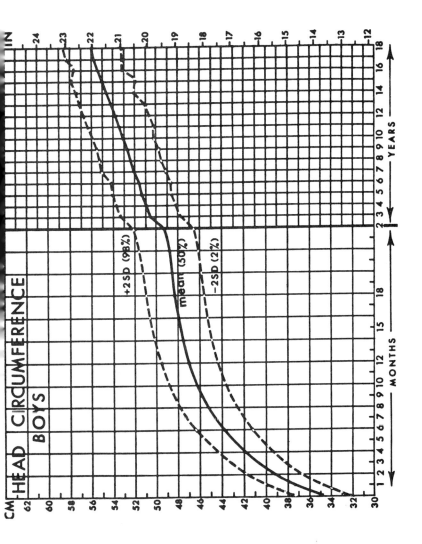

Reproduced with permission from Nellhaus G: Head circumference from birth to eighteen years. Practical composite international and interracial graphs. Pediatrics 41:106, 1968.

Index

A

Abducens nerve, palsy of, 41, 218
Acidemia, organic, 56
Acidosis, metabolic, in coma, 289
respiratory, in coma, 289
Acoustic neuroma(s), 154, 172
Acuity, visual, 8, 214
normal development of, 216
Adenovirus, as cause of meningitis, 130
Adrenoleucodystrophy, 83
Adrenomyeloneuropathy, 83
Agnosia, visual, 217
Aicardie syndrome, 183
Albright's syndrome, 168
Alexander's disease, 83
Alexia, 216
Alice-in-wonderland syndrome, 248
Alkalosis, metabolic, in coma, 289
respiratory, in coma, 289
Alphafetoprotein, 30
in ataxia-telangiectasia, 177
Alphalipoproteinemia, 95
Amniocentesis, 30
Amaurosis, 216
Leber's, 225, 228
Amino acids, disorders of transport, 64-65
sulphur-containing, disorders of, 62, 64
Aminoacidopathies, 54
Aminoacidurias, 59-65
Amyotrophic lateral sclerosis, 91
Andersen's disease, 71
Anencephaly, 30, 31
Aneurysm, intracranial vascular, 49, 50
Angiokeratoma corporis diffusum, 168
Angioma, venous, cerebral, 49
Anomaly, cerebellar, 258
Anosmia, causes of, 6
Anterior horn cell, disorders of, 89-93
congenital abnormalities, 89
Anticonvulsant drugs, 190-193
for absence spells, 187
interaction of, 187
for partial & generalized tonic/clonic seizures, 187

Apert's syndrome, 47
Apgar score, 195, 197
Apnea, neonatal, 205
Apraxia, gaze, 219
Arborvirus, as cause of encephalitis, 130
Archicerebellum, signs of dysfunction of, 259
Arcuate scotoma, 215
Arginase deficiency of, 54
Argininemia, 67
Arginosuccinate lyase, deficiency of, 54
synthetase, deficiency of, 54
Arginosuccinic aciduria, 66
Arnold-Chiari malformation, 33, 34
Arteriovenous malformations, 46, 48, 49
occult, 49 *See also specific malformations.*
Arthrogryposis, 93
Arylsulfatase A, deficiency of, 77
Asphyxia, fetal & neonatal, causes of, 196
perinatal, 197
Astrocytoma, cerebral hemisphere, 147, 154
cerebellar, 147, 149, 150
intraspinal, 161
spinal cord, 162
Ataxia, 23
acute, 260
acute cerebellar, 261
of childhood, 257-265
in Dandy-Walker syndrome, 45
evaluation of, 23
Friedreich's, 264
sensory, 22, 257
-telangiectasia, 176-178
secondary to toxic disorders, 262
caused by trauma, 263
caused by vertebrobasilar occlusive disease, 265
Athetosis, 24, 267, 268
Atrophy, dentatorubral, 264
muscular, scapuloperoneal/facioscapulohumeral, 92
spinal, 89-92
olivopontocerebellar, 264

Atrophy, *(continued)*
  optic, nerve, 224
    heritable, 226
    in craniopharyngioma, 227
    in diabetes, 226
    in hydrocephalus, 226
    in optic nerve glioma, 227
    in meningioma, 227
    in pituitary tumors, 227
    metabolic causes of, 227
Axonal degeneration, 95

B

Babinski sign, 21
Ballism, 24, 268
Battered child syndrome, 142
Battle's sign, 137
Becker's muscular dystrophy, 112
Behr's optic atrophy, 226
Bell's palsy, 98
Benedict's test, 63
Betalipoproteinemia, 95
Birth trauma, 201-203
Blindness, cortical, 216
  day, 8, 216
  night, 8, 216
Bloch-Sulzberger syndrome, 168
Bobble-head-doll syndrome, 272
Bonnet-Dechaume-Blanc syndrome, 168
Brachial plexus palsy, congenital, 106, 107, 203
Brachycephaly, 46
Brain death, 300
Brain-stem glioma, 147, 151, 152
Breath-holding spells, 184, 185
Brudzinski sign, 4, 122

C

Canavan's disease, 83
Carbamyl phosphate synthetase, deficiency of, 55, 66
Carbohydrate, defects of, 56
Carcinoma, intraspinal, 161
Carpenter's syndrome, 47
Cat-scratch disease, as cause of meningitis/encephalitis, 130
Caudal regression syndrome, 36
Cell migration, disorders of, 36-45
Central core disease, 116
Central scotoma, 215
Centrocecal scotoma, 215
Centronuclear myopathy, 116
Cephalohematoma, 137
Cerebellum, functional regions of, 260
  phylogenetic regions, 260
Cerebral, edema, therapy for, 290
  perfusion pressure, 280, 281

Cerebrospinal fluid, formation of, 40
  in bacterial meningitis, 124
  in viral meningitis/encephalitis, 132
  pathways of, 41
  pigmentation following intracranial hemorrhage, 299
  xanthochromic, 298
  in full-term & premature neonates, 301
Cherry-red spot, macular, 225
Chamberlain's line, 259
Chiari malformation, 32, 33
  in hydrocephalus, 44
Chin quivering, 272, 273
Chorea, 24, 268-271
  benign familial, 270
  causes of, 269
Choreoathetosis, familial paroxysmal, 185, 270, 271
Choroid plexus papilloma, 147, 153
Chotzen's syndrome, 47
Citrullinemia, 66
Cobb's syndrome, 168
Coloboma, of optic nerve, 225
Color, blindness, 8
  desaturation, 7
  vision, 214
Coma, 287-301
  emergency management, 288
  mass lesion causing, 291, 294, 295
  metabolic, 291, 296-299
  prognosis, 299, 300
Concussion, spinal cord, 143
Consciousness, anatomy of, 289
Contrecoup injury, craniocerebral, 135
Contusion, cerebral, 136
Convulsive disorders, 179-194. *See also Seizures.*
Cori's disease, 70
Corpus callosum, agenesis of, 36, 37, 45
Cortical blindness, 216
Craniopharyngioma, 147, 155, 156
Craniostenosis, 2, 45
Craniosynostosis, 45-46
Cranium bifida, 31
Crouzen's disease, 47
CTAB test, 63
Cutaneomeningeal angiomatosis, 168
Cyanide-nitroprusside test, 67
Cyst, leptomeningeal, 138
Cystathioninuria, 64
Cystinuria, 65
Cystithionine synthetase, defect of, 62

D

Dandy-Walker syndrome, 2, 44, 45
Dejerine-Sottas disease, 97
Dentatorubral atrophy, 264
Dermatomes, sensory, 25, 26
Dermatomyositis, 120, 121
Dermoid, tumor, intracranial, 153
    intraspinal, 161
    cysts, spinal cord, 163
De Santis Cacchione syndrome, 168
Devic's disease, 93
Diastematomyelia, 34
Dinitrophenylhydrazine, (DNPH)
    test, 63
Diplomyelia, 35
Diplopia, 218
Divry-van Bogaert syndrome, 168
Dolichocephaly, 46
Doll's-head eye phenomenon, 293
Duchenne's muscular dystrophy,
    110-112
Dysautonomia familial, 96
Dyslexia, 216
Dysmetria, ocular, 220
Dysmorphic, child, 207-213
    neurologic features, 212
    features, 208, 209
        prenatal, 208
    patient, diagnostic categoriza-
        tion, 210
Dysmorphism, method of diagnosis,
    209
    types of, 209
Dystonia, 24, 271, 272
Dystonic states, classification of,
    272

E

Echinococcosis, 261, 262
Edema, cerebral, therapy for, 290
Effusions, subdural, in bacterial
    meningitis, 126
Electroencephalography, in neo-
        natal hypoxemic-ischemic
        encephalopathy, 198
    in seizures, 180
Electrodiagnostic studies, in neuro-
        muscular diseases, 88, 89
Encephalitis, postinfectious, 131
    viral, 130-132
        prognosis in, 134
Encephaloceles, 31
Encephalopathy, asphyxia & hyp-
        oxemic-ischemic neonatal,
        195-199
    metabolic, 51-58
        aminoacidopathies, 52
        carbohydrate defects, 52
        as cause of coma, 291
        treatment, 56
        symptoms, 53

Enteroviruses, as cause of menin-
        gitis, 130
Enzymes, in glycogen storage dis-
        eases, 70, 71
    in mucopolysaccharidoses, 74, 75
    in myopathies, 86, 87
    in urea cycle disorders, 66, 67
Eosinophilic granuloma, 158
Ependymoma, cerebral, 147, 151
    intraspinal, 161
    spinal cord, 162
Epidermoid, intraspinal, 161
    cysts, spinal cord, 163
    tumors, 153, 157, 158
Epstein-Barr virus, as cause of
        meningitis, 130
Exencephaly, 31
Extraocular muscles, action of, 9
Eye movements, fusion, 218
    gaze palsies, 219, 220
    pursuit, 218
    saccadic, 217, 218
    vergences, 218
    vestibular, 218

F

Fabry's disease, 73, 95, 168
Facioscapulohumeral muscular
        atrophy, 92
Fasciculation(s), 18, 19
    lingual, 85
Fazio-Londe syndrome, 92
Febrile convulsions, 194
Ferric chloride test, 61, 63
Fetal heart rate abnormalities, 197
Fiber type disproportion, congeni-
        tal, 116
Fibers, intrafusal, muscle spindle,
        250, 251
Fibrous dysplasia, 159
    polyostotic, 168
Fingerprint body myopathy, 117
Fisher syndrome, 99, 261
Fistula, cerebrospinal, 139
Fracture, skull, 137
    complications of, 138, 139
    neonatal, 201
    dislocation, spine, 144, 145
Friedreich's ataxia, 264, 265
Fungal infections, meningitis/en-
        cephalitis, 130
Fusion of eye movements, 218

G

Gait, ataxic, 22
    evaluation of, 22
Galactokinase, deficiency of, 69
Galactose 1-phosphate uridyl trans-
        ferase, deficiency of, 68
Galactosemia, 68, 69

Galactosidase A, deficiency of, 73, 76
Galactosylceramide β-galactosidase, deficiency of, 76
Ganglioneuroma, intraspinal, 161
Gangliosidoses, 73, 78, 79
  adult form, 79
  infantile form, 78
  juvenile form, 78
Gaucher's disease, 76, 77
Gaze apraxia, 219
Germinomas, suprasellar, 157
Glasgow coma score, in cranio-cerebral tumor, 136
  in traumatic coma, 278
Glioblastoma, intraspinal, 161
Glioma(s), hypothalamic, 155
  intraspinal, 161
  optic nerve, 154
Glucocerebrosidase, deficiency of, 77
Glucuronidase, defect of, 75
Glycogen storage diseases, 69-71
Grand mal seizures, 183
Graphesthesia, 27
Growth charts, 302-304
Gruber's syndrome, 168
Guillain-Barre syndrome, 99
Guthrie test, 61

H

Hallucinations, visual, 216
Hamartomas, hypothalamic, 157
Hand-Schuller-Christian disease, 158
Hartnup disease, 64
Head, circumference charts, 304, 305
  nodding, 218
    in spasmus nutans, 273
Headache, 241-249
Hearing impairment in infants, risk factors, 236, 237
Heart rate, fetal, abnormalities of, 197
Hemangioblastoma(s), cerebellar, 153, 154
  in Hippel-Lindau disease, 175
  spinal cord, 162, 163
Hemangioma, skull, 159
Hematoma, epidural, 141
  intracerebral, 141, 142
  subdural, acute, 139, 140
    chronic, 140
Hemeralopia, 8, 216
Hemianopsia, 215
Hemiatrophy, 19
Hemispheres, cerebral, development of, 29
Hemorrhage, epidural, neonatal, 200

Hemorrhage, (continued)
  extracranial, neonatal, 201, 202
  intracranial, neonatal, 199-201
  periventricular, neonatal, 199,
    intraventricular, neonatal, 202
  subarachnoid, neonatal, 200
Hemorrhagic telangiectases, 169
Herpesviruses, as cause of encephalitis, 130
Her's disease, 71
Hippel-Lindau disease, 175-176
Histidase, 62
Histidinemia, 62
Histiocytosis, 158, 159
Homocystinuria, 62, 64
Huntington's chorea, 270
Hunter's syndrome, 74
Hurler syndrome, 74
Hydranencephaly, 37
Hydrocephalus, 35, 39-44
  causes of, 40
  congenital communicating, 43
  intracranial pressure monitoring in, 280
  normal pressure, 42, 43
  pathogenesis of, 44
  shunting procedures in, 43
  treatment of, 42
Hydromyelia, 35
Hygroma(s), subdural, 140
  subgaleal, 138
Hyperammonemia, 55
  exchange transfusion in, 57
  peritoneal dialysis in, 57
Hypoxic-ischemic encephalopathy, neonatal, ECG in, 198
  neonatal management of, 198
  pathology of, 196
Hypotonia, benign congenital, 256
Hypotonia, causes of, 255
Hypotonic infant, 250-256
Hypothalamic glioma, 155
Hypsarrhythmia, 53
  in PKU, 60
Hysteria & coma, 299
  & ataxia, 259, 260

I

Iminoglycinuria, 65
Incontinentia pigmenti, 168
Infantile spasms, 37, 182, 183
Influenza virus, as cause of meningitis, 130
Internuclear ophthalmoplegia, 219
Intracranial, hypertension, 277-286
  emergency treatment of, 282-86
  pressure monitoring in hydrocephalus, 277-280

J

Jansky-Bielschowsky-Batten disease, 82
Jaw jerk, 10
Jaw winking, Marcus-Gunn, 223

K

Klippel-Trenaunay-Weber syndrome, 169
    macrocephaly in, 39
Kempe syndrome, 142
Krabbe's disease, 76
Krabbe-Bartels syndrome, 169
Kugelberg-Welander disease, 91
Kuskokwim disease, 93
Kernig sign, 4, 122

L

Lagophthalmos, 223
Language acquisition, problems in, 229-240
    delayed, 231-235
        motor impairment in, 233
        structural deficits in, 234
        treatment, 238-240
    hearing impairment in, 233, 234
    linguistic/cognitive impairment, 232
    normal stages of, 230, 231
Latent nystagmus, 220
Leber's amaurosis, 225, 228
    optic atrophy, 226
Lennox-Gastaut syndrome, 184
Leptospirosis, causing meningitis/encephalitis, 130
Leucodystrophy, globoid cell, 76
    metachromatic, 77, 81, 84
        adult type, 81
        infantile type, 81
        juvenile type, 81
Letterer-Siwe disease, 158, 159
Lid retraction, 223
Linear nevus syndrome, 169
Lipomatosis, multiple circumscribed, 169
Lipid metabolism, disorders of, 72
Lipidosis, 82
    sphingomyelin, 76
    sulfatide, 77, 81, 84
    of unknown cause, 84
Lipoma, intraspinal, 161
    spinal cord, 164
Lissencephaly, 36
Lovejoy criteria, clinical staging in Reye's syndrome, 278
Louis-Bar syndrome, 176-178
Lumbar puncture, 300
    headache following, 243
    in brain tumors, 130

Lymphatic choriomeningitis virus, causing meningitis, 130
Lymphoma, intraspinal, 161

M

MacEwen's sign, 1, 41
Macrocephaly, 38, 39
    differential diagnosis, 39
Macular, cherry red spot, 225
    lesions in ceroid lipofuscinosis, 225
Maffucci's syndrome, 169
Malformations, congenital, 28-50. *See also specific malformations.*
    vascular, 46, 48-50
Maple syrup urine disease, 62
    exchange transfusion in, 57
    peritoneal dialysis in, 57
Marcus-Gunn jaw winking, 223
McArdle's disease, 71
Maroteaux-Lamy syndrome, 75
Medulloblastoma(s), cerebral, 147, 150
    intraspinal, 161
Megalencephaly, 38, 39
Melkersson syndrome, 98
Meningioma, intracranial, 147, 156
    intraspinal, 161
Meningitis, bacterial, 122-128
    causes of, 123
    clinical characteristics of, 125
    lumbar puncture in, 123, 124
    neuropathology in, 124, 125
    treatment of, 126-128
    mumps, 129
    viral, 129, 130. *See also specific infections.*
    prognosis in, 134
Meningocele, 32
Meningoencephalitis, mumps, 129
Meningomyelocele, 32
Metabolic, coma, 296-299
    acid-base abnormalities, 289
    encephalopathy, causing coma, 291
Metabolism, inborn errors of, 59-84
Microcephaly, 2, 38
    in PKU, 60
Migraine, 246-249
Mitochondrial myopathies, 116
Monocular nystagmus, 220
Morquio's syndrome, 75
Motor, nystagmus, congenital, 220
    system, evaluation of, 18-24
    unit, findings in lesions of, 86
Movement disorders, 266-276
Mucolipidoses, 72
Mucopolysaccharidoses, 69, 72
Multicore disease, 117

Muscle, atrophy of, 19
    biopsy of, 87, 88
    bulk, 19
    primary diseases of, 110-119
    power, 20
        infants, evaluation of, 20
    spindle, 250, 251
    tone, 20
        developmental aspects of 252
        regulatory mechanisms of, 250
Muscular, atrophy, peroneal, 97
    dystrophy, Becker type, 112
        congenital, 118
        distal, 115
        Duchenne type, 110-112
        facioscapulohumeral, 112
        limb-girdle, 114, 115
        myotonic, 113, 114
            congenital, 114
        ocular, 115
        oculopharyngeal, 115
        scapuloperoneal, 113
Myasthenia gravis, congenital, 108
    juvenile, 108
    neonatal, 107, 108
Myasthenic syndrome, 108, 109
Mycoplasma, causing meningitis/
        encephalitis, 130
Myelopathy, transverse, 92, 93
Myokymia, 223
Myoneural junction, disorders of,
        107-110
Myopathy, congenital, 116-118
Myositis, 120, 121
Myotonia, 21
    congenita, 118, 119
    lingual, percussion, 18
Myotonic, chondrodystrophy, 119
    dystrophy, 113, 114
        congenital, 114
Myotubular myopathy, 110

N

Nemaline myopathy, 117
Neocerebellum, signs of dysfunc-
        tion of, 259
Neonatal, apnea, 205
    intracranial hemorrhage, 199
    periventricular hemorrhage, 199
    seizures, 203-205
    visual testing, 216
Nerve(s), abducens, 8
        palsy of, 41, 45
    acoustic, 13
    cutaneous, segmental distri-
        bution, 25, 26
    facial, 10
    glossopharyngeal, 15
    hypoglossal, 18
    oculomotor, 8
    olfactory, 6

Nerve(s), (continued)
    optic, 6
        colobomas of, 225
        hypoplasia of, 224, 225
        neural pathway, 7
    peripheral, disorders, 94-107
        motor conduction velocities
            in, 89
        pathology, 94, 95
    spinal accessory, 17
    trigeminal, 9
    trochlear, 8
    vagus, 16
    vestibular, 14
Neural, crest, formation of, 29
    tube, formation of, 29
Neurinoma, intraspinal, 161
    spinal cord, 164
Neuritis, optic, 224
Neuroblastoma, cerebral, 156
    intraspinal, 161
    occult, in acute ataxia, 261
Neurocutaneous melanosis, 169
Neuroenteric cyst, spinal cord, 163
Neurofibromatosis, 171-173
    macrocephaly in, 39
Neurologic examination, 1-27
Neuroma, acoustic, 154
Neuromuscular disorders, 85-121
Neuromyelitis optica, 93
Neuronal, ceroid lipofuscinosis, 82
    proliferation & migration, 28, 29
Neuropathy, hereditary, sensori-
        motor, 97
    sensory, 96
    hypertrophic interstitial, 97
    infectious, herpes simplex, 106
        herpes zoster, 106
    & tumors, 107
    & vascular disease, 107
Neuropore, 28
Neurulation, disorders of, 30-36
Niemann-Pick disease, 76, 80
Night terrors, 185
Nyctalopia, 8, 216
Nystagmus, 220, 221

O

Obscurations, visual, 216
Ocular, flutter, 220
    fundus, abnormalities of, 223-228
    motor system, 217-221
Oculocephalic reflex, 293
Oculomotor nerve, aberrant
        regeneration, 223
    palsy of, 218
Oculovestibular reflex, 293
Olivocerebellar degeneration, 264
Olivopontocerebellar atrophy, 264
Ophthalmic problems of childhood,
        214-228

Ophthalmoplegia, internuclear, 219
Opsoclonus, 220
    & occult neuroblastoma, 261
Optic, atrophy, 41, 224
        Behr's, 226
        in craniopharyngioma, 227
        in diabetes, 226
        heritable, 226
        in hydrocephalus, 226
        in meningioma, 227
        in optic nerve glioma, 227
        in pituitary tumor, 227
        Leber's, 226
    disc, tilting of, 225
    nerve, glioma, 147, 154
        hypoplasia, 224, 225
    neuritis, 224
Ornithine, carbamyl transferase,
        deficiency, 67
    transcarbamylase, deficiency, 64
Ornithinemia, 67
Oscillopsia, 218
Osler-Weber-Rendu syndrome, 169
Osteoma, skull, 159, 160
Oxycephaly, 46

P

Pachygyria, 36
Paleocerebellum, signs of dys-
        function of, 259
Palsy, abducens nerve, 41, 45, 218
        Bell's, 98
        brachial plexus, congenital, 106,
            207
        bulbar progressive, 92
        facial nerve, idiopathic, 98
            recurrent, 98
        gaze, 219, 220
        oculomotor nerve, 218
        trochlear, 218
Papilledema, 41, 223, 224
Papillitis, 224
Paramyotonia congenita, 119
Paraplegia, familial spastic, 97, 264
Pavor nocturnus, 185
Pelizaeus-Merzbacher disease, 83
Petit mal seizures, 181
Periodic alternating nystagmus, 221
Peroneal muscular atrophy, 97
Pfeiffer's syndrome, 47
Phenylalanine, hydroxylase, 59
        metabolic pathways, 60
        traits of hyperphenylalanemia, 61
Phenylketonuria, 59-62
        clinical characteristics, 60, 61
        treatment, 61, 62
Phosphofructokinase, muscle,
        defect of, 71
Phosphorylase kinase, hepatic,
        defect of, 71
Photopsia, 216

Pineal tumor, 147
Pituitary tumor, 157
Plagiocephaly, 46
Platybasia, 259
Pneumocephalus, 138
Polymyositis, 120
Polyneuritis, idiopathic, 99
Polyneuropathy, & adverse effects
        of drugs, 102, 103
    hereditary, 95-98
        sensory, 96
        sensorimotor, 97
    in heritable metabolic diseases,
        100, 101
    secondary to toxic agents, 104
Pompe's disease, 70
Postconcussion syndrome, 142
Postinfectious viruses, causing
        encephalitis, 130
Posttramatic syndrome, 245
Prader-Willi syndrome, 256
Proprioception, 27
Pseudopapilledema, 224
Pseudoseizures, 185
Ptosis, 222
Pupils & lids, defects of, 221-223
Pursuit movements, eye, 218
Pyknolepsy, 181

Q

Quadrantopsia, 215

R

Rachischisis, 30
Ramsay-Hunt syndrome, 98, 99, 106
Reducing body myopathy, 117
Reflex(es), corneal, 10
    cough, 17
    jaw-jerk, 10
    Moro, 106, 107
    neck righting, 14
    oculocephalic, 293
    oculovestibular, 293
    plantar, 21
    tendon, 20
    tonic-neck, 14
    vomiting, 17
Refsum's disease, 97
Retinal lesions, in subacute sclero-
        sing panencephalitis, 228
Reye's syndrome, 279
    clinical staging of, Lovejoy
        criteria, 278
    causing coma, 298, 299
Riley-Day syndrome, 96
Riley-Smith syndrome, macro-
        cephaly in, 39
Ring scotoma, 215
Rinne test, 14

Rocky Mountain spotted fever, causing meningitis/encephalitis, 130
Romberg sign, 22
Roussy-Levy syndrome, 264

S

Saccadic eye movements, 217, 218
Sacral agenesis, 35
Sandhoff's disease, 79
Sanfillipo's syndrome, 74
Sarcoma, intraspinal, 161
    primary, 161
Sarcotubular myopathy, 117
Scaphocephaly, 46
Scapuloperoneal muscular atrophy, 92
Scheie's syndrome, 75
Schilder's disease, 83
Schirmer test, 12
Schizencephaly, 36
Schwabach test, 13
Sclerosis, diffuse, 83
    tuberous, 166, 167, 170
Schwartz-Jampel syndrome, 119
Scotoma, 215
See-saw nystagmus, 220
Segmental demyelination, 95
Sensory system, evaluation, 24-27
Seizure(s), absence, 181
    akinetic, 184
    atonic, 183, 184
    in bacterial meningitis, 125
    classification of, 180-184
    complex partial, 181
    differential diagnosis, 184-185
    duration of treatment, 189
    electroencephalography in, 180
    febrile, 194
    generalized, 181-184
    incidence of, 179
    infantile spasm, 182, 183
    myoclonic, 181, 182
    partial, with simple symptoms, 180
    in PKU, 60
    prognosis of, 189
    tonic, 183
    tonic/clonic, 183
    treatment of, 186-188, 190-193
    in tuberous sclerosis, 166
    unilateral, 184
Signs. See specific signs.
Skew deviation, ocular, 219
Skull, examination of, 1
Soto syndrome, macrocephaly in, 39
Spasm, hemifacial, 223
    infantile, 182, 183
Spasmus nutans, 220, 273
Speech/language evaluation, 235-38
Spielmeyer-Vogt disease, 82

Spine, abnormal curvature of, 2
Spina bifida, 31
Spinal, cord, & meningeal coverings 95
    muscular atrophy, 89-91
Splanchnocystic dysencephaly, 169
Station, evaluation of, 21
Status epilepticus, 188, 189
Stereognosis, 27
Stupor, 287
Sturge-Weber syndrome, 173-175
    macrocephaly in, 39
Subdural hematoma, chronic, 2
Subluxation, atlantoaxial, transient, 145
Sunset sign, 41
Sydenham's chorea, 268-270
Syncope, 185
Syndrome. See specific syndrome.
Syphilis causing meningitis/encephalitis, 130
Syringobulbia, 35
Syringomyelia, 35

T

Taste, evaluation of, 12
Tay-Sachs disease, 78
Temporal lobe seizures, 181
Teratoma, intraspinal, 161
Test. See specific tests & disorders.
Thrombosis, venous sinus, cerebral, 139
Tics, 273-275
    eyelid, 223
Toe walking, 23
Torsion dystonia, 271, 272
Tourette syndrome, 274, 275
Toxic reactions, causing ataxia, 262
Toxoplasma causing meningitis/encephalitis, 130
Transillumination, skull, 2
Trauma, birth, 201-203
    brain & spinal cord, 135-145
    cerebral contusion, 136
    cranial, cephalohematoma, 137
    craniocerebral, blunt, 135
        diffuse, 142
    spinal cord, 143-145
        perinatal, 143, 201, 203
Tremors, 276
Trigonocephaly, 46
Trilaminar neuromuscular disease, 117
Trochlear nerve, palsy of, 218
Tuberous sclerosis, 166, 167, 170
    macrocephaly in, 39
    tumors in, 157
Tumor(s), brain, 146-157
    See also specific types.
    clinical manifestations, 146-8
    metastatic, 164, 165
    neurodiagnostic tests, 147-9

Tumor(s), *(continued)*
  spinal cord, 160-164
    metastatic, 165
    radiographic changes of, 163

U

Urea cycle, disorders of, 52, 65-67

V

Vascular, malformations, 46, 48-50
    See also specific malformations.
    arteriovenous, occult, 49
      intracranial aneurysm, 49, 50
      vein of Galen, 48
    tumors, intraspinal, 161
Vein of Galen, malformation of, 48
Venous angioma, cerebral, 49
Ventrigulomegaly, posthemorrhagic
      neonatal, 202
Vergences, eye movements, 218
Vertebrobasilar occlusive disease,
      265
Vertical nystagmus, 220
Vertigo, benign paroxysmal, 185,
      248
Vestibular eye movements, 218
Vision, color, 214

Visual, acuity, 8, 214
    agnosia, 217
    fields, 7, 214
      abnormalities of, 215
      color desaturation, 7
      defects of, 7
    hallucinations, 216
    obscurations, 216
    pathways, 7
    testing in neonate, 216
Vomiting, cyclical, 248
von Gierke's disease, 70
von Recklinghausen's disease, 171-3

W

Walking, toe, 23
Wallerian degeneration, 94
Weber test, 13
Werdnig-Hoffmann disease, 89-91
West syndrome, 182, 183
White matter, disorders of, 83, 84
Wyburn-Mason syndrome, 168

X

Xanthochromia, cerebrospinal
      fluid, 298
Xeroderma pigmentosum, 169